Emergency and Intensive Care Medicine

nova
Medicine & Health
New York

Emergency and Intensive Care Medicine

Environmental Emergencies and Injuries in Nature
Murat Yücel, MD (Editor)
Murat Güzel, MD (Editor)
İbrahim İkizceli, MD (Editor)
2022. ISBN: 978-1-68507-833-1 (Hardcover)
2022. ISBN: 978-1-68507-917-8 (eBook)

Multidisciplinary Approach to Trauma
Mehmet Cenk Turgut, MD (Editor)
Asli Turgut, MD (Editor)
2022. ISBN: 978-1-68507-761-7 (Hardcover)
2022. ISBN: 978-1-68507-915-4 (eBook)

Peritonitis: Causes, Diagnosis and Treatment
David F. Walker (Editor)
2021. ISBN: 978-1-53619-624-5 (Softcover)
2021. ISBN: 978-1-53619-641-2 (eBook)

Pediatric Critical Care: A Primer for All Clinicians
Jason Kane, MD (Editor), Joseph R. Hageman, MD (Editor), Rachel Wolfson, MD (Editor) and Stuart Berger, MD (Editor)
2019. ISBN: 978-1-53614-837-4 (Hardcover)
2019. ISBN: 978-1-53614-838-1 (eBook)

Gastrointestinal Bleeding: Symptoms, Treatment and Prognosis
Ahmed Kamel Abdel Aal, MD, PhD and Souheil Saddekni, MD (Editors)
2014. ISBN: 978-1-63117-333-2 (Hardcover)
2014. ISBN: 978-1-63117-334-9 (eBook)

More information about this series can be found at
https://novapublishers.com/shop/peritonitis-causes-diagnosis-and-treatment/

Seda Özkan
and Afsin Ipekci
Editors

Carbon Monoxide Poisoning

Prevention, Treatment and Outcomes

nova
Medicine & Health
New York

NOTICE TO THE READER

Library of Congress Cataloging-in-Publication Data

Names: Özkan, Seda, editor. | Ipekci, Afsin, editor.
Title: Carbon monoxide poisoning: prevention, treatment and outcomes / Seda Özkan, editor, Professor, Department of Emergency Medicine, Cerrahpasa Faculty of Medicine, Istanbul University-Cerrahpasa, Istanabul, Turkey, Afsin Ipekci, editor, Department of Emergency Medicine, Cerrahpasa Faculty of Medicine, Istanbul University-Cerrahpasa, Istanbul, Turkey.
Description: New York : Nova Science Publishers, [2023] | Series: Emergency and intensive care medicine | Includes bibliographical references and index. |
Identifiers: LCCN 2023045969 (print) | LCCN 2023045970 (ebook) | ISBN 9798891132177 (hardcover) | ISBN 9798891132764 (adobe pdf)
Subjects: LCSH: Carbon monoxide--Toxicology.
Classification: LCC RA1247.C2 C3955 2023 (print) | LCC RA1247.C2 (ebook) | DDC 615.9/1--dc23/eng/20231103
LC record available at https://lccn.loc.gov/2023045969
LC ebook record available at https://lccn.loc.gov/2023045970

Published by Nova Science Publishers, Inc. † New York

Contents

Preface

Poisoning and dramatic deaths due to "colorless, odorless, tasteless and non-irritating carbon monoxide gas" is a common public health problem worldwide. Carbon monoxide gas is a silent killer because it poisons people without being noticed. The pathophysiology of the acute and late effects of this poisoning, which has been seen for centuries, is still not fully known. As new information about the pathophysiology of carbon monoxide poisoning is discovered, new treatment methods are also being investigated.

The first place of admission for carbon monoxide poisoning, which mimics the symptoms of many diseases, is the emergency departments. Diagnosis and treatment are done in emergency departments. Physicians working in emergency medicine are expected to know and manage poisoning due to carbon monoxide gas well. However, since carbon monoxide gas causes poisoning by affecting different systems of the body, a multidisciplinary approach is important in the clinic. Valuable authors from different clinics contributed to the writing of the book due to the importance of the multidisciplinary approach.

In our book, we aimed to present the most up-to-date information in detail by covering all aspects of carbon monoxide poisoning.

Professor Seda Özkan, MD
Associate Professor Afşın İpekci, MD

Chapter 1

The Properties, Epidemiology, and Physiopathology of Carbon Monoxide Gas

Ali Halıcı[1,*], MD
Kerim Abatay[2], MD
İzzettin Hür[3], MD
and Eren Usul[4], MD

[1]Department of Emergency Medicine, Kutahya Health Science University, Kutahya, Turkey
[2]Department of Emergency Medicine, Muş Public Hospital, Muş, Turkey
[3]Department of Emergency Medicine, Mehmet Akif İnan Research Hospital, Şanlıurfa, Turkey
[4]Department of Emergency Medicine, Ankara Etlik City Hospital, Ankara, Turkey

Abstract

Carbon monoxide gas is a deadly gas that is produced by carbon monoxide molecules that are released due to the combustion of hydrocarbon molecules. The fact that this gas is colorless and odorless and there are no clear symptoms following poisoning by inhalation, complicates the diagnosis of such cases when they are admitted to the hospital. The history of the patient is vital for an accurate diagnosis since it can provide evidence of the patient has been exposed. Although its diagnosis is technically simple, carbon monoxide poisoning usually provides clinicians with little or no clues regarding the patient's history and symptomatology, which are essential for the diagnosis of any patient.

Since the carbon monoxide molecule competes with oxygen to bind to hemoglobin and prevents the transport of oxygen and its transfer to

[*] Corresponding Author's Email: ali.halici@ksbu.edu.tr.

In: Carbon Monoxide Poisoning
Editors: Seda Özkan and Afsin Ipekci
ISBN: 979-8-89113-217-7

tissues, adequate tissue oxygenation forms the basis of treatment for carbon monoxide poisoning. This treatment begins with the removal of the patient from the environment where carbon monoxide exposure occurred, after which rapid diagnosis and evaluation of end-organ damage following hospital admission are crucial. Since a delayed neuropsychiatric syndrome may occur days after exposure, follow-up of the patient after acute treatment is also important.

Keywords: carbon monoxide toxicity, delayed neuropsychiatric syndrome, carboxyhemoglobin

Introduction

Carbon monoxide gas is called a silent killer, because it affects victims serially and without any sign of presence in the environment. Patients quickly lose their consciousness and so cannot escape from exposure. Diagnosis is also difficult for healthcare professionals because of the low chance of taking sufficient anamnesis.

Properties of Carbon Monoxide Gas

Carbon monoxide is a simple compound that is formed by one carbon joined by a single oxygen. Carbon and oxygen share three electron pairs and bind to each other with three covalent bonds. Each atom has one free electron pair. The electronegativity of oxygen is higher than that of carbon, and so oxygen has a partial negative charge. The carbon monoxide molecule has a linear shape (Wu & Wang 2005).

The specific gravity of the CO gas is 0.967 and its density is 1.25 g/L under normal pressure. This means that CO is slightly lighter than air and diffuses evenly in the air. The solubility of CO gas in water is very low. CO reacts very slowly with O2 (Wu & Wang 2005). In normal inhaled air CO is around 0.01 to 1 ppm and at 100 ppm levels it causes poisoning symptoms (Hanley & Patel, 2022; Schallner et al., 2012).

Carbon monoxide is a tasteless, odorless, and non-irritant through inhalation by the lungs. Carbon monoxide gas poisoning is a common cause of fatal poisoning (Ernst & Zibrak, 1998) and constitutes a large portion of poisoning cases admitted to emergency departments (Kao & Nanagas, 2006).

History of carbon monoxide poisoning; The first known documentation of carbon monoxide in history was written by Aristotle. He stated "Coal fumes lead to heavy head and death" at 350 BC. At 275 BC, Erasistratus claimed that coal fumes affect normal breathing. Most of the trace evidence relevant to CO that had emerged in the ancient history period focused on the toxicity of coal fumes. Although not specifically relevant to therapeutic origins, ancient events are presented to illustrate progress in humankind's understanding of CO. Cassius was the first scientist who published the symptoms of CO poisoning in "Medical Questions" at 130 AD. After that at 150 AD, Galen realized that coal fume changed the composition of the air, making it harmful to inhalation. Marcellinus discussed the symptoms of head swelling by referring to the neurotoxic effects of coal fumes on the brain in 350 AD. The earliest reported incident of CO poisoning occurred in Nuceria, where the Romans are said to have drowned in baths due to leaks in hypocaust heating technology; similarly, the fumes may have been used militarily to execute Roman prisoners by invading the Carthaginian armies led by Hannibal in the second Punic War. More evidence of CO poisoning emerged under Julius Caesar (about 70 BC), in accounts recorded by Cicero and Livy showing that the fumes from coal were well understood to be deadly and served both i) as a suicide agent and ii) as a death sentence. The method used "the greenest possible wood that can produce the most smoke;" such executions were carried out by Emperor Lucius Verus (172 AD) (Hopper et al., 2021). When we came to modern times, at 1857 Bernard first recognized the reversible binding of CO with hemoglobin as a potent chemical reaction that could cause asphyxia. After then at 1895, Haldane calculated the oxygen–hemoglobin dissociation curve and showed the antagonistic effect of high partial pressure of O2 on the binding of CO hemoglobin (Koçyiğit & Benay, 2021).

CO poisoning is often observed in cold climates and during the winter months. Carbon monoxide poisoning can occur as a result of carbon monoxide gas being produced as a result of combustion in fires, coal and wood stoves, motor vehicle exhaust, hookah, and cigarette smoke (Retzky, 2017; Nguyen et al., 2020). Although less common, carbon monoxide poisoning may also be caused by the inhalation of waste gases from kerosene heaters, charcoal grills, camping stoves, gasoline-powered electricity generators, or exposure to motorboat exhaust fumes in the open air (Thomassen et al., 2004; CDC, 2005; Hampson & Dunn, 2015; CDC, 2004). The most common causes of CO poisoning in the USA are inhalation of exhaust gases or industrial waste gases that were not adequately evacuated from the environment (Wolf et al., 2008). In Türkiye, the most common causes of CO poisoning are household accidents, usually caused by wind disrupting the waste gas removal mechanisms of space or water heating systems (Uysalol et al., 2011).

CO poisoning should be suspected in fire victims, patients with flu-like symptoms in cold climates, and patients with unexplained changes in their mental state. Blood COHb levels below 3% are considered normal in non-smokers, while COHb levels up to 10% are considered normal in smokers. COHb measurements are required to determine the level of exposure to CO. However, COHb levels are not fully correlated with the degree of intoxication, as higher carbon monoxide levels confirm exposure, they may not indicate the degree of exposure. In addition, hydroxocobalamin treatment may affect COHb measurements and cause erroneous results (Livshits et al., 2012; Lee et al., 2007; Borron et al., 2007; Baud, 2007; Pace et al., 2014). The degree of intoxication is related to the duration of exposure to carbon monoxide. Treatment is planned according to patient symptoms and findings, rather than CO levels.

Carbon monoxide (CO) is a colorless, odorless, tasteless, and non-irritating gas produced by the combustion of hydrocarbons. CO gas poisoning is a common cause of fatal poisoning (Ernst&Zibrak,1998) and constitutes a large portion of poisoning cases admitted to emergency departments (Kao & Nanagas, 2006). It should be noted that patients may sometimes be admitted with nonspecific symptoms, therefore CO poisoning should be considered a differential diagnosis when evaluating the detailed physical history and physical examination of the patient (Hardy & Thom, 1994). CO poisoning can lead to permanent neurological impact, and patients with CO poisoning may be admitted to the emergency room exhibiting flu-like symptoms. This may lead to delays in, or even failure to correctly diagnose cases of CO intoxication. CO binds to hemoglobin with much greater affinity than oxygen, forming carboxyhemoglobin (COHb) and causing a disruption in the transportation of oxygen through the blood and its use in tissues. This means that carbon monoxide gas may lead to permanent neurological impact or can even be fatal.

The most common causes of CO poisoning in the USA are inhalation of exhaust gases or industrial waste gases that were not adequately evacuated from the environment (Wolf et al., 2008). In Türkiye, the most common causes of CO poisoning are household accidents, usually caused by wind disrupting the waste gas removal mechanisms of space or water heating systems (Uysalol et al., 2011).

CO poisoning is often observed in cold climates and during the winter months. Carbon monoxide poisoning can occur as a result of carbon monoxide gas being produced as a result of combustion in fires, coal and wood stoves, motor vehicle exhaust, hookah, and cigarette smoke (Retzky, 2017; Nguyen et al., 2020). Although less common, carbon monoxide poisoning may also be caused by the inhalation of waste gases from kerosene heaters, charcoal grills, camping stoves, gasoline-powered electricity generators, or exposure to motorboat exhaust fumes in the open air (Thomassen et al., 2004; CDC, 2005; Hampson & Dunn, 2015; CDC, 2004).

Epidemiology of Carbon Monoxide Poisoning

The incidences of carbon monoxide poisoning increase dramatically during and after disasters that occur in winter (Tintinalli, 2013). Carbon monoxide poisoning can be described as a public health problem whose actual incidence cannot be determined with certainty, as its clinical symptoms vary from person to person. However, carbon monoxide poisoning is a preventable cause of death in both our country and globally.

The number of studies conducted on carbon monoxide poisoning in our country is limited. In a study conducted by Koyuncu et al., in the emergency department of Kayseri Training and Research Hospital, 4,073 visits to the emergency department between November 2012 and May 2013 were evaluated, and 106 (2.6%) carbon monoxide poisonings were recorded (Koyuncu et al., 2020). In another study, Metin et al., determined that there were a total of 10,154 cases of carbon monoxide poisoning in Türkiye in 2010, with the incidence frequency of 14/100000. They determined that the mortality rate of CO poisoning was 5/10000000 (Metin et al., 2011).

It has been found that the incidence of CO poisoning varies between communities according to socioeconomic status and geography. Kinoshita et al., reported that between 2000 and 5000 people die every year in Japan due to carbon monoxide poisoning and that this number corresponds to more than half of the poisoning cases that occur in Japan (Kinoshita et al., 2020).

The World Health Organization reported that 1,365 people in England and Wales, and more than 3,800 people in the USA, died from carbon monoxide poisoning in 1,985. It was also reported that more than 10000 people received medical treatment for CO poisoning (Raub et al., 1999).

In a study conducted in Iran, Hosseininejad et al., analyzed 10 epidemiological studies conducted between 1999 and 2016 and found that the incidence of carbon monoxide poisoning was 38.91/100000, the mortality rate being 11.6/1000 for the 6372 cases analyzed (Hosseininejad et al., 2018).

Simosen et al., examined 22,930 cases of carbon monoxide poisoning between 1995 and 2015 in Denmark and found that 9.2% of the cases died in the first 30 days of poisoning (Simonsen et al., 2019).

In a recent study conducted in Türkiye by Temrel, 1,896 CO-related deaths were examined through data obtained from the Turkish Statistical Institute between 2013-2017, and the mortality rate was found to be 3.84 per 100,000 people (Temrel, 2021).

In another study conducted in Türkiye by Can et al., 27,881 news articles from 2008 to 2017 containing the keywords poisoning, death, and carbon monoxide were evaluated, and 2,667 deaths were analyzed. According to the aforementioned study, the risk of death due to carbon monoxide was 0.35/100,000 (Can et al., 2019).

In a study conducted in Timişoara, Romania by Mureşan et al., (2019) at the Institute of Forensic Medicine, 298 autopsies conducted between 2000-2018 were examined and the rate of carbon monoxide poisoning was found to be 79.18%. The reports in the literature regarding deaths from carbon monoxide vary. It is reported that males are more susceptible to death due to CO poisoning (Mureşan et al., 2019), and this finding is supported by other studies which concluded that of the CO poisoning cases that resulted in death, 53.3% of the cases were male and 46.7% were female (Hosseininejad et al., 2018), and that 51.4% of the CO poisoning victims were male and 48.6% of them were female (Can et al., 2019). In another study, the ratio of male victims to female victims was found to be 1.83 (M/F:68/37) (Temrel, 2021).

On average, 4% to 10% of cases of carbon monoxide poisoning were observed to occur in children (Gozubuyuk et al., 2017). In one study examining deaths due to CO poisoning, the average age of the victims was found to be 30 years (Hosseininejad et al., 2018). In contrast, another study found that the average age of CO poisoning deaths was 51.8 (Temrel, 2021).

It was reported that CO poisoning in domiciles is observed more frequently in winter months and in windy weather (Can et al., 2019; Gozubuyuk, et al., 2017). Most cases of CO poisoning were observed to occur in January (n:30, 28.6%), February (n:14, 13.3%), and December (n:15, 14.3%). When the locations where CO poisoning occurs are examined, it is observed that the most common occurrence is in domiciles (n:75, 71.4%). It was also reported that the most common source of CO poisoning was heating stoves (n:32, 30.5%) (Temrel, 2021).

A study analyzing CO poisoning cases in terms of occupational groups and literacy reported that 36.37% of the cases were middle school graduates, 52.74% were single, and most of the cases were working as cleaners

(Hosseininejad et al., 2018). In another study that analyzed 4,754 cases of carbon monoxide that occurred between July 2009 and June 2019, using data obtained from the US armed forces military health system, it was found that the highest incidence of CO poisoning was observed in soldiers working in maintenance and engineering units (Williams et al., 2020).

The reports of studies conducted in Türkiye also vary according to the provinces examined. In one study, the province with the highest incidence of CO poisoning was determined to be Manisa (n:266, 14%), followed by Balıkesir (3.84/100,000), Niğde (4.8/100,000) and Nevşehir (4.6/100,000). The mortality rates were determined to be 0.37/100,000 in Ankara and 0.12/100,000 in Istanbul [63]. In another study, Kilis (1.81/100000), Kırıkkale (1.78/100000), and Karabük (1.31/10000) were found to be the 3 provinces with the highest risk of mortality on the mortality risk map (Can et al., 2019).

In most cases of CO poisoning, victims do not aware that they have been exposed to carbon monoxide. When the current literature is examined, it is apparent that the mortalities and morbidities due to CO exposure are clearly higher than expected, which only underlines the seriousness of the problem.

Pathophysiology of Carbon Monoxide Poisoning

Carbon monoxide gas exhibits its toxic effects mainly through three mechanisms (Ernst & Zibrak, 1998):

- By binding to hemoglobulin, preventing oxygen transport and the delivery of oxygen to tissues by shifting the hemoglobulin dissociation curve to the left, causing hypoxia and ischemia
- By disrupting the normal energy production of cells via hemeproteins such as myoglobulin, cytochrome, and guanylate cyclase
- Increasing the activity of nitric oxide and causing oxidative damage through superoxide radicals

Carbon monoxide gas inhaled from the air passes through the alveoli of the lungs by diffusion and directly enters the bloodstream. Since carbon monoxide has a 200-fold greater affinity for hemoglobin compared to oxygen, about 85% of the carbon monoxide diffused into the bloodstream quickly binds to hemoglobin (Ernst & Zibrak, 1998; Engel et al., 1969). The binding of CO to hemoglobin is very strong, and evidence for this is provided by the fact that the partial pressure of carbon monoxide in the bloodstream is very low compared to the external environment (Prockop et al., 2007). The binding carbon monoxide to the heme proteins on hemoglobin replaces oxygen and thus reduces the oxygen-carrying capacity of hemoglobin. Under regular conditions, the hemoglobin protein consists of 4 globular proteins, with each globular protein carrying one oxygen molecule via the iron atom in its center. The first oxygen atom binds to hemoglobin with lower affinity, and as more oxygen molecules bind to hemoglobin, the affinity of subsequent oxygen molecules increases due to the structure of the protein. When the carbon monoxide molecule binds to hemoglobin (COHb), it not only replaces oxygen and reduces oxygen capacity but also stabilizes hemoglobin in the R-state. Since hemoglobulin has a high affinity for oxygen while in the R-state, it cannot release oxygen to tissues when it reaches them (Hardy & Thom, 1994).

The binding carbon monoxide gas to hemoglobin exerts its toxic effects, not only by reducing the oxygen-carrying capacity of the blood but also by preventing the transfer of oxygen from the blood to the tissues. The presence of COHb shifts the hemoglobin oxygen dissociation curve to the left.

However, although the effects of carbon monoxide on oxygen transport are more prominent, the mortal and morbid effects of carbon monoxide occur via disruption of intra-cellular mitochondria function or via direct destruction of tissues. Approximately 10-15% of the carbon monoxide taken after exposure binds to extravascular proteins (Coburn, 1970). In a study conducted by Goldbaum et al., in dogs, one group of dogs received blood transfusions containing 80% COHb, while the other group inhaled air with 13% CO. Although the blood CO levels of both groups were close to each other and no symptoms were observed in the transfused dogs, the group of dogs that inhaled air with 13% CO died (Goldbaum et al., 1975).

The inhibition of oxidative phosphorylation in mitochondria causes carbon monoxide to bind irreversibly, not only to hemoglobin but also to other heme proteins. Cytochrome enzymes and myoglobin are heme proteins responsible for intracellular respiration and the transport of oxygen within the cell. Cytochrome C is involved in the last step of the electron transport chain. Carbon monoxide binding to cytochrome c oxidase disrupts the function of the molecule and, as a result, ceases ATP production in the cell. Since energy production is higher in organs such as the brain and heart, symptoms are first observed in these organs (Ernst & Zibrak, 1998).

The probable direct toxic effect of CO on brain tissue is to cause reperfusion damage, especially by causing nucleic acids free oxygen radicals to be formed during re-oxygenation after hypoxia due to carbon monoxide. In addition, carbon monoxide toxicity causes demyelination in the central nervous system through peroxidation of lipids (Ernst & Zibrak, 1998). Nitric oxide is the most prominent actor responsible for these effects. Elevated levels of carbon monoxide increase nitric oxide activity, leading to cerebral vasodilation and decreased cerebral blood flow. Loss of consciousness and increased nitric oxide levels are strongly correlated. The addition of probable hypotension secondary to the effects of peripheral vasodilation to this clinical picture may also cause syncope (Ischiropoulos et al., 1996; Meyer-Witting et al., 1991). Nitric oxide also affects neutrophil adhesion molecules, such as the B2-integrin, and prevents neutrophil adhesion to the endothelium. As a result, neutrophils infiltrating the intercellular space generate free oxygen radicals and cause both oxidative damage and lipid peroxidation in the brain. Ultimately, this creates a clinical picture of delayed neuropsychiatric syndrome (DNS) (Thom et al., 1994).

Conclusion

Carbon monoxide poisoning has been a life-threatening disease throughout human history. When we look at the form of poisoning, it is a type of poisoning that is easy to protect but also overlooked. Especially in winter, people living in rural areas are at high risk for carbon monoxide poisoning. In this regard, studies should be organized by state institutions to increase social awareness. Equipment used for rapid diagnosis should be expanded.

References

Baud, F. (2007). Clarifications regarding interference of hydroxocobalamin with carboxyhemoglobin measurements in victims of smoke inhalation. *Annals of emergency medicine*, *50*(5), 625-626. https://doi.org/10.1016/j.annemergmed.2007.05.026.

Borron, S. W., Uhl, W., Nolting, A., Hostalek, U., & Serono, M. (2007). Interference of the cyanide antidote hydroxocobalamin with carboxyhemoglobin measurements should not limit clinical use in suspected or confirmed cyanide poisoning. *Annals of emergency medicine*, *50*(5), 624-625. https://doi.org/10.1016/j.annemergmed.2007.05.027.

Can, G., Sayılı, U., Aksu Sayman, Ö., Kuyumcu, Ö. F., Yılmaz, D., Esen, E., Yurtseven, E., & Erginöz, E. (2019). Mapping of carbon monoxide related death risk in Turkey: a ten-year analysis based on news agency records. *BMC Public Health*, *19*, 1-7.

CDC (Centers for Disease Control and Prevention) (2004). Carbon monoxide poisonings resulting from open air exposures to operating motorboats--Lake Havasu City, Arizona, 2003. *MMWR Morb. Mortal Wkly Rep.,* 53, 314-318. https://doi.org/10.1001/jama.291.22.2692.

CDC (Centers for Disease Control and Prevention) (2005). Carbon monoxide poisoning from hurricane-associated use of portable generators--Florida, 2004. *MMWR Morb. Mortal Wkly Rep.,* 54, 697-700. https://doi.org/10.1001/jama.294.12.1482.

Coburn, R. F. (1970). The carbon monoxide body stores. *Annals of the New York Academy of Sciences, 174*(1), 11-22. https://doi.org/10.1111/j.1749-6632.1970.tb49768.x.

Engel, R. R., Rodkey, F. L., O'NEAL, J. D., & Collison, H. A. (1969). Relative affinity of human fetal hemoglobin for carbon monoxide and oxygen. *Blood, 33*(1), 37-45. https://doi.org/10.1182/blood.v33.1.37.37.

Ernst, A., & Zibrak, J. D. (1998). Carbon monoxide poisoning. *New England journal of medicine, 339*(22), 1603-1608. https://doi.org/10.1056/nejm199811263392206.

Goldbaum, L. R., Ramirez, R. G., & Absalon, K. B. (1975). What is the mechanism of carbon monoxide toxicity?. *Aviation, space, and environmental medicine, 46*(10), 1289-1291.

Gozubuyuk, A. A., Dag, H., Kaçar, A., Karakurt, Y., & Arica, V. (2017). Epidemiology, pathophysiology, clinical evaluation, and treatment of carbon monoxide poisoning in child, infant, and fetus. *Northern clinics of Istanbul, 4*(1), 100.

Hampson, N. B., & Dunn, S. L. (2015). Carbon monoxide poisoning from portable electrical generators. *The Journal of emergency medicine, 49*(2), 125-129. https://doi.org/10.1016/j.jemermed.2014.12.091.

Hanley, M. E., & Patel, P. H. (2022). Carbon Monoxide Toxicity. *StatPearls [Internet].* Treasure Island (FL): StatPearls Publishing.

Hardy, K. R., & Thom, S. R. (1994). Pathophysiology and treatment of carbon monoxide poisoning. *Journal of Toxicology: Clinical Toxicology, 32*(6), 613-629. https://doi.org/10.3109/15563659409017973.

Hopper, C. P., Zambrana, P. N., Goebel, U., & Wollborn, J. (2021). A brief history of carbon monoxide and its therapeutic origins. *Nitric Oxide, 111*, 45-63.

Hosseininejad, S. M., Aminiahidashti, H., Khatir, I. G., Ghasempouri, S. K., Jabbari, A., & Khandashpour, M. (2018). Carbon monoxide poisoning in Iran during 1999–2016: A systematic review and meta-analysis. *Journal of forensic and legal medicine, 53*, 87-96. https://doi.org/10.1016/j.jflm.2017.11.008.

Ischiropoulos, H., Beers, M. F., Ohnishi, S. T., Fisher, D., Garner, S. E., & Thom, S. R. (1996). Nitric oxide production and perivascular nitration in brain after carbon monoxide poisoning in the rat. *The Journal of clinical investigation, 97*(10), 2260-2267. https://doi.org/10.1172/jci118667.

Kao, L. W., & Nañagas, K. A. (2004). Carbon monoxide poisoning. *Emergency Medicine Clinics, 22*(4), 985-1018. https://doi.org/10.1016/j.emc.2004.05.003.

Kao, L. W., & Nanagas, K. A. (2006). Toxicity associated with carbon monoxide. *Clinics in laboratory medicine, 26*(1), 99-125. https://doi.org/10.1016/j.cll.2006.01.005.

Kinoshita, H., Türkan, H., Vucinic, S., Naqvi, S., Bedair, R., Rezaee, R., & Tsatsakis, A. (2020). Carbon monoxide poisoning. *Toxicology reports, 7*, 169-173. https://doi.org/10.1016/j.toxrep.2020.01.005.

Koçyiğit, A., & Benay, C. A. N. (2021). Karbonmonoksit Zehirlenmelerinde Postmortem Değişiklikler [Postmortem Changes in Carbon Monoxide Poisoning]. *Journal of Faculty of Pharmacy of Ankara University*, *45*(3), 722-735.

Koyuncu, S., Bol, O., Ertan, T., Günay, N., & Akdogan, H. İ. (2020). The detection of occult CO poisoning through noninvasive measurement of carboxyhemoglobin: A cross-sectional study. *The American journal of emergency medicine*, *38*(6), 1110-1114. https://doi.org/10.1016/j.ajem.2019.158383.

Lee, J., Mukai, D., Kreuter, K., Mahon, S., Tromberg, B., & Brenner, M. (2007). Potential interference by hydroxocobalamin on cooximetry hemoglobin measurements during cyanide and smoke inhalation treatments. *Annals of emergency medicine*, *49*(6), 802-805. https://doi.org/10.1016/j.annemergmed.2006.11.016.

Livshits, Z., Lugassy, D. M., Shawn, L. K., & Hoffman, R. S. (2012). Falsely low carboxyhemoglobin level after hydroxocobalamin therapy. *New England Journal of Medicine*, *367*(13), 1270-1271. https://doi.org/10.1056/nejmc1114820.

Metin, S., Yıldız, Ş., Çakmak, T., & Demirbaş, Ş. (2011). Frequency of carboxyhemoglobin poisoning in Turkey in 2010. *TAF Preventive Medicine Bulletin*, *10*(5), 587-592. https://doi.org/10.5455/pmb.20110417125648.

Meyer-Witting, M., Helps, S., & Gorman, D. F. (1991). Acute carbon monoxide exposure and cerebral blood flow in rabbits. *Anaesthesia and intensive care*, *19*(3), 373-377. https://doi.org/10.1177/0310057x9101900311.

Mureşan, C. O., Zăvoi, R. E., Dumache, R. O., Precup, C. V., Ciocan, V., Bulzan, O. Ş., Florou, C. & Enache, A. (2019). Co-morbidities in the multiple victims of the silent killer in carbon monoxide poisoning. *Rom J Morphol Embryol*, *60*(1), 125-131.

Nguyen, V., Salama, M., Fernandez, D., Sperling, J. D., Regina, A., Rivera, R., Wang, J., Friedman, B. W. & Smith, S. W. (2020). Comparison between carbon monoxide poisoning from hookah smoking versus other sources. *Clinical toxicology*, *58*(12), 1320-1325. https://doi.org/10.1080/15563650.2020.1745225.

Pace, R., Bon Homme, M., Hoffman, R. S., & Lugassy, D. (2014). Effects of hydroxocobalamin on carboxyhemoglobin measured under physiologic and pathologic conditions. *Clinical Toxicology*, *52*(7), 647-650. https://doi.org/10.3109/15563650.2014.939659.

Prockop, L. D., & Chichkova, R. I. (2007). Carbon monoxide intoxication: an updated review. *Journal of the neurological sciences*, *262*(1-2), 122-130. https://doi.org/10.1016/j.jns.2007.06.037.

Raub, J, World Health Organization & International *Programme on Chemical Safety. (1999). Carbon monoxide* (2nd ed.). World Health Organization. https://apps.who.int/iris/handle/10665/42180.

Retzky, S. S. (2017). Carbon monoxide poisoning from hookah smoking: an emerging public health problem. *Journal of medical toxicology*, *13*(2), 193-194. https://doi.org/10.1007/s13181-017-0617-5.

Schallner, N., Fuchs, M., Schwer, C. I., Loop, T., Buerkle, H., Lagrèze, W. A., van Oterendorp, C., Biermann, J., & Goebel, U. (2012). Postconditioning with inhaled carbon monoxide counteracts apoptosis and neuroinflammation in the ischemic rat retina. *PLoS One,* 7, e46479. https://doi.org/10.1371/journal.pone.0046479.

Simonsen, C., Thorsteinsson, K., Mortensen, R. N., Torp-Pedersen, C., Kjærgaard, B., & Andreasen, J. J. (2019). Carbon monoxide poisoning in Denmark with focus on mortality and factors contributing to mortality. *PLoS one*, *14*(1), e0210767. https://doi.org/10.1371/journal.pone.0210767.

Temrel, T. A. (2021). Mortality rate associated with carbon monoxide poisoning in Turkey: A national database study. *JPMA. The Journal of the Pakistan Medical Association*, *71*(1 (B)), 262-266. https://doi.org/10.47391/jpma.637.

Thom, S. R., Ohnishi, S. T., & Ischiropoulos, H. (1994). Nitric oxide released by platelets inhibits neutrophil B2 integrin function following acute carbon monoxide poisoning. *Toxicology and applied pharmacology*, *128*(1), 105-110. https://doi.org/10.1006/taap.1994.1186.

Thomassen, Ø., Brattebø, G., & Rostrup, M. (2004). Carbon monoxide poisoning while using a small cooking stove in a tent. *The American journal of emergency medicine*, *22*(3), 204-206. https://doi.org/10.1016/j.ajem.2004.02.011.

Tintinalli, E. (2013). *Tintinalli Emergency Medicine, A Comprehensive Study Guide*. (Çete, Y., Denizbaşı, A., Çevik, A.A., Oktay, C., Atilla, A., Trnsl. Eds.). İstanbul: Nobel Tıp Kitabevi

Uysalol, M., Paslı Uysalol, E., Saraçoğlu Varol, G., & Kayaoğlu, S. (2011). A retrospective analysis of pediatric patients admitted to the pediatric emergency service for carbon monoxide intoxication. *Balkan Medical Journal*, 28, 237-243. https://doi.org/10.5174/tutfd.2010.03766.1.

Williams, V. F., Fedgo, A., & Stahlman, S. (2020). Carbon monoxide poisoning, active and reserve component service members and non-service member beneficiaries of the Military Health System, US Armed Forces, July 2009-June 2019. *Medical surveillance monthly report*, *27*(1), 2-16.

Wolf, S. J., Lavonas, E. J., Sloan, E. P., & Jagoda, A. S. (2008). Clinical policy: critical issues in the management of adult patients presenting to the emergency department with acute carbon monoxide poisoning. *Journal of Emergency Nursing*, *34*(2), e19-e32. https://doi.org/10.1016/j.jen.2008.02.009.

Wu, L., & Wang, R. (2005). Carbon monoxide: endogenous production, physiological functions, and pharmacological applications. *Pharmacological reviews*, *57*(4), 585-630. https://doi.org/10.1124/pr.57.4.3.

Chapter 2

Acute Clinical Effects of Carbon Monoxide Poisoning

Ali Duman[1,*], MD
Ayhan Aköz[1], MD
Selçuk Eren Çanakçı[1], MD
and Çağaç Yetiş[2], MD

[1]Department of Emergency Medicine, Aydın Adnan Menderes University, Aydın, Turkey
[2]Emergency Medicine, Aydın Söke Fehime Faik Kocagöz State Hospital, Söke, Aydın, Turkey

Abstract

Carbon monoxide (CO) is an odorless, tasteless, colorless, and nonirritating gas, and it is produced by inadequate hydrocarbon combustion. CO poisoning is common. It is a preventable cause of mortality, it can cause permanent neurological damage and is likely to be underdiagnosed because of its atypical flu-like symptoms. CO poisoning is common during winter; poorly functioning heating systems, generators, poorly ventilated heating and cooking appliances, and inhaled smoke may cause poisoning. After inhalation of CO, it diffuses rapidly through the pulmonary capillary membrane, and, with a higher affinity for Hb than oxygen, it is the leading cause of poisoning. The clinical findings of CO intoxication are often nonspecific and inconsistent. Headache, nausea, and dizziness were the most frequently reported complaints. Physical findings in CO poisoning usually consist of tachypnea, tachycardia, and changes in mental status, unless there is an

* Corresponding Author's Email: aliduman3489@gmail.com.

In: Carbon Monoxide Poisoning
Editors: Seda Özkan and Afsin Ipekci
ISBN: 979-8-89113-217-7

accompanying burn or trauma. Patients may be in a state of consciousness such as confusion, stupor, and coma. Treatment begins with oxygen. HBO Therapy aims to prevent delayed neurologic sequelae. Patients with mild symptoms can be treated in the emergency room and safely discharged. Patients with severe poisoning symptoms and/or with other additional medical or social causes should be hospitalized.

Keywords: emergency, carbon monoxide, clinical effects, poisoning

Introduction

The so-called "silent killer" carbon monoxide (CO) is an odorless, tasteless, colorless, nonirritating gas, and it is produced by inadequate hydrocarbon combustion (Can et al., 2019). While endogenous CO production by hemoglobin (Hb) catabolism is a component of normal biochemical processes, exogenous CO sources such as motor vehicle exhaust fumes, generators, poorly functioning heating systems, poorly ventilated heating and cooking appliances, and inhaled smoke may cause poisoning (Ernst & Zibrak, 1998). Volatile anesthetic agents can also be a source of CO in operating rooms (OR), especially when used with carbon dioxide absorbents, and may cause CO poisoning in the operating room (OR) (Coppens et al., 2006). The concentration of CO in the atmosphere is less than 0.001%, but can rise to 20% in vehicle exhaust, up to 30% in gas heating circuits, and up to 60% in smoke from explosions and fires (Sinkovič et al., 2006). Some occupations, such as firefighters and steelworkers, are at high risk of accidental CO poisoning. Suicide is the most common cause of intentional CO poisoning, and it often appears to be the result of inhaling car exhaust fumes indoors (Ernst & Zibrak, 1998; Gorman et al., 2003). Recently, cases of CO poisoning due to waterpipe (hookah) smoking have also been reported (Nguyen et al., 2020; Retzky, 2017). In physiological amounts, endogenous CO acts as a neurotransmitter (Boehning et al., 2003). Low levels of CO can positively modulate apoptosis, inflammation, and cell proliferation and regulate biogenesis in mitochondria. However, as exposure increases, symptoms of poisoning occur (Mannaioni et al., 2006; Suliman et al., 2007; Taillé et al., 2003; Zhang et al., 2003). Two-thirds of deaths from CO poisoning are intentional, while unintended CO poisonings cause the rest (Rose et al., 2017). While unintentional poisonings are more common in cold climates during winter, these seasonal and regional differences are not seen in intentional poisonings (Manaker & Perry, 2023).

CO poisoning is still the most common cause of poisoning-related mortality in the United States (USA), although it is preventable (Shin et al., 2023). It is estimated to occur in 50.000 people annually in the US with an overall mortality rate of 1 to 3 percent (Manaker & Perry, 2023). CO can also precipitate irreversible delayed neurologic sequela (DNS), expanding its importance as a public health concern (Manaker & Perry, 2023).

Pathophysiology

After inhalation of CO, it immediately diffuses through the pulmonary capillary membrane, and with a higher affinity for Hb than oxygen, it is the leading cause of the toxicity. The affinity of CO for Hb is about 200 times greater than that of oxygen (Weaver, 2009). CO binds to HB with high affinity, and the resulting carboxyhemoglobin (CO-Hb) complex becomes incapable of delivering adequate oxygen to the tissues and the cells. Thus, the arterial oxygen content is decreased despite adequate partial oxygen pressures in the blood. More damage occurs when CO causes the oxyhemoglobin dissociation curve to move leftwards. Therefore, the delivery of oxygen from hemoglobin to the tissue is reduced (Roughton & Darling, 1944). Even exposure to low levels of CO (10 ppm) may result in measurable COHb levels of about 2% (Raub et al., 2000). The World Health Organization (WHO) claims that prolonged exposure to levels higher than 6 ppm is potentially toxic (Penny et al., 2010). Smokers have a higher basal CO level than non-smokers. While 10% or more COHb level is abnormal in smokers and 2% or more in non-smokers and may cause symptoms (Hampson et al., 2012; Penny et al., 2010). COHb-related hypoxia is not the only cause of CO toxicity. The symptoms of intoxicants as well as complications such as the DNS phenomenon cannot be predicted by the degree of binding between CO and Hb. Also, this cannot explain cognitive damage even at COHb levels as low as 4-5% (Tomaszewski, 2015). What is inherent in CO toxicity is its transmission to vital organs like the heart and brain. Although the COHb level is easily measurable, its contribution to clinical toxicity is rare. CO can reach tissue not by binding to Hb but by dissolving in plasma (Tomaszewski, 2015). About 10-15% of CO is extravascular and bound to extravascular proteins such as myoglobin, NADPH reductase, and cytochromes that cause impairment of oxidative phosphorylation (Hardy & Thom, 1994). CO causes superoxide generation and oxidative stress, possibly contributing to lipid peroxidation and neurological damage (Manaker & Perry, 2023).

Clinical Effects

Subacute CO exposure defines long-term exposure that lasts more than 24 hours. This exposure usually occurs sporadically, including weeks, months, or even years. The incidence of chronic exposure has not been revealed. Symptoms of subacute intoxication may differ from acute intoxication and include emotional distress, chronic fatigue, difficulty working, memory deficits, vertigo, sleep disturbances, neuropathy, paresthesias, polycythemia, abdominal pain, recurrent infections, and diarrhea (Penny, 2007). The clinical findings of acute CO poisoning are usually nonspecific and inconstant. Patients with mild or moderate CO intoxication usually present with simple symptoms and may be misdiagnosed with the viral syndrome (Weaver, 2009). Headache, nausea, and dizziness were the most frequently reported complaints in exposure calls made to poison centers in the US (Table 1) (Shin et al., 2023). These typical complaints and the fact that exposure is most common during the winter months explain why these patients were misdiagnosed with influenza (Dolan et al., 1987). CO exposure values and the resulting COHb level determine the severity of symptoms (Mattiuzzi & Lippi, 2020). If the CO concentration is between 10-20%, patients usually experience tachypnea, fatigue, nausea, confusion, emotionality, and clumsiness. CO levels between 21% and 30% are accompanied by exertional dyspnea, angina, headache, mild muscular weakness, visual impairment, difficulty adapting to the environment, lack of reaction to danger and decreased sensory perception. Nausea, vomiting, dizziness, troubled decision-making, fainting, and confusion are common symptoms when the CO concentration rises between 31% and 50%. At >51% CO values, severe acidosis, coma, seizures, and death are common symptoms (Gözübüyük, 2017). The most common reports of CO exposure to poison centers are usually for children and young adults; however, deaths from CO poisoning occur more frequently among men and older adults (≥80 years) (Shin et al., 2023). Children and the elderly are more prone to CO poisoning because their metabolic demands are increased, they cannot express symptoms, and their mobility is limited (Wolkin et al., 2012). Headache, the most common symptom, is often expressed as frontal, continuous, and dull. CO poisoning is often misdiagnosed with colic in infants, gastroenteritis, and food poisoning as well. Children, as adults, have nonspecific symptoms that make diagnosis difficult (Tomaszewski, 2015). In the absence of concomitant trauma or burns, findings of CO poisoning are often limited to tachypnea, tachycardia, and changes in mental status. Patients may be in a state of consciousness ranging from mild confusion to coma (Manaker & Perry, 2023).

Table 1. Symptoms reported to poison centers and their frequency

Headache	58%
Nausea	33%
Dizziness	29%
Drowsiness	14%
Vomiting	14%
Cough/choking	6%
Confusion	5%
Shortness of breath	5%
Syncope	5%
Throat or eye irritation Chest pain Weakness	<5%

Critical Illness

CO poisoning is more critical in some patients and these patients and therefore require special intensive and supportive care. Severe acute CO poisoning is associated with progressive brain damage and edema and cognitive dysfunction that can progress quickly (Weaver, 2009). The parameters related to high early mortality are fire as a source of CO poisoning, unconsciousness, high levels of COHb, pH values less than 7.2, and the need for endotracheal intubation (Hampson & Hauff, 2008).

Effects on the Central Nervous System

The central nervous system (CNS) is the organ system most susceptible to CO intoxication. In patients without comorbid disease, headache, dizziness, and ataxia can be seen acutely, even at COHb levels as low as 15-20%. Patients with higher levels of COHb and a longer exposure history may experience syncope, seizures, or coma (Weaver, 2009). Patients can present with focal neurological symptoms that may be confused with a stroke. Decreases in oxygen delivery and mitochondrial oxidative phosphorylation mediated by

CO exposure cause anoxic and ischemic brain damage leading to cognitive impairments in survivors (Geocadin et al., 2008). Brain injury due to ischemia may result from acidosis, excitotoxicity, oxidative stress, ionic imbalance, and depolarization, inflammation, and apoptosis. A large influx of intracellular calcium aggravates brain injury due to the inactivation of the plasma membrane Ca^{2+} ATPase resulting from a decrease in oxidative phosphorylation and ATP synthesis (Doyle et al., 2008). Eventually, there is an activation of excitatory amino acids that may be mainly responsible for the subsequent loss of neurons (Thom et al., 2004). In a study, it was shown that the concentrations of glutamate, an excitatory amino acid, increased in the rat brain after CO intoxication. Glutamate binds to N methyl-D-aspartate (NMDA) receptors and causes intracellular calcium release, resulting in an effect that ends in delayed neuron death. This increase in glutamate concentrations is then followed by an increase in hydroxyl radicals (Piantadosi et al., 1997). Eventually, at 1-3 weeks, rats show histological evidence of both neuronal necrosis and apoptosis in the cerebellum, frontal cortex, and globus pallidus, accompanied by a lack of learning and memory (Tomaszewski, 2015). The electroencephalogram (EEG) may show diffuse frontal slow wave activity. On a day of coma-inducing exposure, computed tomography (CT) and magnetic resonance imaging (MRI) can show a decrease in density in the globus pallidus and central white matter (Lo et al., 2007). Involvement in several other areas, including the cerebellum, cerebral cortex, substantia nigra, and hippocampus, has been demonstrated in autopsies (Lapresle & Fardeau, 1967).

Effects on Cardiovascular System

Continuous exposure to CO can lead to symptoms related to decreased oxygen delivery to the myocardium. CO poisoning can aggravate angina and cause myocardial damage, even in people with normal coronary arteries (Kalay et al., 2007; Satran et al., 2005). Therefore, patients with CO exposure should undergo a cardiovascular examination that includes electrocardiography (ECG) and measurement of cardiac enzymes (Weaver, 2009). In volunteers with stable angina, low-level exposures resulting in COHb levels between 2-4% cause signs and symptoms of myocardial ischemia with reduced exercise tolerance (Allred et al., 1989). At higher CO levels (6% COHb), the frequency of premature ventricular contractions increases during exercise. Arrhythmias and acute myocardial infarction can occur in poisoned patients, and acute death from CO intoxication is often the result of ventricular arrhythmias (Allred et al., 1989, 1991). Impairment of repolarization and prolongation of the QT interval appear to be the most common CO-related electrophysiological disorder (Dallas et al., 2012; Macmillan et al., 2001). Reduced access to ATP due to inhibition of oxidative phosphorylation causes changes in calcium gradients, resulting in increased diastolic intracellular calcium, increased calcium sensitivity of myofilaments, and a hyperadrenergic state (Andre et al., 2010). Long-term exposure to CO is usually related to transient myocardial stunning lasting around 24 hours and accompanied by a reduction in left ventricular ejection fraction (LVEF) (Kalay et al., 2007). The increase in β-type natriuretic peptide seen in these patients is associated with a decrease in LVEF. Troponin levels may also be elevated without signs of coronary artery disease or changes in ECG or echocardiography (Cha et al., 2014; Davutoglu et al., 2006). There is an increased risk of cardiac mortality associated with the death of approximately one-third of these patients within 8 years of severe CO intoxication (Henry et al., 2006). There may be multiple mechanisms that cause cardiac dysfunction and myocardial ischemia in CO intoxication. Animal studies have shown that the decreased systemic oxygen delivery associated with CO poisoning is initially compensated by oxygen extraction and increased cardiac output (Smithline et al., 2003). CO has been shown to increase the risk of arterial and venous thrombosis presumably due to CO-binding fibrinogen-heme and increased platelet aggregation (Dziewierz et al., 2013; Lippi et al., 2012). It has been claimed that CO-induced increased free radical production and global endothelial dysfunction escalate coronary vasoconstriction (Lippi et al., 2012). CO increases the expression of inducible NO synthase leading to NO-related myocardial damage (Meyer et al., 2015). The direct binding of CO with high affinity to myoglobin in myocytes and the inhibition of oxidative phosphorylation cause acute myocardial infarction and cardiac dysfunction even without an underlying coronary artery disease (Lippi et al., 2012; Prockop & Chichkova, 2007).

Metabolic Effects

Metabolic changes can show the toxic effects of CO more than the COHb level itself. In mild CO poisoning, respiratory alkalosis can occur to compensate for decreased oxygen transport capacity and oxygen delivery. Severe exposures cause metabolic acidosis with high lactate levels accompanied by tissue hypoxia (Sokal & Kralkowska, 1985).

Effects on Other Organ Systems

While the heart and brain are the most susceptible organs, other organs can experience the effects of CO intoxication as well. 20-30% of patients with severe CO intoxication (requiring advanced airway management) develop pulmonary edema (Tomaszewski, 2015). The development of pulmonary edema may be due to cardiac depression directly from CO or acute respiratory distress syndrome (ARDS) from smoke inhalation (Grabowska et al., 2012; Kalay et al., 2007). Patients rarely develop acute renal failure (ARF) even though myonecrosis and compartment syndromes can occur. Retinal hemorrhages can develop in exposures lasting 12 hours. Cherry-red skin color, a postmortem finding, occurs only after overexposure due to CO-induced vasodilation, inability to extract oxygen from arterial blood, and accompanying tissue ischemia. Severe exposure may cause another uncommon phenomenon in which cutaneous bullae appear. These are presumed to be caused by a combination of the direct effects of CO on the epidermis and pressure necrosis (Tomaszewski, 2015).

Effects on Pregnant Women, Fetuses, and Infants

Pregnant women should be hospitalized after exposure to CO and intensive monitoring should be provided for both pregnant women and fetuses. The affinity of CO for fetal Hb is stronger. Fetal COHb level is higher than maternal and clearance is 5 times slower (Gözübüyük, 2017). Fetal COHb level returns to normal 40 hours after maternal COHb level (Ernst & Zibrak, 1998; Turner et al., 1999). Another important issue at this point is that fetal exposure may occur, even if the maternal CO level is not toxic. Thus, compared to other cases of CO poisoning, hyperbaric oxygen (HBO) treatment is initiated at lower maternal CO levels and is longer-lasting and more aggressive in protecting the fetus (Gözübüyük, 2017). There is no correlation between maternal COHb level and fetal death (Levasseur et al., 1996). In addition, CO exposure may have teratogenic effects, such as miscarriage and physical and/or psychomotor deformities. In cases of CO poisoning, adverse effects have been reported on the fetal brain in the third trimester, despite the administration of HBO therapy (Gözübüyük, 2017). CO intoxication in infants is often reported when the mother is exposed (Salam et al., 2005). The normal CO level is 4% in infants. The longer half-life of fetal COHb, the higher affinity of CO for fetal Hb, immature CNS, and increased consumption of oxygen escalate the risks of CO intoxication in infants (Chou et al., 2000).

Delayed Neurologic Sequelae

Delayed neurological sequelae (DNS) syndrome includes personality changes, varying degrees of cognitive impairment, movement disorders, and neurological defects (Manaker & Perry, 2023). This syndrome occurs in 15-40% of patients with severe CO exposure (Rose et al., 2017). DNS usually occurs within 20 days after CO-poisoning but is reported to occur 3 to 240 days after apparent recovery. Deficits may persist for a year or more (Choi, 1983; Thom et al., 1995). Thirty-three years after a mining accident involving 156 CO-poisoning miners, 68.6% of survivors had mental disorders and 48.7% had neurological symptoms, which shows the irreversible nature of this situation (Mimura et al., 1999). Patients older than 30 years of age are more sensitive to the development of DNS. Most cases are related to loss of consciousness in acute toxicity (Choi, 1983). The severity of initial symptoms is not associated with the development of long-term neurological problems (Chambers et al., 2008). Even though DNS has been associated with deformities in deep white matter and the globus pallidus, these findings are typically not present in acute poisoning on CT and MRI (Choi, 1983; Kim et al., 2003; Teksam et al., 2002; Zagami et al., 1993).

Management

Treatment begins with oxygen. The half-life of COHb is in contrariwise proportional to PO_2. While it is about 5 hours in room air, it can be reduced to 1 hour by providing 100% oxygen and 30 minutes with HBO treatment in 3 atmospheres (Christopher & Lewis, 2022). Without functioning Hb, an adequate PO_2 can be obtained with the administration of HBO therapy to keep the patient alive. However, this only helps when the COHb level is too high. Therefore, the primary indication for HBO therapy is not to prevent mortality, but to prevent delayed neurological sequelae. There are differing perspectives on the benefit of HBO therapy because the effect is not immediate and evaluation needs close follow-up and complicated testing (Lin et al., 2018). HBO therapy should be administered within 6 hours after CO exposure, and its effectiveness appears to decrease as this period is delayed. HBO therapy helps prevent the development of delayed neuropsychiatric and neurological sequelae, and its use has been shown to reduce DNS from approximately 12% to less than 1% (Christopher & Lewis, 2022). A patient with a neurological abnormality or cardiovascular instability is a candidate for HBO therapy. When deciding on HBO Therapy, evaluating the COHb level alone is insufficient. However, HBO Therapy is recommended for asymptomatic patients with a COHb level of 25% or higher and pregnant women with a COHb level of 15% or higher regardless of symptoms. Patients with low-level long-term CO exposure may exhibit a "soaking" phenomenon characterized by extremely high tissue CO concentrations despite low levels of COHb. Therefore, if clinical signs thought to be associated with CO poisoning are present, HBO Therapy should be given despite relatively low COHb levels (Christopher & Lewis, 2022).

Disposition

Patients with mild symptoms and whose complaints improve can be discharged with special follow-up. Patients with signs of end-organ damage, such as altered mental status or chest pain, should be hospitalized for observation if they are not eligible for HBO therapy. All patients exposed to CO should be closely followed for the DNS (Christopher & Lewis, 2022).

Conclusion

CO is a toxic gas that is released by the inadequate combustion of carbon-containing materials and can damage the heart, brain, and lungs. Exposure to this gas decreases the ability of the blood to deliver oxygen to tissues and vital organs. Pregnant women and fetuses, infants, the elderly, and people with a history of respiratory or heart disease and/or anemia are more sensitive to poisoning. In addition, it can cause delayed irreversible neurological sequela, which poses an important public health problem. Headache, dizziness, and nausea are the most common complaints. Patients are often misdiagnosed with influenza because of the most common exposure in winter and those typical complaints. Treatment begins with oxygen. HBO Therapy aims to prevent DNS. Patients with mild symptoms can be treated in the emergency room and discharged safely. Patients with severe poisoning symptoms and/or other additional medical or social causes should be hospitalized.

References

Allred, E. N., Bleecker, E. R., Chaitman, B. R., Dahms, T. E., Gottlieb, S. O., Hackney, J. D., Pagano, M., Selvester, R. H., Walden, S. M., & Warren, J. (1989). Short-Term Effects of Carbon Monoxide Exposure on the Exercise Performance of Subjects with Coronary Artery Disease. *New England Journal of Medicine*, *321*(21), 1426–1432. https://doi.org/10.1056/NEJM198911233212102.

Allred, E. N., Bleecker, E. R., Chaitman, B. R., Dahms, T. E., Gottlieb, S. O., Hackney, J. D., Pagano, M., Selvester, R. H., Walden, S. M., & Warren, J. (1991). Effects of carbon monoxide on myocardial ischemia. *Environmental Health Perspectives*, *91*(1), 89–132. https://doi.org/10.1289/ehp.919189.

Andre, L., Boissière, J., Reboul, C., Perrier, R., Zalvidea, S., Meyer, G., Thireau, J., Tanguy, S., Bideaux, P., Hayot, M., Boucher, F., Obert, P., Cazorla, O., & Richard, S. (2010). Carbon monoxide pollution promotes cardiac remodeling and ventricular arrhythmia in healthy rats. *American Journal of Respiratory and Critical Care Medicine*, *181*(6), 587–595. https://doi.org/10.1164/rccm.200905-0794OC.

Boehning, D., Moon, C., Sharma, S., Hurt, K. J., Hester, L. D., Ronnett, G. V., Shugar, D., & Snyder, S. H. (2003). Carbon monoxide neurotransmission activated by CK2 phosphorylation of heme oxygenase-2. *Neuron*, *40*(1), 129–137. https://doi.org/10.1016/S0896-6273(03)00596-8.

Can, G., Saylll, U., Aksu Sayman, Ö., Kuyumcu, Ö. F., Yllmaz, D., Esen, E., Yurtseven, E., & Erginöz, E. (2019). Mapping of carbon monoxide related death risk in Turkey: A ten-year analysis based on news agency records. *BMC Public Health*, *19*(1), 1–7. https://doi.org/10.1186/s12889-018-6342-4.

Cha, Y. S., Cha, K. C., Kim, O. H., Lee, K. H., Hwang, S. O., & Kim, H. (2014). Features and predictors of myocardial injury in carbon monoxide poisoned patients. *Emergency Medicine Journal*, *31*(3), 210–215. https://doi.org/10.1136/emermed-2012-202152.

Chambers, C. A., Hopkins, R. O., Weaver, L. K., & Key, C. (2008). Cognitive and affective outcomes of more severe compared to less severe carbon monoxide poisoning. *Brain Injury*, *22*(5), 387–395. https://doi.org/10.1080/02699050802008075.

Choi, S. (1983). Delayed Neurologic Sequelae in Carbon Monoxide Intoxication. *Archives of Neurology*, *40*(7), 433–435. https://doi.org/10.1001/archneur.1983.04050070063016.

Chou, K. J., Fisher, J. L., & Silver, E. J. (2000). Characteristics and outcome of children with carbon monoxide poisoning with and without smoke exposure referred for hyperbaric oxygen therapy. *Pediatric Emergency Care*, *16*(3), 151–155. https://doi.org/10.1097/00006565-200006000-00002.

Christopher, W. M., & Lewis, S. N. (2022). Inhaled Toxins. In R. M. Walls, R. S. Hockberger, M. Gausche-Hill, T. B. Erickson, S. R. Wilcox, K. Bakes, C. A. Brown III, D. F. M. Brown, J. Davis, A. Jagoda, A. H. Kaji, L. D. Sanchez, J. A. Tyndall, &

M. VanRooyen (Eds.), *Rosen's Emergency Medicine - Concepts and Clinical Practice 10th Edition* (10th ed., pp. 1940–1947). Elsevier.

Coppens, M. J., Versichelen, L. F. M., Rolly, G., Mortier, E. P., & Struys, M. M. R. F. (2006). The mechanisms of carbon monoxide production by inhalational agents. *Anaesthesia*, *61*(5), 462–468. https://doi.org/10.1111/j.1365-2044.2006.04536.x.

Dallas, M. L., Yang, Z., Boyle, J. P., Boycott, H. E., Scragg, J. L., Milligan, C. J., Elies, J., Duke, A., Thireau, J., Reboul, C., Richard, S., Bernus, O., Steele, D. S., & Peers, C. (2012). Carbon monoxide induces cardiac arrhythmia via induction of the late Na+ current. *American Journal of Respiratory and Critical Care Medicine*, *186*(7), 648–656. https://doi.org/10.1164/rccm.201204-0688OC.

Davutoglu, V., Gunay, N., Kocoglu, H., Gunay, N. E., Yildirim, C., Cavdar, M., & Tarakcioglu, M. (2006). Serum levels of NT-ProBNP as an early cardiac marker of carbon monoxide poisoning. *Inhalation Toxicology*, *18*(2), 155–158. https://doi.org/10.1080/08958370500305885.

Dolan, M. C., Haltom, T. L., Barrows, G. H., Short, C. S., & Ferriell, K. M. (1987). Carboxyhemoglobin levels in patients with flu-like symptoms. *Annals of Emergency Medicine*, *16*(7), 782–786. https://doi.org/10.1016/S0196-0644(87)80575-9.

Doyle, K. P., Simon, R. P., & Stenzel-Poore, M. P. (2008). Mechanisms of ischemic brain damage. *Neuropharmacology*, *55*(3), 310–318. https://doi.org/10.1016/j.neuropharm.2008.01.005.

Dziewierz, A., Ciszowski, K., Gawlikowski, T., Rakowski, T., Kleczyński, P., Surdacki, A., & Dudek, D. (2013). Primary angioplasty in patient with st-segment elevation myocardial infarction in the setting of intentional carbon monoxide poisoning. *Journal of Emergency Medicine*, *45*(6), 831–834. https://doi.org/10.1016/j.jemermed.2013.05.061.

Ernst, A., & Zibrak, J. D. (1998). Carbon Monoxide Poisoning. *New England Journal of Medicine*, *339*(22), 1603–1608. https://doi.org/10.1056/NEJM199811263392206.

Geocadin, R. G., Koenig, M. A., Jia, X., Stevens, R. D., & Peberdy, M. A. (2008). Management of Brain Injury After Resuscitation From Cardiac Arrest. *Neurologic Clinics*, *26*(2), 487–506. https://doi.org/10.1016/j.ncl.2008.03.015.

Gorman, D., Drewry, A., Huang, Y. L., & Sames, C. (2003). The clinical toxicology of carbon monoxide. *Toxicology*, *187*(1), 25–38. https://doi.org/10.1016/S0300-483X(03)00005-2.

Gözübüyük, A. A. (2017). Carbon monoxide intoxication epidemiology, pathophysiology, clinical evaluation and treatment during childhood, in newborn and fetus. *Northern Clinics of Istanbul*, *4*(1), 100–107. https://doi.org/10.14744/nci.2017.49368.

Grabowska, T., Skowronek, R., Nowicka, J., & Sybirska, H. (2012). Prevalence of hydrogen cyanide and carboxyhemoglobin in victims of smoke inhalation during enclosed-space fires: A combined toxicological risk. *Clinical Toxicology*, *50*(8), 759–763. https://doi.org/10.3109/15563650.2012.714470.

Hampson, N. B., & Hauff, N. M. (2008). Risk factors for short-term mortality from carbon monoxide poisoning treated with hyperbaric oxygen. *Critical Care Medicine*, *36*(9), 2523–2527. https://doi.org/10.1097/CCM.0b013e31818419d8.

Hampson, N. B., Piantadosi, C. A., Thom, S. R., & Weaver, L. K. (2012). Practice recommendations in the diagnosis, management, and prevention of carbon monoxide poisoning. *American Journal of Respiratory and Critical Care Medicine*, *186*(11), 1095–1101. https://doi.org/10.1164/rccm.201207-1284CI.

Hardy, K. R., & Thom, S. R. (1994). Pathophysiology and Treatment of Carbon Monoxide Poisoning. *Journal of Toxicology: Clinical Toxicology*, *32*(6), 613–629. https://doi.org/10.3109/15563659409017973.

Henry, C. R., Satran, D., Lindgren, B., Adkinson, C., Nicholson, C. I., & Henry, T. D. (2006). Myocardial injury and long-term mortality following moderate to severe carbon monoxide poisoning. *Jama*, *295*(4), 398–402. https://doi.org/10.1001/jama.295.4.398.

Kalay, N., Ozdogru, I., Cetinkaya, Y., Eryol, N. K., Dogan, A., Gul, I., Inanc, T., Ikizceli, I., Oguzhan, A., & Abaci, A. (2007). Cardiovascular Effects of Carbon Monoxide Poisoning. *American Journal of Cardiology*, *99*(3), 322–324. https://doi.org/10.1016/j.amjcard.2006.08.030.

Kim, J. H., Chang, K. H., Song, I. C., Kim, K. H., Kwon, B. J., Kim, H. C., Kim, J. H., & Han, M. H. (2003). Delayed encephalopathy of acute carbon monoxide intoxication: Diffusivity of cerebral white matter lesions. *American Journal of Neuroradiology*, *24*(8), 1592–1597.

Lapresle, J., & Fardeau, M. (1967). *The Central Nervous System and Carbon Monoxide Poisoning II. Anatomical Study of Brain Lesions following Intoxication with Carbon Monoxide (22 cases)* (Vol. 6, pp. 31–74). https://doi.org/10.1016/S0079-6123(08)60181-8.

Levasseur, L., Galliot-Guilley, M., Richter, F., Scherrmann, J., & Baud, F. (1996). Effects of mode of inhalation of carbon monoxide and normobaric oxygen administration on carbon monoxide elimination from the blood. *Human & Experimental Toxicology*, *15*(11), 898–903. https://doi.org/10.1177/096032719601501106.

Lin, C.-H., Su, W.-H., Chen, Y.-C., Feng, P.-H., Shen, W.-C., Ong, J.-R., Wu, M.-Y., & Wong, C. S. (2018). Treatment with normobaric or hyperbaric oxygen and its effect on neuropsychiatric dysfunction after carbon monoxide poisoning. *Medicine*, *97*(39), e12456. https://doi.org/10.1097/md.0000000000012456.

Lippi, G., Rastelli, G., Meschi, T., Borghi, L., & Cervellin, G. (2012). Pathophysiology, clinics, diagnosis and treatment of heart involvement in carbon monoxide poisoning. *Clinical Biochemistry*, *45*(16–17), 1278–1285. https://doi.org/10.1016/j.clinbiochem.2012.06.004.

Lo, C. P., Chen, S. Y., Lee, K. W., Chen, W. L., Chen, C. Y., Hsueh, C. J., & Huang, G. S. (2007). Brain injury after acute carbon monoxide poisoning: early and late complications. *AJR. American Journal of Roentgenology*, *189*(4), 205–211. https://doi.org/10.2214/AJR.07.2425.

Macmillan, C. S. A., Wildsmith, J. A. W., & Hamilton, W. F. D. (2001). Reversible increase in QT dispersion during carbon monoxide poisoning. *Acta Anaesthesiologica Scandinavica*, *45*(3), 396–397. https://doi.org/10.1034/j.1399-6576.2001.045003396.x.

Manaker, S., & Perry, H. (2023). *Carbon Monoxide Poisoning*. UpToDate. https://www.uptodate.com/contents/carbon-monoxide-poisoning/print.

Mannaioni, P. F., Vannacci, A., & Masini, E. (2006). Carbon monoxide: The bad and the good side of the coin, from neuronal death to anti-inflammatory activity. *Inflammation Research*, *55*(7), 261–273. https://doi.org/10.1007/s00011-006-0084-y.

Mattiuzzi, C., & Lippi, G. (2020). Worldwide epidemiology of carbon monoxide poisoning. *Human and Experimental Toxicology*, *39*(4), 387–392. https://doi.org/10.1177/0960327119891214.

Meyer, G., André, L., Kleindienst, A., Singh, F., Tanguy, S., Richard, S., Obert, P., Boucher, F., Jover, B., Cazorla, O., & Reboul, C. (2015). Carbon monoxide increases inducible nos expression that mediates co-induced myocardial damage during ischemia-reperfusion. *American Journal of Physiology-Heart and Circulatory Physiology*, *308*(7), 759–767. https://doi.org/10.1152/ajpheart.00702.2014.

Mimura, K., Harada, M., Sumiyoshi, S., Tohya, G., Takagi, M., Fujita, E., Takata, A., & Tatetsu, S. (1999). Long-term follow-up study on sequelae of carbon monoxide poisoning; serial investigation 33 years after poisoning. *Seishin Shinkeigaku Zasshi = Psychiatria et Neurologia Japonica*, *101*(7), 592–618. http://www.ncbi.nlm.nih.gov/pubmed/10502996.

Nguyen, V., Salama, M., Fernandez, D., Sperling, J. D., Regina, A., Rivera, R., Wang, J., Friedman, B. W., & Smith, S. W. (2020). Comparison between carbon monoxide poisoning from hookah smoking versus other sources. *Clinical Toxicology*, *58*(12), 1320–1325. https://doi.org/10.1080/15563650.2020.1745225.

Penny, D. (2007). Carbon Monoxide Poisoning. In D. G. Penney (Ed.), *Carbon monoxide poisoning* (1st ed.). CRC Press. https://doi.org/10.1201/9780849384189.

Penny, D., Benignus, V., Kephalopoulos, S., Kotzias, D., Kleinman, M., & Verrier, A. (2010). Carbon monoxide. In *WHO guidelines for indoor air quality: selected pollutants* (pp. 55–103). http://www.ncbi.nlm.nih.gov/books/NBK138710/.

Piantadosi, C. A., Zhang, J., Levin, E. D., Folz, R. J., & Schmechel, D. E. (1997). Apoptosis and delayed neuronal damage after carbon monoxide poisoning in the rat. *Experimental Neurology*, *147*(1), 103–114. https://doi.org/10.1006/exnr.1997.6584.

Prockop, L. D., & Chichkova, R. I. (2007). Carbon monoxide intoxication: An updated review. *Journal of the Neurological Sciences*, *262*(1–2), 122–130. https://doi.org/10.1016/j.jns.2007.06.037.

Raub, J. A., Mathieu-Nolf, M., Hampson, N. B., & Thom, S. R. (2000). Carbon monoxide poisoning - A public health perspective. *Toxicology*, *145*(1), 1–14. https://doi.org/10.1016/S0300-483X(99)00217-6.

Retzky, S. S. (2017). Carbon Monoxide Poisoning from Hookah Smoking: An Emerging Public Health Problem. *Journal of Medical Toxicology*, *13*(2), 193–194. https://doi.org/10.1007/s13181-017-0617-5.

Rose, J. J., Wang, L., Xu, Q., McTiernan, C. F., Shiva, S., Tejero, J., & Gladwin, M. T. (2017). Carbon monoxide poisoning: Pathogenesis, management, and future directions of therapy. *American Journal of Respiratory and Critical Care Medicine*, *195*(5), 596–606. https://doi.org/10.1164/rccm.201606-1275CI.

Roughton, F. J. W., & Darling, R. C. (1944). The Effect Of Carbon Monoxide On The Oxyhemoglobin Dissociation Curve. *American Journal of Physiology-Legacy Content*, *141*(1), 17–31. https://doi.org/10.1152/ajplegacy.1944.141.1.17.

Salam, M. T., Millstein, J., Li, Y. F., Lurmann, F. W., Margolis, H. G., & Gilliland, F. D. (2005). Birth outcomes and prenatal exposure to ozone, carbon monoxide, and particulate matter: Results from the Children's Health Study. *Environmental Health Perspectives*, *113*(11), 1638–1644. https://doi.org/10.1289/ehp.8111.

Satran, D., Henry, C. R., Adkinson, C., Nicholson, C. I., Bracha, Y., & Henry, T. D. (2005). Cardiovascular manifestations of moderate to severe carbon monoxide poisoning. *Journal of the American College of Cardiology*, *45*(9), 1513–1516. https://doi.org/10.1016/j.jacc.2005.01.044.

Shin, M., Bronstein, A. C., Glidden, E., Malone, M., Chang, A., Law, R., Boehmer, T. K., Strosnider, H., & Yip, F. (2023). Morbidity and Mortality of Unintentional Carbon Monoxide Poisoning: United States 2005 to 2018. *Annals of Emergency Medicine*, *81*(3), 309–317. https://doi.org/10.1016/j.annemergmed.2022.10.011.

Sinkovič, A., Smolle-Juettner, F. M., Krunic, B., & Marinšek, M. (2006). Severe carbon monoxide poisoning treated by hyperbaric oxygen therapy - A case report. *Inhalation Toxicology*, *18*(3), 211–214. https://doi.org/10.1080/08958370500434289.

Smithline, H. A., Ward, K. R., Chiulli, D. A., Blake, H. C., & Rivers, E. P. (2003). Whole body oxygen consumption and critical oxygen delivery in response to prolonged and severe carbon monoxide poisoning. *Resuscitation*, *56*(1), 97–104. https://doi.org/10.1016/S0300-9572(02)00272-1.

Sokal, J. A., & Kralkowska, E. (1985). The relationship between exposure duration, carboxyhemoglobin, blood glucose, pyruvate, and lactate and the severity of intoxication in 39 cases of acute carbon monoxide poisoning in men. *Archives of Toxicology*, *57*(3), 196–199. https://doi.org/10.1007/BF00290887.

Suliman, H. B., Carraway, M. S., Tatro, L. G., & Piantadosi, C. A. (2007). A new activating role for CO in cardiac mitochondrial biogenesis. *Journal of Cell Science*, *120*(2), 299–308. https://doi.org/10.1242/jcs.03318.

Taillé, C., Almolki, A., Benhamed, M., Zedda, C., Mégret, J., Berger, P., Lesèche, G., Fadel, E., Yamaguchi, T., Marthan, R., Aubier, M., & Boczkowski, J. (2003). Heme oxygenase inhibits human airway smooth muscle proliferation via a bilirubin-dependent modulation of ERK1/2 phosphorylation. *Journal of Biological Chemistry*, *278*(29), 27160–27168. https://doi.org/10.1074/jbc.M300364200.

Teksam, M., Casey, S. O., Michel, E., Liu, H., & Truwit, C. L. (2002). Diffusion-weighted MR imaging findings in carbon monoxide poisoning. *Neuroradiology*, *44*(2), 109–113. https://doi.org/10.1007/s002340100639.

Thom, S. R., Fisher, D., Zhang, J., Bhopale, V. M., Cameron, B., & Buerk, D. G. (2004). Neuronal nitric oxide synthase and N-methyl-D-aspartate neurons in experimental carbon monoxide poisoning. *Toxicology and Applied Pharmacology*, *194*(3), 280–295. https://doi.org/10.1016/j.taap.2003.09.017.

Thom, S. R., Taber, R. L., Mendiguren, I. I., Clark, J. M., Hardy, K. R., & Fisher, A. B. (1995). Delayed Neuropsychologic Sequelae After Carbon Monoxide Poisoning: Prevention by Treatment With Hyperbaric Oxygen. *Annals of Emergency Medicine*, *25*(4), 474–480. https://doi.org/10.1016/S0196-0644(95)70261-X.

Tomaszewski, C. (2015). Carbon Monoxide. In R. S. Hoffman, M. A. Howland, N. A. Lewin, L. S. Nelson, & L. R. Goldfrank (Eds.), *Goldfranks Toxicologic Emergencies 10th Edition* (10th ed., pp. 2681–2700). McGraw Hill.

Turner, M., Hamilton-Farrell, M. R., & Clark, R. J. (1999). Carbon monoxide poisoning: An update. *Journal of Accident and Emergency Medicine*, *16*(2), 92–96. https://doi.org/10.1136/emj.16.2.92.

Weaver, L. K. (2009). Carbon Monoxide Poisoning. *New England Journal of Medicine*, *360*(12), 1217–1225. https://doi.org/10.1056/NEJMcp0808891.

Wolkin, A. F., Martin, C. A., Law, R. K., Schier, J. G., & Bronstein, A. C. (2012). Using poison center data for national public health surveillance for chemical and poison exposure and associated illness. *Annals of Emergency Medicine*, *59*(1), 56–61. https://doi.org/10.1016/j.annemergmed.2011.08.004.

Zagami, A. S., Lethlean, A. K., & Mellick, R. (1993). Delayed neurological deterioration following carbon monoxide poisoning: MRI findings. *Journal of Neurology*, *240*(2), 113–116. https://doi.org/10.1007/BF00858727.

Zhang, X., Shan, P., Otterbein, L. E., Alam, J., Flavell, R. A., Davis, R. J., Choi, A. M. K., & Lee, P. J. (2003). Carbon monoxide inhibition of apoptosis during ischemia-reperfusion lung injury is dependent on the p38 mitogen-activated protein kinase pathway and involves caspase 3. *Journal of Biological Chemistry*, *278*(2), 1248–1258. https://doi.org/10.1074/jbc.M208419200.

Chapter 3

Carbon Monoxide and Its Cardiovascular Effects

Eser Durmaz, MD
and Gündüz İncesu*, MD
Department of Cardiology,
Istanbul University-Cerrahpasa Cerrahpasa Medical Faculty, İstanbul, Turkey

Abstract

The effects of carbon monoxide on the cardiovascular system are diverse. Intoxication by the aforementioned substance is a common entity in the emergency units and is responsible for more than 400 deaths per year. The patient can present with various clinical symptoms, from acute myocardial ischemia to decompensated heart failure. Because of that, it is very important to suspect such a possibility for the right patient. It is a known risk factor for the progression of atherosclerosis, although its therapeutic implications have been studied for a long time. The cardiovascular effects of CO poisoning can include myocardial ischemia, arrhythmias, and cardiac arrest. Treatment of CO poisoning involves the removal of the patient from the source of CO exposure, the administration of high-flow oxygen, and the consideration of hyperbaric oxygen therapy (HBOT) in severe cases.

Keywords: carbon monoxide, cardiac effects, intoxication, heart failure, hyperbaric oxygen therapy, myocardial ischemia

* Corresponding Author's Email: gunduzincesu@gmail.com.

In: Carbon Monoxide Poisoning
Editors: Seda Özkan and Afsin Ipekci
ISBN: 979-8-89113-217-7

Introduction

The effects of carbon monoxide (CO) on the cardiovascular system have long been studied both in clinical and preclinical settings. CO is recognized as having toxic side effects on many organ systems. It is the most common cause of death from poisoning in the United States. It can be responsible for more than 400 deaths, 2,000 hospitalizations, and 21,000 emergency department (ER) visits per year (Yoon et al., 1998). It is an odorless, tasteless, and colorless gas. It has the capacity to bind human hemoglobin with more than 200 times greater affinity than oxygen (O2). It can block the binding of oxygen and therefore its transportation. It is recognized that CO binding to one heme molecule can cause an increase in the affinity of other heme molecules for O2. It can, therefore, cause a shift to the left in the hemoglobin-O2 dissociation curve. At the cellular level, the main reason for its toxicity is that in mitochondria, it causes inhibition of cytochrome c oxidase, which is the reason for the cessation of ATP synthesis and increase of the production of reactive oxygen species (Young & Caughey, 1990).

CO is present in natural air. Its concentration is <2 parts per million (ppm), which is very low. In comparison, near gas stoves, the CO concentration increases up to 15 ppm. Wood fires can cause a concentration of about 5000 ppm. Car exhaust can contain about 7000 ppm. There is no cut-off for one person who gets intoxicated, but the duration and intensity of CO exposure can significantly change the clinical picture. It depends mostly on the amount of carboxyhemoglobin that is generated during this exposure (Young & Caughey, 1990).

CO poisoning is considered one of the most crucial health concerns. Very few studies are present in the field and have investigated its cardiovascular risks. It has the nickname "silent killer" because of its odorless, colorless, and tasteless properties. The main mechanism of its pathophysiology is tissue-level hypoxia as mentioned above. The two most oxygen-demanding systems, the central nervous system, and the cardiovascular system are greatly affected in an intoxication case, although it can affect every single cell whose continuation of function is dependent on the supply of O2. However, to describe the clinical picture, these two systems characterize the clinical features of an intoxicated patient. Although there are very few studies on the topic of the effects of CO poisoning on the cardiovascular system, it is well-known that myocardial injury is inevitable when the oxygen supply is damaged. This can translate into an increased risk of heart failure, myocardial ischemia, arrhythmia, etc. (Barret et al., 2008; Hampson & Hauff, 2008).

Despite the fact that studies showing its cardiovascular effects are very few, there are epidemiological studies showing that it can cause an increase in the frequency of coronary artery disease, cardiac arrhythmia, and even in the frequency of atherosclerosis, possibly through increased inflammation. Another possible suggested mechanism is that it may cause coronary vasospasm and through this vasospasm, it can cause harm to the relevant myocardium (Barret et al., 2008).

Although its cardiovascular effects are, regarding mainly the endpoint of congestive heart failure, not greater than 10% in cohorts, these effects can be devastating in the elderly population. They are more prone to develop serious cardiac adverse events in a CO poisoning scenario (Barret et al., 2008).

Congestive Heart Failure

CO poisoning is a significant public health concern, as it can cause a variety of acute and chronic health effects, including congestive heart failure (CHF). It is not an uncommon complication of CO poisoning, and it occurs when the heart is unable to pump enough blood to meet the body's needs. In this section, we will try to describe the relationship between CO poisoning and CHF, including the pathophysiology, clinical presentation, and management of this condition (F. Y. Lee et al., 2015).

CO poisoning can lead to CHF through a variety of mechanisms. First, CO binds to hemoglobin in the blood, reducing the amount of oxygen that can be carried to the tissues of the body. This hypoxia can lead to damage to the heart muscle, causing impaired cardiac function and CHF. Additionally, CO can directly affect heart muscle by increasing oxidative stress and causing mitochondrial dysfunction. This can cause inflammation and cell death in the heart muscle, further affecting cardiac function and contributing to the development of CHF (Kuniavsky et al., 2018).

The clinical presentation of CO poisoning and CHF can vary widely depending on the severity and duration of exposure (Hampson & Hauff, 2008). Acute exposure to high levels of CO can cause symptoms such as headache, dizziness, nausea, and confusion, while prolonged exposure to lower levels can lead to fatigue, shortness of breath, and chest pain. CHF can present with classical symptoms such as fatigue, shortness of breath, swelling of the legs and ankles, and rapid or irregular heartbeats. In severe cases, CHF can cause pulmonary edema that can be life-threatening (Hampson & Hauff, 2008).

The treatment of CO poisoning and CHF depends on the severity of the condition and the general health status of the patient. In cases of acute CO poisoning, the first step in treatment is to remove the patient from the source of exposure and administer high-flow oxygen therapy. In severe cases, hyperbaric oxygen therapy may be necessary to rapidly remove CO from the patient's bloodstream and tissues. In cases where CHF has developed as a complication of CO poisoning, the management involves a multidisciplinary approach, including medications such as diuretics and ACE inhibitors to reduce fluid accumulation and improve cardiac function. Cardiac rehabilitation and lifestyle changes such as weight loss, smoking cessation, and exercise, can also be helpful in managing CHF in patients with a history of CO poisoning (Hampson & Hauff, 2008).

Prevention of CO poisoning and its complications is critical, as it is a preventable condition. The use of CO detectors in homes and workplaces can help alert individuals to the presence of CO and prevent exposure. Proper ventilation of fuel-burning appliances and regular maintenance of these devices can also reduce the risk of CO poisoning. Public education and awareness campaigns can also play a role in preventing CO poisoning by promoting safe practices when using fuel-burning appliances (Hampson & Hauff, 2008).

In conclusion, CO poisoning is a significant public health concern that can lead to a range of acute and chronic health effects, including CHF. The pathophysiology of CO poisoning and CHF involves a complex interaction between hypoxia, oxidative stress, inflammation, and cell death in the heart muscle. The clinical presentation of CO poisoning and CHF can vary widely, and the management of treatment depends on the severity and duration of exposure. Prevention of CO poisoning and its complications is critical and can be achieved through the use of CO detectors, proper ventilation of fuel-burning appliances, and public education campaigns. Healthcare providers should be aware of the relationship between CO poisoning and CHF and be prepared to manage these complications in patients with a history of CO exposure (Hampson & Hauff, 2008).

Arrhythmias

Cardiac arrhythmias refer to abnormal heart rhythms that can arise from disturbances in the electrical conduction system of the heart. Arrhythmias can cause symptoms such as palpitations, dizziness, chest pain, and syncope, and can lead to serious complications such as heart failure and sudden cardiac arrest (Nanavati et al., 2020).

Carbon monoxide poisoning has been associated with a variety of cardiovascular effects, including the potential to cause arrhythmias. Studies reported that CO exposure was associated with an increased risk of ventricular tachycardia, a type of arrhythmia characterized by a rapid and irregular heartbeat that originates from the ventricles of the heart (Nanavati et al., 2020).

The mechanisms by which CO can cause arrhythmias are not fully understood but may involve both direct and indirect effects on the heart. CO can directly affect electrical properties of cardiac myocytes, the cells that make up the heart muscle. CO has been shown to increase the duration of action potentials, which are the electrical signals that trigger the contraction of the heart muscle. Prolonged duration of the action potential can lead to delayed repolarization and increased susceptibility to arrhythmias (Dallas et al., 2012; Gürkan et al., 2002).

In addition to direct effects on cardiac myocytes, CO can also indirectly affect the heart by reducing the availability of oxygen. Hypoxia, or reduced oxygen supply to tissues, can lead to cellular dysfunction and death. The heart is particularly susceptible to hypoxia, as it requires a constant supply of oxygen to function properly. In the case of CO poisoning, the formation of carboxyhemoglobin can displace oxygen from hemoglobin and reduce the amount of oxygen available to the heart (Dahms et al., 1993b).

Carbon monoxide poisoning can also result in the production of reactive oxygen species (ROS), which are highly reactive molecules that can damage cellular components, including the heart. ROS can induce oxidative stress, inflammation, and apoptosis, which can lead to cellular dysfunction and death (Dahms et al., 1993b).

The clinical manifestations of CO-induced arrhythmias can vary depending on the severity of the poisoning and the duration of exposure. Acute CO poisoning can result in sudden cardiac arrest, which is a medical emergency that requires immediate treatment with cardiopulmonary resuscitation (CPR) and defibrillation (Al-Owais et al., 2021; Dahms et al., 1993a, 1993b).

The diagnosis of CO-induced arrhythmias can be challenging, as symptoms may be nonspecific and mimic other cardiovascular conditions. Patients with suspected CO poisoning should undergo a thorough medical evaluation, including a detailed history, physical examination, and laboratory tests. The diagnosis of CO poisoning can be confirmed by measuring carboxyhemoglobin levels in the blood (Piantadosi, 1999).

Treatment of CO-induced arrhythmias depends on the severity of the arrhythmia and the degree of CO poisoning. It is not very different from current practice, but the elimination of the underlying cause, in this case, CO poisoning, is the most beneficial and is the main pillar. In cases of acute CO poisoning with severe arrhythmias, prompt treatment with CPR and defibrillation is necessary. In less severe cases of CO poisoning, treatment may involve oxygen therapy, hyperbaric oxygen therapy, and supportive care (Dahms et al., 1993b).

Coronary Artery Disease

Coronary artery disease (CAD) is a common cardiovascular disease that is characterized by the accumulation of plaque in the arteries that supply blood to the heart. The clinical presentation can vary from the progression of preexisting CAD to acute coronary syndromes which include Myocardial Infarction both with ST-segment elevation (STEMI) and without NSTEMI. CAD can result in symptoms such as chest pain, shortness of breath, and myocardial infarction, and can lead to serious complications such as heart failure and sudden cardiac arrest (K. K. Lee et al., 2020; Marius-Nunez, 1990; Mustafić et al., 2012).

Carbon monoxide has been implicated in the development of CAD through several mechanisms. One mechanism involves the formation of carboxyhemoglobin, which reduces the amount of oxygen available to the heart muscle. The heart muscle requires a constant supply of oxygen to function properly, and a reduction in oxygen supply can lead to cellular dysfunction and death. In addition, CO can induce oxidative stress and inflammation, which are key processes involved in the development of CAD (K. K. Lee et al., 2020).

Studies have shown that CO can promote the development of atherosclerosis, the underlying process of CAD. Atherosclerosis is a chronic inflammatory disease that involves the accumulation of lipid-rich plaques in the arterial walls. CO can promote the development of atherosclerosis by inducing endothelial dysfunction, a condition characterized by impaired endothelial cell function and reduced nitric oxide bioavailability. Nitric oxide is a key regulator of vascular tone and reduced nitric oxide bioavailability can lead to vasoconstriction and impaired blood flow Young & Caughey, 1990).

CO can also promote the development of atherosclerosis by activating immune cells and promoting inflammation. CO has been shown to activate macrophages, a type of immune cell involved in the development of atherosclerosis. Activated macrophages release pro-inflammatory cytokines, chemokines, and reactive oxygen species, which can induce endothelial dysfunction and promote plaque formation (Young & Caughey, 1990).

Another mechanism by which CO can promote the development of CAD is through the induction of proliferation and migration of the vascular smooth muscle cell. Vascular smooth muscle cells are key players in the development of atherosclerosis, as they contribute to plaque formation and stabilization. CO has been shown to stimulate the proliferation and migration of the vascular smooth muscle cell, which can contribute to plaque formation (Young & Caughey, 1990).

The clinical manifestations of CO-induced CAD can vary depending on the severity of the poisoning and the duration of exposure. Acute CO poisoning can result in sudden cardiac arrest, which is a medical emergency requiring immediate treatment with cardiopulmonary resuscitation (CPR) and defibrillation. Chronic exposure to low levels of CO can lead to progressive cardiovascular disease, including CAD, hypertension, and heart failure (Young & Caughey, 1990).

The diagnosis of CO-induced CAD can be challenging, as symptoms may be nonspecific and can mimic other cardiovascular conditions. Patients with suspected CO poisoning should undergo a thorough medical evaluation, including a detailed history, physical examination, and laboratory tests. In addition, imaging tests such as coronary angiography and computed tomography angiography can be used to diagnose CAD (Young & Caughey, 1990).

Treatment of CO-induced CAD depends on the severity of the disease and the degree of CO poisoning. In the cases of acute CO poisoning with severe CAD, prompt treatment with CPR and defibrillation is necessary. Acute coronary syndromes should be managed as described in the current guidelines (Collet et al., 2021; Ibanez et al., 2018). Regarding antithrombotic therapy, there is no consensus on the subject and each patient should be treated with a tailored approach. In less severe cases of CO poisoning and CAD, treatment may involve lifestyle modifications, such as reducing smoking, regular exercise, and a healthy diet. In addition, medications such as aspirin, statins, and beta-blockers may be used to manage CAD and reduce the risk of cardiovascular events (Collet et al., 2021; Ibanez et al., 2018).

In conclusion, carbon monoxide poisoning can lead to the development of CAD through several mechanisms and this effect can be at several levels from very mild progression of already existing CAD at a subclinical level to acute myocardial infarction. It is essential to recognize each clinical picture and start appropriate treatment as necessary.

Progression of Atherosclerosis

Atherosclerosis is a chronic inflammatory disease that involves the accumulation of fatty plaques in the arterial walls. Atherosclerosis is a major cause of cardiovascular disease, leading to death worldwide. Emerging evidence suggests that carbon monoxide may contribute to the progression of atherosclerosis through several mechanisms (Piantadosi, 2008).

One mechanism by which CO may contribute to the progression of atherosclerosis is through the induction of oxidative stress. Oxidative stress is a condition in which there is an imbalance between the production of reactive oxygen species (ROS) and the antioxidant defense system. ROS can react with lipids, proteins, and DNA, leading to cellular damage and dysfunction. Several studies have shown that CO can induce oxidative stress in endothelial cells, smooth muscle cells, and macrophages, which are key players in the development of atherosclerosis. Oxidative stress can promote the activation of inflammatory pathways and the production of pro-inflammatory cytokines, chemokines, and adhesion molecules, which can contribute to the progression of atherosclerosis (Piantadosi, 2008; Zuckerbraun et al., 2007).

Another mechanism by which CO may contribute to the progression of atherosclerosis is through the induction of endothelial dysfunction. Endothelial dysfunction is a condition in which endothelial cell function is impaired, which can lead to reduced nitric oxide (NO) bioavailability, vasoconstriction, and inflammation. NO is a key regulator of vascular tone and plays a critical role in the prevention of atherosclerosis. Studies have shown that CO can induce endothelial dysfunction by reducing NO bioavailability, promoting the expression of adhesion molecules and pro-inflammatory cytokines, and stimulating the proliferation of smooth muscle cells. Endothelial dysfunction can contribute to the development of atherosclerosis by promoting the adhesion and infiltration of inflammatory cells and the accumulation of lipid-rich plaques in the arterial walls (Piantadosi, 2008).

CO can also contribute to the progression of atherosclerosis by activating immune cells and promoting inflammation. CO has been shown to activate macrophages, which are immune cells involved in the development of atherosclerosis. Activated macrophages release pro-inflammatory cytokines, chemokines, and ROS, which can promote the activation of other immune cells and the production of extracellular matrix proteins, leading to the formation of atherosclerotic plaques. In addition, CO can promote the migration and proliferation of smooth muscle cells, which can contribute to plaque formation (Piantadosi, 2008; Zuckerbraun et al., 2007).

Emerging evidence suggests that CO may also contribute to the progression of atherosclerosis by promoting the formation of foam cells, which are hallmarks of atherosclerosis. Foam cells are macrophages that have engulfed modified low-density lipoprotein (LDL) particles. Foam cells contribute to the formation of fatty plaques and the development of atherosclerosis. Studies have shown that CO can promote the formation of foam cells by improving the uptake of modified LDL particles and stimulating the expression of scavenger receptors in macrophages. (Piantadosi, 2008; Zuckerbraun et al., 2007).

The clinical implications of the CO-induced progression of atherosclerosis are significant. Atherosclerosis is a major cause of cardiovascular disease, leading to death worldwide. CO-induced progression of atherosclerosis can lead to the development of serious complications such as heart attack, stroke, and peripheral artery disease. Patients with chronic CO poisoning may be at increased risk of developing atherosclerosis and cardiovascular disease and may require close monitoring and aggressive treatment of cardiovascular risk factors.

Smoking and CO Poisoning

Carbon monoxide (CO) is a toxic gas that can be produced by the incomplete combustion of hydrocarbons, such as tobacco smoke. Smoking is a major source of CO exposure and is associated with a wide range of cardiovascular diseases, including coronary artery disease, stroke, peripheral artery disease, and heart failure. Emerging evidence suggests that CO may contribute to the harmful effects of smoking on the cardiovascular system through several mechanisms (Marius-Nunez, 1990).

CO has a high affinity for hemoglobin and can reduce the oxygen-carrying capacity of the blood, leading to tissue-level hypoxia. Chronic exposure to CO can lead to the development of carboxyhemoglobinemia, which is a condition in which there is an increased level of CO bound to hemoglobin. Carboxyhemoglobinemia can impair oxygen delivery to the tissues and promote oxidative stress, inflammation, and endothelial dysfunction, which are key mechanisms involved in the development of cardiovascular disease (Lee et al., 2020).

One mechanism by which CO may contribute to the harmful effects of smoking on the cardiovascular system is through the induction of oxidative stress. Oxidative stress is a condition in which there is an imbalance between the production of reactive oxygen species (ROS) and the antioxidant defense system. ROS can react with lipids, proteins, and DNA, leading to cellular damage and dysfunction. Several studies have shown that CO can induce oxidative stress in endothelial cells, smooth muscle cells, and macrophages, which are key players in the development of cardiovascular disease. Oxidative stress can promote the activation of inflammatory pathways and the production of pro-inflammatory cytokines, chemokines, and adhesion molecules, which can contribute to the development of atherosclerosis, hypertension, and other cardiovascular diseases (Piantadosi, 2008).

Another mechanism by which CO may contribute to the harmful effects of smoking on the cardiovascular system is through the induction of endothelial dysfunction. Endothelial dysfunction is a condition in which endothelial cell function is impaired, which can lead to reduced nitric oxide (NO) bioavailability, vasoconstriction, and inflammation. NO is a key regulator of vascular tone and plays a critical role in the development of cardiovascular disease. Studies have shown that CO can induce endothelial dysfunction by reducing NO bioavailability, promoting the expression of adhesion molecules and pro-inflammatory cytokines, and stimulating the proliferation of smooth muscle cells. Endothelial dysfunction can contribute to the development of atherosclerosis, hypertension, and other cardiovascular diseases by promoting adhesion and infiltration of inflammatory cells and accumulation of lipid-rich plaques in arterial walls (Piantadosi, 2008).

CO can also contribute to the harmful effects of smoking on the cardiovascular system by promoting platelet activation and thrombosis. Platelets are small circulating blood cells that play a critical role in the formation of blood clots. Studies have shown that CO can promote platelet activation and aggregation, leading to the formation of blood clots and the occlusion of blood vessels. CO can also promote the expression of tissue factors, which is a key initiator of the coagulation cascade. Platelet activation and thrombosis can contribute to the development of cardiovascular diseases such as coronary artery disease, stroke, and peripheral artery disease (Zuckerbraun et al., 2007).

The harmful effects of CO on the cardiovascular system may be exacerbated by other cardiovascular risk factors, such as hypertension, diabetes, and dyslipidemia. CO can promote the development of hypertension by inducing vasoconstriction, promoting the proliferation of smooth muscle cells, and impairing endothelial function. CO can also promote the development of diabetes by impairing glucose metabolism and promoting insulin resistance. In addition, CO can promote dyslipidemia by promoting the accumulation of lipid-rich plaques in arterial walls and promoting the formation of foam cells.

In conclusion, emerging evidence suggests that CO may contribute to the harmful effects of smoking on the cardiovascular system through several mechanisms, including oxidative stress, endothelial dysfunction, platelet activation, and reducing NO bioavailability.

Treatment and Prevention of Adverse Cardiovascular Effects

The cardiovascular effects of CO poisoning can include myocardial ischemia, arrhythmias, and cardiac arrest. The treatment of CO poisoning involves the removal of the patient from the source of CO exposure, the administration of high-flow oxygen, and the consideration of hyperbaric oxygen therapy (HBOT) in severe cases (Kuniavsky et al., 2018).

The primary goal of treatment for CO poisoning is the rapid removal of CO from the patient's body. The first step in the management of CO poisoning is the identification and removal of the source of CO exposure. Patients should be removed from the area of exposure and taken to a well-ventilated area as soon as possible. The second step is the administration of high-flow oxygen therapy. Oxygen therapy increases the availability of oxygen to tissues, which can help displace CO from hemoglobin and promote its elimination from the body. Patients with CO poisoning should receive high-flow oxygen therapy through a non-rebreather mask or intubation according to the clinical picture until their symptoms resolve and their carboxyhemoglobin levels return to normal (Ilano & Raffin, 1990; Piantadosi, 1999).

HBOT is a treatment option that can be considered in severe cases of CO poisoning. HBOT involves the administration of 100% oxygen at a pressure greater than atmospheric pressure. HBOT can help quickly eliminate CO from the body by promoting the diffusion of oxygen into tissues that are poorly perfused due to CO-induced vasoconstriction. HBOT has been shown to reduce the risk of neurologic sequelae and mortality in severe cases of CO poisoning. However, HBOT is not without risks and its use should be carefully considered in each case (Hampson & Little, 2005; Kuniavsky et al., 2018).

Myocardial ischemia is a potential complication of CO poisoning that can result from the reduced oxygen-carrying capacity of the blood. Myocardial ischemia can present as chest pain, ST-segment changes on the electrocardiogram (ECG), or elevated cardiac biomarkers. Treatment of myocardial ischemia in CO poisoning involves the administration of high-flow oxygen therapy, which can help increase oxygen delivery to the heart muscle. In appropriate cases, nitroglycerin and aspirin can also be administered to alleviate chest pain and prevent thrombotic complications.

Arrhythmias are another potential complication of CO poisoning that can result from the direct toxic effects of CO on the heart. Arrhythmias can present as palpitations, lightheadedness, or syncope. Treatment of arrhythmias in CO poisoning involves the administration of high-flow oxygen therapy, which can help to improve cardiac oxygen delivery and reduce the risk of arrhythmias. In severe cases, anti-arrhythmic medications or electrical cardioversion may be necessary (Nanavati et al., 2020).

Cardiac arrest is a rare but potentially fatal complication of CO poisoning that can result from severe myocardial ischemia or arrhythmias. Treatment of cardiac arrest in CO poisoning involves standard advanced cardiac life support (ACLS) protocols, including chest compressions, defibrillation, and administration of high-flow oxygen therapy. In severe cases, extracorporeal membrane oxygenation (ECMO) may be necessary to support the patient's cardiovascular system until CO elimination can be achieved (Ilano & Raffin, 1990).

In summary, CO poisoning is a serious medical emergency that can result in significant cardiovascular morbidity and mortality. Treatment of CO poisoning involves the rapid removal of CO from the patient's body, the administration of high-flow oxygen therapy, and the consideration of HBOT in severe cases.

Conclusion

In conclusion, carbon monoxide poisoning is a potentially life-threatening condition that can cause significant cardiovascular morbidity and mortality. The cardiovascular effects of CO poisoning can include myocardial ischemia, arrhythmias, and cardiac arrest. Early recognition and prompt treatment of CO poisoning are critical to prevent these complications and improve outcomes (Barret et al., 2008). Treatment of CO poisoning involves the rapid removal of CO from the patient's body, administration of high-flow oxygen therapy, and consideration of hyperbaric oxygen therapy in severe cases. Healthcare providers should be aware of the cardiovascular effects of CO poisoning and be prepared to manage these complications in the event of an emergency CO poisoning. Public education and awareness campaigns can also play a role in preventing CO poisoning by promoting the use of CO detectors and safe practices when using fuel-burning appliances. Overall, a comprehensive approach to the prevention and management of CO poisoning can help reduce the burden of this preventable and potentially deadly condition on individuals and communities.

References

Al-Owais, M. M., Steele, D. S., Holden, A. V., & Benson, A. P. (2021). Deterministic and Stochastic Cellular Mechanisms Contributing to Carbon Monoxide Induced Ventricular Arrhythmias. *Frontiers in Pharmacology*, *12*, 936. https://doi.org/10.3389/FPHAR.2021.651050/BIBTEX.

Barret, L., Danel, V., & Faure, J. (2008). Carbon Monoxide Poisoning, a Diagnosis Frequently Overlooked. *Journal of Toxicology: Clinical Toxicology*, *23*(4–6), 309–313. https://doi.org/10.3109/15563658508990638.

Collet, J.-P., Thiele, H., Barbato, E., Barthélémy, O., Bauersachs, J., Bhatt, D. L., Dendale, P., Dorobantu, M., Edvardsen, T., Folliguet, T., Gale, C. P., Gilard, M., Jobs, A., Jüni, P., Lambrinou, E., Lewis, B. S., Mehilli, J., Meliga, E., Merkely, B., Siontis, G. C. M., & ESC Scientific Document Group. (2021). 2020 ESC Guidelines for the management of acute coronary syndromes in patients presenting without persistent ST-segment elevationThe Task Force for the management of acute coronary syndromes in patients presenting without persistent ST-segment elevation of the European Society of Cardiology (ESC). *European Heart Journal*, *42*(14), 1289–1367. https://doi.org/10.1093/EURHEARTJ/EHAA575.

Dahms, T. E., Younis, L. T., Wiens, R. D., Zarnegar, S., Byers, S. L., & Chaitman, B. R. (1993a). Effects of carbon monoxide exposure in patients with documented cardiac arrhythmias. *Journal of the American College of Cardiology*, *21*(2), 442–450. https://doi.org/10.1016/0735-1097(93)90687-V.

Dahms, T. E., Younis, L. T., Wiens, R. D., Zarnegar, S., Byers, S. L., & Chaitman, B. R. (1993b). Effects of carbon monoxide exposure in patients with documented cardiac arrhythmias. *Journal of the American College of Cardiology*, *21*(2), 442–450. https://doi.org/10.1016/0735-1097(93)90687-V.

Dallas, M. L., Yang, Z., Boyle, J. P., Boycott, H. E., Scragg, J. L., Milligan, C. J., Elies, J., Duke, A., Thireau, J., Reboul, C., Richard, S., Bernus, O., Steele, D. S., & Peers, C. (2012). Carbon Monoxide Induces Cardiac Arrhythmia via Induction of the Late Na+ Current. *American Journal of Respiratory and Critical Care Medicine*, *186*(7), 648–656. https://doi.org/10.1164/RCCM.201204-0688OC.

Gürkan, Y., Canatay, H., Toprak, A., Ural, E., & Toker, K. (2002). Carbon monoxide poisoning − a cause of increased QT dispersion. *Acta Anaesthesiologica Scandinavica*, *46*(2), 180–183. https://doi.org/10.1034/J.1399-6576.2002.460210.X.

Hampson, N. B., & Hauff, N. M. (2008). Carboxyhemoglobin levels in carbon monoxide poisoning: do they correlate with the clinical picture? *The American Journal of Emergency Medicine*, *26*(6), 665–669. https://doi.org/10.1016/J.AJEM.2007.10.005.

Hampson, N. B., & Little, C. E. (2005). Hyperbaric treatment of patients with carbon monoxide poisoning in the United States *HBO 2 in CO patients in US*. *32*(1), 21-26.

Ibanez, B., James, S., Agewall, S., Antunes, M. J., Bucciarelli-Ducci, C., Bueno, H., Caforio, A. L. P., Crea, F., Goudevenos, J. A., Halvorsen, S., Hindricks, G., Kastrati, A., Lenzen, M. J., Prescott, E., Roffi, M., Valgimigli, M., Varenhorst, C., Vranckx, P., Widimský, P., & ESC Scientific Document Group (2018). 2017 ESC Guidelines for the management of acute myocardial infarction in patients presenting with ST-segment elevationThe Task Force for the management of acute myocardial infarction in patients presenting with ST-segment elevation of the European Society of Cardiology (ESC). *European Heart Journal*, *39*(2), 119–177. https://doi.org/10.1093/EURHEARTJ/EHX393.

Ilano, A. L., & Raffin, T. A. (1990). Management of Carbon Monoxide Poisoning. *Chest*, *97*(1), 165–169. https://doi.org/10.1378/CHEST.97.1.165.

Kuniavsky, M., Bechor, Y., Leitman, M., & Efrati, S. (2018). Carbon monoxide poisoning in a young, healthy patient: A case study of heart failure recovery after Hyperbaric Oxygenation Treatment. *Intensive and Critical Care Nursing*, *47*, 85–88. https://doi.org/10.1016/J.ICCN.2018.04.008.

Lee, F. Y., Chen, W. K., Lin, C. L., & Kao, C. H. (2015). Carbon Monoxide Poisoning and Subsequent Cardiovascular Disease Risk: A Nationwide Population-based Cohort Study. *Medicine*, *94*(10). https://doi.org/10.1097/MD.0000000000000624.

Lee, K. K., Spath, N., Miller, M. R., Mills, N. L., & Shah, A. S. V. (2020). Short-term exposure to carbon monoxide and myocardial infarction: A systematic review and meta-analysis. *Environment International*, *143*, 105901. https://doi.org/10.1016/J.ENVINT.2020.105901.

Marius-Nunez, A. L. (1990). Myocardial Infarction with Normal Coronary Arteries After Acute Exposure to Carbon Monoxide. *Chest*, *97*(2), 491–494. https://doi.org/10.1378/CHEST.97.2.491.

Mustafić, H., Jabre, P., Caussin, C., Murad, M. H., Escolano, S., Tafflet, M., Périer, M. C., Marijon, E., Vernerey, D., Empana, J. P., & Jouven, X. (2012). Main Air Pollutants and Myocardial Infarction: A Systematic Review and Meta-analysis. *JAMA*, *307*(7), 713–721. https://doi.org/10.1001/JAMA.2012.126.

Nanavati, S., Vora, A., Samuel, A., Patel, K., Sharma, H., Sharaan, A., Kalatoudis, H., Upadhyay, S., & Mathew, J. (2020). A Case Of Carbon Monoxide Poisoning-Induced Atrial Fibrillation. *Chest*, *158*(4), A148–A149. https://doi.org/10.1016/j.chest.2020.08.165.

Piantadosi, C. A. (1999). Diagnosis and treatment of carbon monoxide poisoning. *Respiratory Care Clinics of North America*, *5*(2), 183–202. https://europepmc.org/article/med/10333448.

Piantadosi, C. A. (2008). Carbon monoxide, reactive oxygen signaling, and oxidative stress. *Free Radical Biology and Medicine*, *45*(5), 562–569. https://doi.org/10.1016/J.FREERADBIOMED.2008.05.013.

Yoon, S. S., Macdonald, S. C., & Parrish, R. G. (1998). Deaths From Unintentional Carbon Monoxide Poisoning and Potential for Prevention With Carbon Monoxide Detectors. *JAMA*, *279*(9), 685–687. https://doi.org/10.1001/JAMA.279.9.685.

Young, L. J., & Caughey, W. S. (1990). Pathobiochemistry of CO poisoning. *FEBS Letters*, *272*(1–2), 1–6. https://doi.org/10.1016/0014-5793(90)80436-M.

Zuckerbraun, B. S., Chin, B. Y., Bilban, M., d'Avila, J. de C., Rao, J., Billiar, T. R., & Otterbein, L. E. (2007). Carbon monoxide signals via inhibition of cytochrome c oxidase and generation of mitochondrial reactive oxygen species. *The FASEB Journal*, *21*(4), 1099–1106. https://doi.org/10.1096/FJ.06-6644COM.

Chapter 4

The Neurological Aspects of Carbon Monoxide Poisoning

Furkan Asan*, **MD**
and Mehmet Sakir Delil, MD
Department of Neurology, Istanbul University-Cerrahpasa, Istanbul, Turkey

Abstract

Carbon monoxide (CO) poisoning is significant due to its high incidence in emergency departments. In addition to neurological conditions detected during the acute stage, it can be considered a specific toxicity due to the various neurological symptoms that can develop in the following weeks or even months. While the mortality rate is between 1-3%, approximately one-third of surviving patients experience neurocognitive disorders. Parkinsonism, chorea, dystonia, and affective disorders are also observed in patients following the acute stage of poisoning. The most effective treatment for acute CO poisoning, for which there is no antidote, is hyperbaric oxygen therapy. However, there is no clear evidence that hyperbaric oxygen therapy is successful in preventing delayed neurological syndrome. In this section, our aim is to describe the neurological aspect of CO poisoning in detail.

Keywords: carbon monoxide poisoning, delayed neurological syndrome, parkinsonism, movement disorders

* Corresponding Author's Email: furkan61asan@gmail.com.

In: Carbon Monoxide Poisoning
Editors: Seda Özkan and Afsin Ipekci
ISBN: 979-8-89113-217-7

Introduction

In the US, approximately 50,000 people (annual incidence 16/100,000) are affected annually by carbon monoxide (CO) poisoning, and more than a thousand people die as a result (Sircar et al., 2015). About half of all fatal poisoning cases worldwide are due to CO poisoning (Raub et al., 2000). Approximately 15,000 cases of carbon monoxide poisoning detected in the US are caused by intentional exposure, and two-thirds of deaths occur in this way (Hampson, 2016). While there are few epidemiological studies related to CO poisoning in Turkey, the annual incidence has been reported to be 14/100,000 (Demirbaş et al., 2011). Unlike in the US, intentional exposure is very rare in these cases.

The majority of carbon monoxide poisoning cases are non-fatal, but in about one-third of those who survive, neurological and psychiatric disorders develop despite appropriate treatment. Therefore, education programs and precautions are of great importance in carbon monoxide poisoning, which is a mostly preventable condition.

In the acute stage of CO poisoning, symptoms such as headache, generalized weakness, nausea, shortness of breath, and changes in consciousness ranging from somnolence to coma are observed. However, delayed neurological sequelae (DNS) can occur up to one year later in some survivors, with impaired attention and executive functions, memory and mood disorders, and movement disorders such as parkinsonism and chorea. In this section, we will try to explain the neurological consequences that occur during and after CO poisoning.

Mechanism of Brain Injury

CO binds to various proteins containing ferrous heme with high affinity. Hemoglobin (Hb) shows 250 times more affinity for CO than for oxygen. The binding of CO to Hb results in conformational changes in the Hb complex and decreases the oxygen-carrying capacity of Hb (Hall & Guyton, 2011). As a result, the amount of oxygen transported to tissues decreases significantly, leading to tissue hypoxia.

CO toxicity not only disrupts oxygen transport to tissues, but also binds to various proteins containing heme, such as myoglobin and mitochondrial cytochrome c oxidase, and impairs their functions. Inhibition of the cytochrome c oxidase enzyme results in mitochondrial dysfunction, which leads to an inability to meet cellular energy demands. (Goldbaum et al., 1976). This disruption of aerobic metabolism leads to increased lactic acid production and systemic acidosis.

In addition to ischemic and hypoxic conditions, CO triggers an inflammatory response by enhancing the release of nitric oxide from endothelial cells, which leads to platelet and subsequently neutrophil activation (Thom et al., 1997). CO poisoning also causes myelin loss in the central nervous system through lipid peroxidation, ultimately exacerbating the extent of neuronal damage (Thom, 1990).

In the acute stages of CO poisoning, vasorelaxation occurs in the cerebral arteries through cerebral autoregulation mechanisms, resulting in increased cerebral blood flow (Komuro et al., 2001). However, in cases where toxicity is severe, along with impaired cardiac function, decreased cardiac output leads to systemic hypotension and, ultimately, to decreased in cerebral blood flow. This leads to a faster activation of the hypoxia-anoxia cascade at the neuronal level (Komuro et al., 2001).

CO primarily causes more severe functional impairments in organs with high energy demands, such as the heart and brain, due to its disruption of the transport and utilization of oxygen in tissues. It is known that brain regions such as watershed areas, basal ganglia, second and third layers of the cortex, and cerebellar purkinje cells, which have a high energy demand, are more susceptible to hypoxia, and are also more susceptible to CO toxicity (Lapresle & Fardeau, 1967). Post-mortem examinations of individuals exposed to CO toxicity have also revealed widespread microinfarctions at the level of the basal ganglia and petechial hemorrhages in the basal ganglia, along with cerebellar purkinje cells (Lapresle & Fardeau, 1967). In addition to these findings, myelin loss in the deep cerebral white matter has also been demonstrated in pathology specimens (Kobayashi et al., 1984).

Neurological Consequences of Carbon Monoxide Poisoning

Acute Stage of the Poisoning

There is a relationship between neurological symptoms in the acute stage of carbon monoxide poisoning and the level of carboxyhemoglobin (COHb) in the blood. However, it is not possible to determine sharp limits based on COHb levels (Hampson et al., 2012; Weaver, 2020). Nevertheless, the likelihood of more severe neurological signs such as coma and seizures are higher at COHb concentrations above 50%. For example, the rate of loss of consciousness was found to be 90% when the COHb level was above 50%, while it was 45% in patients with COHb levels between 10-20% (Hampson et al., 2012).

The most common neurological symptom in cases of carbon monoxide poisoning is headache, which is observed in approximately 80% of patients (Hampson et al., 2012; Handa & Tai, 2005). The headache is usually located in the frontal region and has a dull character. The severity of headache is not correlated with COHb levels, and it often improves prior to hyperbaric oxygen therapy (Hampson & Hampson, 2002). Dizziness is seen in about half of the patients. Depending on the severity and duration of CO exposure, changes in consciousness ranging from somnolence to coma, focal neurological deficits due to ischemic infarctions, and epileptic seizures may also occur (Jankovic et al., 2021).

The frequency of epileptic seizures in CO poisoning is reported to be between 1-4% (Hampson et al., 1996; Sloan et al., 1989). Seizures are more common in patients with higher COHb concentrations. Seizures are generally generalized, but focal motor seizures are also observed less frequently (Sloan et al., 1989). Epileptic seizures can also occur during hyperbaric oxygen (HBO) treatment, which is used in the treatment of CO poisoning. Seizures are among the complications of HBO treatment, but the frequency of epileptic seizures is much higher in patients receiving HBO treatment due to CO poisoning compared to other indications (Sanders et al., 2012). Therefore, the likelihood that seizures are associated with HBO treatment is controversial. Due to the low frequency, low probability of recurrence and ease of management of seizures during the acute stage of CO poisoning, routine use of prophylactic antiepileptic treatment is a subject of debate (Sloan et al., 1989).

Neuroimaging findings in carbon monoxide poisoning vary depending on the stages of poisoning. Abnormalities are most commonly detected in the globus pallidus on magnetic resonance imaging (MRI). Additionally, abnormalities can also be perceived in the medial temporal lobe, cerebral white matter, cerebellum, and cortex. The signal changes observed on MRI typically show an increase in T2 and fluid-attenuated inversion recovery (FLAIR) signals, along with a decrease in the T1 signal (O'donnell et al., 2000). In the early stages, particularly within the first 24 hours, lesions that have not yet been established on T2-FLAIR can be detected earlier on diffusion-weighted images (DWI), providing early data on possible central nervous system involvement (Beppu, 2014). Additionally, hemorrhagic foci can be detected in the early stages, mostly in the globus pallidus (Bianco & Floris, 1996; Silverman et al., 1993).

Delayed Neurologic Syndrome

Delayed neurologic syndrome (DNS) is a rapid neurological deterioration that occurs following complete recovery from the acute phase of CO poisoning. This pseudo-well-being state that precedes the onset of DNS can last from 2-40 days and up to several months (S. Choi, 1983; Kitamoto et al., 2016; Min, 1986). Patients present with different combinations of symptoms such as parkinsonism, chore, dystonia, cognitive decline, incontinence, psychiatric disorders, and memory impairment, following complete recovery.

The pathophysiology of DNS has not yet been clearly identified. Studies based on a limited number of pathological examinations have formed some hypotheses on this subject. The most important of these studies is the one by Lapresle et al., who stated that demyelination is a widespread finding and the most significant difference from patients in the acute stage of CO poisoning in those who develop DNS (Lapresle & Fardeau, 1967). The neurological improvement in the following years in most patients who develop DNS may indicate that a demyelination-remyelination process occurs rather than axonal damage. In fact, in patients followed by MRI spectroscopy and diffusion tensor imaging, it has been found that DNS occurs together with radiological findings of the demyelination, and radiological findings of the demyelination also regress with clinical improvement (Terajima et al., 2008).

DNS can occur in 3-30% of patients who have experienced CO poisoning (I. S. Choi & Cheon, 1999; S. Choi, 1983; Hsiao et al., 2004; Min, 1986; Thom et al., 1995). The different rates reported in various studies may be related to differences in the duration and severity of CO exposure, as well as demographic differences among patients. Studies aimed at identifying risk factors for DNS development have found that longer time for CO exposure, lower Glasgow Coma Scale score at initial presentation, and older age are among the risk factors (Pepe et al., 2011; Weaver et al., 2007). However, there is no correlation between the COHb level at presentation and DNS development (Kitamoto et al., 2016; Weaver et al., 2007). Another potential marker that has been proposed to predict DNS development is a molecule called myelin basic protein (MBP). High levels of MBP in cerebrospinal fluid (CSF) have been shown to predict DNS development, as its high concentration in CSF indicates demyelination in the central nervous system (Kuroda et al., 2015).

Cognitive impairment develops in approximately one-third of patients following CO poisoning (Pages et al., 2014). This cognitive impairment has been observed in frontal-executive, working memory, and verbal memory function, indicating that the cognitive impairment occurs in a multi-domain fashion. Approximately 20-40% of patients develop depression and anxiety disorders after 6 weeks of the acute stage of CO poisoning (Chambers et al., 2008; Jasper et al., 2005). These affective disorders persist at high rates even one year after the poisoning, and patients should be monitored accordingly. Some of these patients also experience suicidal attempts along with depressive disorders during the follow-up period (Jasper et al., 2005).

Parkinsonism is the most common movement disorder that develops after CO poisoning. It is assumed to develop as a result of demyelination that occurs after the acute stage, particularly affecting the basal ganglia, especially the globus pallidus. Although its frequency is reported at variable rates, it can reach up to 10% (I. S. Choi & Cheon, 1999). In most patients, gait disorders, hypokinesia, and bradymimia develop. Unlike idiopathic Parkinson's disease, sphincter defects accompany it in 80% of cases, and rest tremor is generally not observed. In some patients, intention tremor is observed (I. S. Choi, 2002; I. S. Choi & Cheon, 1999). Although basal ganglia lesions are detected in significant proportions of patients who develop parkinsonism, basal ganglia lesions are also found in patients without parkinsonism. Therefore, it should be kept in mind that the detection of basal ganglia lesions on neuroimaging does not predict the development of parkinsonism.

Dystonia and chorea can also develop after CO poisoning, although they are less common. Dystonia typically appears approximately 50 weeks after exposure, which is different from other movement disorders in this manner (I. S. Choi & Cheon, 1999). It has been reported that the use of neuroleptics worsens chorea, and discontinuation of neuroleptics improves chorea (Park & Choi, 2004). Both dystonia and chorea that develop after CO poisoning have been reported to self-limit within a few months (I. S. Choi & Cheon, 1999; Park & Choi, 2004).

Neuroimaging abnormalities detected in the chronic stage of CO poisoning are similar to those seen in the acute stage, but with some differences. The most frequently affected areas are the basal ganglia (especially the globus pallidus) and the cerebral white matter (CWM) (Beppu, 2014). In addition, widespread brain atrophy can also be observed in the chronic stage (Pavese et al., 1999). It has been found that cognitive impairment is more pronounced in patients with brain atrophy and widespread involvement of the cerebral white matter (Parkinson et al., 2002). In patients without CWM involvement in the acute stage, the development of DNS has been associated with the appearance of CWM lesions in later periods (Pavese et al., 1999). These observations may indicate that the widespread demyelination process that occurs sometime after CO poisoning may be responsible for the clinical findings.

Treatment Options for Delayed Neurological Syndrome

The most effective treatment for acute CO poisoning is believed to be HBO therapy. HBO implicates the application of 100% oxygen at a pressure of 2.5-3 atmospheres. While the half-life of COHb with 100% normobaric oxygen drops from 4 hours to 1 hour, it drops to 20 minutes with this treatment method. However, randomized controlled studies on the effectiveness of HBO therapy in preventing DNS development have yielded conflicting results. A meta-analysis of randomized controlled studies found that HBO therapy did not prevent DNS development (Buckley et al., 2011). However, due to the heterogeneity of the studies and patient groups, as well as the different study designs, these results should be interpreted with caution. It seems that further studies are needed to determine whether HBO therapy prevents DNS development.

It has been reported in case studies that cognitive functions significantly improved in patients with DNS by using acetylcholinesterase inhibitors (Yanagiha et al., 2017). In another case study, it was reported that memantine used in combination with methylprednisolone significantly improved cognitive impairment (Iwamoto, 1991). However, since there is limited knowledge on pharmacological treatment, it is difficult to generalize these results.

The most common movement disorder that develops within DNS, as mentioned previously, is parkinsonism. It has been reported that levodopa, dopamine agonists, and anticholinergic agents are not as effective in the treatment of patients with parkinsonism as they are in idiopathic Parkinson's disease (Choi, 2002). However, some anecdotal reports have suggested that dopamine agonists may be more effective than levodopa preparations in symptomatic treatment (Klawans et al., 1982; Yoshii et al., 1998).

Conclusion

Carbon monoxide poisoning is a specific type of toxicity due to the neurological deterioration known as DNS that occurs after a period of temporary improvement, in addition to the neurological deficits brought on during the acute stage. The emerging treatment for CO poisoning, which has no antidote, is hyperbaric oxygen. However, currently there is insufficient evidence on how to prevent or treat the neurological deterioration that occurs after a certain period following poisoning. In the near future, a better understanding of the pathophysiology of DNS will help clarify treatment approaches on this topic.

References

Beppu, T. (2014). The Role of MR Imaging in Assessment of Brain Damage from Carbon Monoxide Poisoning: A Review of the Literature. *AJNR: American Journal of Neuroradiology*, *35*(4), 625–631. https://doi.org/10.3174/ajnr.A3489.

Bianco, F., & Floris, R. (1996). MRI appearances consistent with haemorrhagic infarction as an early manifestation of carbon monoxide poisoning. *Neuroradiology*, *38 Suppl 1*, S70-72. https://doi.org/10.1007/BF02278123.

Buckley, N. A., Juurlink, D. N., Isbister, G., Bennett, M. H., & Lavonas, E. J. (2011). Hyperbaric oxygen for carbon monoxide poisoning. *The Cochrane Database of Systematic Reviews*, *2011*(4), CD002041. https://doi.org/10.1002/14651858.CD002041.pub3.

Chambers, C. A., Hopkins, R. O., Weaver, L. K., & Key, C. (2008). Cognitive and affective outcomes of more severe compared to less severe carbon monoxide poisoning. *Brain Injury*, *22*(5), 387–395. https://doi.org/10.1080/02699050802008075.

Choi, I. S. (2002). Parkinsonism after Carbon Monoxide Poisoning. *European Neurology*, *48*(1), 30–33. https://doi.org/10.1159/000064954.

Choi, I. S., & Cheon, H. Y. (1999). Delayed movement disorders after carbon monoxide poisoning. *European Neurology*, *42*(3), 141–144. https://doi.org/10.1159/000008088.

Choi, S. (1983). Delayed Neurologic Sequelae in Carbon Monoxide Intoxication. *Archives of Neurology*, *40*(7), 433–435. https://doi.org/10.1001/archneur.1983.04050070063016.

Demirbaş, Ş., Metin, S., Çakmak, T., & Yildiz, Ş. (2011). 2010 yılında Türkiye'de karbonmonoksit zehirlenmesinin sıklığı [Frequency of carbon monoxide poisoning in Turkey in 2010.]. *TSK Koruyucu Hekimlik Bülteni*, *10*(5), 587 - 592.

Goldbaum, L. R., Orellano, T., & Dergal, E. (1976). Mechanism of the toxic action of carbon monoxide. *Annals of Clinical and Laboratory Science*, *6*(4), 372–376.

Hall, J. E., & Guyton, A. C. (2011). *Guyton and Hall textbook of medical physiology* (12th ed). Saunders/Elsevier.

Hampson, N. B. (2016). U.S. Mortality Due to Carbon Monoxide Poisoning, 1999-2014. Accidental and Intentional Deaths. *Annals of the American Thoracic Society, 13*(10), 1768–1774. https://doi.org/10.1513/AnnalsATS.201604-318OC.

Hampson, N. B., Dunn, S. L., & UHMCS/CDC CO Poisoning Surveillance Group. (2012). Symptoms of carbon monoxide poisoning do not correlate with the initial carboxyhemoglobin level. *Undersea & Hyperbaric Medicine: Journal of the Undersea and Hyperbaric Medical Society, Inc, 39*(2), 657–665.

Hampson, N. B., & Hampson, L. A. (2002). Characteristics of headache associated with acute carbon monoxide poisoning. *Headache, 42*(3), 220–223. https://doi.org/10.1046/j.1526-4610.2002.02055.x.

Hampson, N. B., Simonson, S. G., Kramer, C. C., & Piantadosi, C. A. (1996). Central nervous system oxygen toxicity during hyperbaric treatment of patients with carbon monoxide poisoning. *Undersea & Hyperbaric Medicine: Journal of the Undersea and Hyperbaric Medical Society, Inc, 23*(4), 215–219.

Handa, P. K., & Tai, D. Y. H. (2005). Carbon monoxide poisoning: A five year review at Tan Tock Seng Hospital, Singapore. *Annals of the Academy of Medicine, Singapore, 34*(10), 611–614.

Hsiao, C.-L., Kuo, H.-C., & Huang, C.-C. (2004). Delayed encephalopathy after carbon monoxide intoxication—Long-term prognosis and correlation of clinical manifestations and neuroimages. *Acta Neurologica Taiwanica, 13*(2), 64–70.

Iwamoto, E. T. (1991). Characterization of the antinociception induced by nicotine in the pedunculopontine tegmental nucleus and the nucleus raphe magnus. *The Journal of Pharmacology and Experimental Therapeutics, 257*(1), 120–133.

Jasper, B. W., Hopkins, R. O., Duker, H. V., & Weaver, L. K. (2005). Affective Outcome Following Carbon Monoxide Poisoning: A Prospective Longitudinal Study. *Cognitive and Behavioral Neurology, 18*(2), 127. https://doi.org/10.1097/01.wnn.0000160820.07836.cf.

Kitamoto, T., Tsuda, M., Kato, M., Saito, F., Kamijo, Y., & Kinoshita, T. (2016). Risk factors for the delayed onset of neuropsychologic sequelae following carbon monoxide poisoning. *Acute Medicine & Surgery, 3*(4), 315–319. https://doi.org/10.1002/ams2.197.

Klawans, H. L., Stein, R. W., Tanner, C. M., & Goetz, C. G. (1982). A Pure Parkinsonian Syndrome Following Acute Carbon Monoxide Intoxication. *Archives of Neurology, 39*(5), 302–304. https://doi.org/10.1001/archneur.1982.00510170044012.

Kobayashi, K., Isaki, K., Fukutani, Y., Kurachi, M., Eboshida, A., Matsubara, R., & Yamaguchi, N. (1984). CT Findings of the Interval Form of Carbon Monoxide Poisoning Compared with Neuropathological Findings. *European Neurology, 23*(1), 34–43. https://doi.org/10.1159/000115675.

Komuro, T., Borsody, M. K., Ono, S., Marton, L. S., Weir, B. K., Zhang, Z.-D., Paik, E., & Macdonald, R. L. (2001). The Vasorelaxation of Cerebral Arteries by Carbon Monoxide. *Experimental Biology and Medicine, 226*(9), 860–865. https://doi.org/10.1177/153537020122600909.

Kuroda, H., Fujihara, K., Kushimoto, S., & Aoki, M. (2015). Novel clinical grading of delayed neurologic sequelae after carbon monoxide poisoning and factors associated with outcome. *Neurotoxicology*, *48*, 35–43. https://doi.org/10.1016/j.neuro.2015.03.002.

Lapresle, J., & Fardeau, M. (1967). The Central Nervous System and Carbon Monoxide Poisoning II. Anatomical Study of Brain Lesions following Intoxication with Carbon Monoxide (22 cases). In H. Bour & McA. Ledingham (Eds.), *Progress in Brain Research* (Vol. 24, pp. 31–74). Elsevier. https://doi.org/10.1016/S0079-6123(08)60181-8.

Jankovic, J., Maziotta, J. C., Pomeroy, S. L., Newman, N. J. (2021). *Bradley and Daroff's Neurology in Clinical Practice, 2-Volume Set* (N. J. N. MD, Ed.; 8th edition). Elsevier.

Min, S. K. (1986). A brain syndrome associated with delayed neuropsychiatric sequelae following acute carbon monoxide intoxication. *Acta Psychiatrica Scandinavica*, *73*(1), 80–86. https://doi.org/10.1111/j.1600-0447.1986.tb02671.x.

O'donnell, P., Buxton, P. J., Pitkin, A., & Jarvis, L. J. (2000). The Magnetic Resonance Imaging Appearances of the Brain in Acute Carbon Monoxide Poisoning. *Clinical Radiology*, *55*(4), 273–280. https://doi.org/10.1053/crad.1999.0369.

Pages, B., Planton, M., Buys, S., Lemesle, B., Birmes, P., Barbeau, E. J., Maziero, S., Cordier, L., Cabot, C., Puel, M., Genestal, M., Chollet, F., & Pariente, J. (2014). Neuropsychological outcome after carbon monoxide exposure following a storm: A case-control study. *BMC Neurology*, *14*, 153. https://doi.org/10.1186/1471-2377-14-153.

Park, S., & Choi, I. S. (2004). Chorea Following Acute Carbon Monoxide Poisoning. *Yonsei Medical Journal*, *45*(3), 363–366. https://doi.org/10.3349/ymj.2004.45.3.363.

Parkinson, R. B., Hopkins, R. O., Cleavinger, H. B., Weaver, L. K., Victoroff, J., Foley, J. F., & Bigler, E. D. (2002). White matter hyperintensities and neuropsychological outcome following carbon monoxide poisoning. *Neurology*, *58*(10), 1525–1532. https://doi.org/10.1212/wnl.58.10.1525.

Pavese, N., Napolitano, A., De Iaco, G., Canapicchi, R., Collavoli, P. L., Lucetti, C., Gambaccini, G., & Bonuccelli, U. (1999). Clinical outcome and magnetic resonance imaging of carbon monoxide intoxication. A long-term follow-up study. *The Italian Journal of Neurological Sciences*, *20*(3), 171–178. https://doi.org/10.1007/s100720050028.

Pepe, G., Castelli, M., Nazerian, P., Vanni, S., Del Panta, M., Gambassi, F., Botti, P., Missanelli, A., & Grifoni, S. (2011). Delayed neuropsychological sequelae after carbon monoxide poisoning: Predictive risk factors in the Emergency Department. A retrospective study. *Scandinavian Journal of Trauma, Resuscitation and Emergency Medicine*, *19*, 16. https://doi.org/10.1186/1757-7241-19-16.

Raub, J. A., Mathieu-Nolf, M., Hampson, N. B., & Thom, S. R. (2000). Carbon monoxide poisoning—A public health perspective. *Toxicology*, *145*(1), 1–14. https://doi.org/10.1016/S0300-483X(99)00217-6.

Sanders, R. W., Katz, K. D., Suyama, J., Akhtar, J., O'Toole, K. S., Corll, D., & Ladenburger, R. N. (2012). Seizure During Hyperbaric Oxygen Therapy for Carbon Monoxide Toxicity: A Case Series and Five-year Experience. *Journal of Emergency Medicine*, *42*(4), e69–e72. https://doi.org/10.1016/j.jemermed.2008.12.017.

Silverman, C. S., Brenner, J., & Murtagh, F. R. (1993). Hemorrhagic necrosis and vascular injury in carbon monoxide poisoning: MR demonstration. *AJNR: American Journal of Neuroradiology*, *14*(1), 168–170.

Sircar, K., Clower, J., Shin, M. kyong, Bailey, C., King, M., & Yip, F. (2015). Carbon monoxide poisoning deaths in the United States, 1999 to 2012. *The American Journal of Emergency Medicine*, *33*(9), 1140–1145. https://doi.org/10.1016/j.ajem.2015.05.002.

Sloan, E. P., Murphy, D. G., Hart, R., Cooper, M. A., Turnbull, T., Barreca, R. S., & Ellerson, B. (1989). Complications and protocol considerations in carbon monoxide-poisoned patients who require hyperbaric oxygen therapy: Report from a ten-year experience. *Annals of Emergency Medicine*, *18*(6), 629–634. https://doi.org/10.1016/S0196-0644(89)80516-5.

Terajima, K., Igarashi, H., Hirose, M., Matsuzawa, H., Nishizawa, M., & Nakada, T. (2008). Serial Assessments of Delayed Encephalopathy after Carbon Monoxide Poisoning Using Magnetic Resonance Spectroscopy and Diffusion Tensor Imaging on 3.0T System. *European Neurology*, *59*(1–2), 55–61. https://doi.org/10.1159/000109262.

Thom, S. R. (1990). Carbon monoxide-mediated brain lipid peroxidation in the rat. *Journal of Applied Physiology*. https://doi.org/10.1152/jappl.1990.68.3.997.

Thom, S. R., Taber, R. L., Mendiguren, I. I., Clark, J. M., Hardy, K. R., & Fisher, A. B. (1995). Delayed neuropsychologic sequelae after carbon monoxide poisoning: Prevention by treatment with hyperbaric oxygen. *Annals of Emergency Medicine*, *25*(4), 474–480. https://doi.org/10.1016/s0196-0644(95)70261-x.

Thom, S. R., Xu, Y. A., & Ischiropoulos, H. (1997). Vascular endothelial cells generate peroxynitrite in response to carbon monoxide exposure. *Chemical Research in Toxicology*, *10*(9), 1023–1031. https://doi.org/10.1021/tx970041h.

Weaver, L. K. (2020). Carbon monoxide poisoning. *Undersea & Hyperbaric Medicine: Journal of the Undersea and Hyperbaric Medical Society, Inc*, *47*(1), 151–169. https://doi.org/10.22462/01.03.2020.17.

Weaver, L. K., Valentine, K. J., & Hopkins, R. O. (2007). Carbon monoxide poisoning: Risk factors for cognitive sequelae and the role of hyperbaric oxygen. *American Journal of Respiratory and Critical Care Medicine*, *176*(5), 491–497. https://doi.org/10.1164/rccm.200701-026OC.

Yanagiha, K., Ishii, K., & Tamaoka, A. (2017). Acetylcholinesterase inhibitor treatment alleviated cognitive impairment caused by delayed encephalopathy due to carbon monoxide poisoning: Two case reports and a review of the literature. *Medicine*, *96*(8), e6125. https://doi.org/10.1097/MD.0000000000006125.

Yoshii, F., Kozuma, R., Takahashi, W., Haida, M., Takagi, S., & Shinohara, Y. (1998). Magnetic resonance imaging and 11C-N-methylspiperone/positron emission tomography studies in a patient with the interval form of carbon monoxide poisoning. *Journal of the Neurological Sciences*, *160*(1), 87–91. https://doi.org/10.1016/S0022-510X(98)00218-4.

Chapter 5

The Late Effects of Carbon Monoxide Poisoning

Hasan Sultanoğlu*, MD
Yasin Haydar Yartaşı, MD
and Ali Can Kara, MD
Department of Emergency Medicine, School of Medicine,
Düzce University, Düzce, Turkey

Abstract

Carbon monoxide is a highly toxic gas for humans, which is formed as a result of the incomplete combustion of carbon-based fuels. It is a difficult gas to detect due to its non-irritant and high diffusion capacity. That is why it is called the "silent killer". While there are complaints of headache, nausea, vomiting, dizziness, and shortness of breath in the acute phase of carbon monoxide poisoning, cardiac ischemic problems, muscle weakness, decreased attention, confusion, convulsions, paralysis, and coma may develop in the chronic period as exposure and severity increase. CO poisoning still remains important because of its mortal course and the fact that it occurs in different people in different ways and at different times, causing difficulties for physicians in the diagnostic process. Although the current technological possibilities are advanced, the suspicion that occurs in the minds of doctors after a good anamnesis is more important than all other methods. The good clinical course of diagnosed patients in the acute period should not mislead doctors. It should be kept in mind that cardiac and neurological findings may occur in the late period and patients should be followed up regularly.

---

* Corresponding Author's Email: drsultanoglu@hotmail.com.

In: Carbon Monoxide Poisoning
Editors: Seda Özkan and Afsin Ipekci
ISBN: 979-8-89113-217-7

Keywords: carbon monoxide, late effects, cardiac effects, neurological effects, neuropsychiatric effects

Introduction

Carbon monoxide (CO) is a colorless, odorless, tasteless, non-irritant gas formed as a result of incomplete combustion of carbon-based fuels, hence called the "silent killer", which is highly toxic to humans (Chenoweth et al., 2021). It is a difficult gas to detect because of being colorless, odorless, tasteless, non-irritant, with a high diffusion capacity. Patients usually do not realize the poisoning until symptoms appear.

CO gas is produced from both man-made and natural sources. Sources of carbon monoxide can be listed as incorrectly adjusted gas appliances, ovens, coal and wood stoves, fireplaces, water heaters, combi boilers, bottled gas, kerosene, and petrol. In industry, it is used in generator gas, water gas, power gas, and air gas. It has been reported that 50% of CO emission in the USA is caused by road transport vehicles and 13% is caused by other transport vehicles. Due to the increasing cases of poisoning due to carbon monoxide from high-speed watercraft used in water sports in the USA, it has been mandatory to install detectors in these vehicles since 1998 (Agency for Toxic Substances and Disease Registry, 2012).

Carbon monoxide can be found endogenously and exogenously in the human body. Endogenous CO is formed during the breakdown of haemoprotein into bile pigments by heme oxygenase and forms carboxyhaemoglobin (COHb) at a rate of 1%. The most important source of exogenous CO is automobile exhaust. This is followed by CO produced by heating and cooking, factories, mining accidents, and fires. Indirect poisoning is seen with increased COHb as a result of inhalation of methylene chloride (dichloromethane, CH2Cl2), the main component of paint strippers, degreasers, and plastic-based adhesives, metabolized to carbon monoxide in the liver, accumulated in adipose tissue, and released slowly (Wilbur et al., 2012).

CO gas with a molar mass of 28.01 g/mol is formed by the combination of one carbon and one oxygen atom with a triple covalent bond. The density of CO gas is 1.25 kg/m^3 at 0°C temperature and 1-atmosphere pressure (Piantadosi, 2002).

Carbon monoxide is a stable gas that can remain in the atmosphere for over two months. Although it is known that carbon monoxide is normally 10 ppm in the air, this rate increases especially in cities, and it has been determined that poisoning starts after 10 ppm. Organs with high oxygen demand and, therefore, dependent on high blood flow can be seriously affected. CO enters the human body by inhalation and since its affinity for the haemoglobin molecule is approximately 200-250 times higher than that of oxygen, it replaces oxygen and forms carboxy haemoglobin, which can cause hypoxia in tissues where oxygen cannot go (Piantadosi, 2002; Megas et al., 2021).

Organs with high oxygen demand and thus dependent on high blood flow can be severely affected. For example, because of its affinity for myoglobin, which is 60 times greater than oxygen, its displacement of oxygen leads to cardiac depression and hypotension. Although the exact pathophysiological mechanism is not yet fully understood, the toxic effect is attributed to the binding of CO to cytochrome oxidase and inhibition of the electron transport chain (Megas et al., 2021).

The symptoms caused by carbon monoxide poisoning are generally nausea (40%), headache (46%), shortness of breath (20%), tachycardia (41%), dizziness and vomiting (Grieb et al., 2011; Garland and Pearce, 1967).

Carbon monoxide poisoning is estimated to be responsible for 30,000 to 50,000 emergency department visits each year. In the USA, this rate is approximately 10.000 to 15.000 per year and almost 500 people die from this cause every year. The mortality rate due to poisoning is highest in individuals aged 65 years and older. Non-fatal poisonings are more common between the ages of 15-34 (Hampson and Weaver, 2007; Janík et al., 2017).

Background

Carbon monoxide poisoning in organisms that need oxygen (O_2) to survive probably dates back to ancient civilizations when humans first learned to control fire around 800.000 BCE to heat their homes, cook food, and make weapons (Choi and Otterbein, 2002; Goren-Inbar et al., 2004). Native Americans are also thought to have experienced the psychoactive effects of CO during fireside rituals, as evidence of CO in native archaeological sites dates back to before 20.000 BCE (Dillehay et al., 2015; Schallner and Otterbein, 2015; Watt et al., 2018). The earliest analytical evidence for the presence of atmospheric CO was detected in ice sheet samples around 500 BCE (Robbins et al., 1973).

In 350 BCE, Aristotle recorded carbon monoxide poisoning for the first time when he stated that smoke from burning coal caused headaches and death (Jain, 2017).

Similarly, Erasistratus suggested that coal fumes affected normal respiration (275 BCE) (Vreman et al., 2000). Symptoms of CO poisoning first appeared in Cassius' (130 AD) book, named Medical Questions (Sayers and Davenport, 1937). Galen recognized that coal altered the composition of the air, thus making it harmful for breathing (ca. 150 AD), and Marcellinus also referred to the neurotoxic effects of coal fumes on the brain when discussing the symptoms of the throbbing of the head (ca. 350 AD). Further recognition of the neurotoxicity of CO came when Caelius Aurelianus observed disturbances in movement and general sensation (ca. 400 AD) (Pankow, 2000; Sayers and Davenport, 1937).

In addition to toxicity, people may have experienced the neuroactive properties of carbon monoxide by performing rituals around fire (Hopper et al., 2021).

The earliest reported case of CO poisoning occurred in Nuceria, where Romans are said to have suffocated in baths due to leaks in hypocaust heating technology; similarly, fumes may have been used militarily to execute Roman prisoners in the second Punic War, invading Carthaginian armies led by Hannibal (ca. 200 BC) (Weaver, 2009; Sayers and Davenport, 1937; Houston, 1989; Sykes and Walker, 2016; Clemens, 1926).

Documented evidence of CO reappeared in the late Middle Ages when Avicenna described a state of paralysis caused by CO fumes (980-1037 AD) (Cooper, 1966). In the late thirteenth century, the Spanish alchemist Arnold of Villanova described a poisonous gas produced by the combustion of wood; the gas he identified was carbon monoxide (Grace, 2014).

Friedrich Hoffmann conducted the first modern scientific investigation of CO poisoning from coal in 1716. Herman Boerhaave conducted the first scientific experiments on the effect of CO on animals in the 1730s (Hopper et al., 2021).

Between 1772 and 1799, Priestley recognized the difference between carbon dioxide (CO_2) and carbon monoxide and explained the properties of carbon monoxide (Schofield, 2005).

Carbon monoxide attracted attention in 1857 when French physiologist Claude Bernard found that the gas causes asphyxia by reversibly binding with haemoglobin (Hb) (Bernard, 1857).

In 1895, J.S. Haldane showed that the binding of CO to haemoglobin could be antagonized by high partial O_2 (PO_2) pressures and that mammals could survive fatal CO poisoning if large amounts of O_2 were dissolved in the blood plasma. He showed that rats suffering from carbon monoxide intoxication could be saved by administering oxygen at 2 atmospheric pressure (Haldane, 1895).

During the 19th century Industrial Revolution, coal was widely used as a fuel for power generation, and the resulting carbon monoxide led to the discovery of its toxic effects. In 1925, American physician Cecil Drinker published a paper describing the symptoms of carbon monoxide poisoning, including headache, dizziness, and nausea (Drinker, 1938). In 1942, End and Long demonstrated the benefits of hyperbaric oxygen therapy for experimental carbon monoxide poisoning in dogs and pigs. In 1960, hyperbaric oxygen (HBO) therapy was successfully used with humans for the first time (Jain, 2017).

During the Second World War, Roughton and Darling reported that carboxyhaemoglobin (COHb) shifted the dissociation curve of oxyhaemoglobin to the left because the empty haem of the haemoglobin tetramer binds to O_2 with greater affinity after the addition of CO to a site (Roughton and Darling, 1944).

At the University of Pennsylvania in the 1960s and 1970s, largely through the physiological research of Coburn, CO storage in the body was measured and CO uptake by tissues, particularly skeletal and cardiac muscle, was demonstrated during ambient exposure (Coburn and Mayers, 1971). Similarly, CO has been shown to diffuse from the maternal circulation into the placenta and bind to fetal haemoglobin in vivo (Hill et al., 1977).

It has been found that CO is oxidised by mitochondria in the body and converted to CO_2. CO alters the mitochondrial redox state as well as the energy supply in the brain, and these effects persist after COHb is cleared from the blood (Piantadosi, 2002).

The first hyperbaric oxygen (HBO) chamber for medical purposes was described in 1622 and, in the 19th century, HBO chambers were used to treat diseases such as tuberculosis, anemia and cholera (Danesh-Sani et al., 2012). However, in the late 19th century, an HBO chamber was first used in connection with CO poisoning. In 1895, Haldane published his study of a rat in a chamber with a high oxygen concentration and a low CO concentration, but HBO was not studied for some time (Haldane, 1895).

Churchill-Davidson first described the benefits of HBO therapy in patients with CO poisoning (Churchill, 1966). The first major studies on this subject were conducted in the 1980s. In a study comparing the use of normobaric oxygen (NBO) with HBO, Raphael et al. showed that HBO therapy was not beneficial regardless of the carboxyhaemoglobin level in patients who did not lose consciousness during carbon monoxide poisoning. In this study, no positive or a negative effect of HBO treatment could be demonstrated (Raphael et al., 1989).

Studies reveal that the vast majority of patients benefit from hyperbaric oxygen therapy, effectively minimizing the development of cerebral oedema and pathological changes in the central nervous system, as well as late neurological sequelae (Sinkovič et al., 2006; Stoller, 2007; Buckley et al., 2011). Currently, there are only a few national guidelines and no international guidelines on how to treat CO poisoning and at what stage to use HBO therapy. In summary, a common perspective at present seems to be that routine HBO therapy cannot be recommended in general but may be beneficial in patients with severe poisoning (Buckley et al., 2011).

Pathophysiology of Carbon Monoxide Poisoning

Carbon monoxide shows its toxic effects through multiple intertwined mechanisms that are not fully understood. Inhaled carbon monoxide shows 200-250 times more affinity for haemoglobin and causes COHb formation. As a result, the oxygen-haemoglobin dissociation curve shifts to the left, leading to tissue hypoxia and increased anaerobic metabolism. Carbon monoxide exposure as low as 10 ppm can lead to COHb levels of approximately 2% (Raub et al., 2000).

The World Health Organization suggests that levels higher than 6 ppm are potentially toxic. COHb levels above 2% in non-smokers and above 10% in heavy smokers are abnormal and signs of toxicity may be observed (World Health Organization, 2010; Hampson et al., 2012).

Carbon monoxide in the human body functions as a neurotransmitter in physiological amounts (Boehning et al., 2003). It modulates inflammation, regulates apoptosis, cell proliferation, and mitochondrial biogenesis (Suliman et al., 2007).

Carbon monoxide binds to iron-containing haemoproteins with high affinity. CO competes with oxygen for binding to haemoglobin and binds to haemoglobin with 250 times more affinity than oxygen. This reduces the oxygen-carrying capacity of the body and increases the amount of COHb in the body. The binding of carbon monoxide to haemoglobin also stabilizes the relaxed and high-affinity quaternary state of haemoglobin (known as the R-state), increasing the oxygen affinity of other regions within the Hb tetramer, further reducing oxygen release and delivery. In addition to Hb, CO binds to myoglobin, mitochondrial cytochrome c oxidase (COX; complex IV), and other haem-containing proteins in cardiac and skeletal muscle. Since the elimination times in tissue and blood are different, tissue damage may also develop with delay (Weaver, 2020; Blumenthal, 2001).

Carbon monoxide disrupts the normal respiratory function of cells. Similar to the effects of cyanide and nitric oxide (NO), CO inhibits mitochondrial respiration by binding to the ferrous haemprotein at the active site of COX and effectively stops oxidative phosphorylation (Goldbaum, 1976; Brown and Piantadosi, 1990; Brown and Piantadosi, 1992; Turner et al., 1999; Shiva et al., 2007). COX binds 3-fold more to CO than to O_2. Due to the competitive binding of O_2 and CO to COX, CO-mediated mitochondrial inhibition is greatest under hypoxic conditions. When COX is inhibited, oxidative phosphorylation slows, reducing ATP production in tissues with high oxygen demand, such as the brain or heart. Other complexes in the electron transport chain continue to transport electrons, producing superoxide, leading to further damage, necrosis, and apoptosis of cells and tissues (Gnaiger et al., 1998; Wald and Allen, 1957; Lo Iacono et al., 2011). Impaired cellular respiration initiates a number of stress responses, including the activation of hypoxia-inducible factor 1a (HIF-1a). This results in carbon monoxide dose-dependent neurological and cardiac protection or damage through gene regulation (Mannaioni et al., 2006).

Excess carbon monoxide in the body activates platelets by displacing nitric oxide from platelet surface haemoproteins. The displaced free nitric oxide reacts with superoxide released by neutrophils into the intravascular space to produce peroxynitrite. Peroxynitrite increases the activation of adhesion molecules on platelets and neutrophils. Activated platelets stimulate neutrophils to degranulate and release myeloperoxidase (MPO) (Thom et al., 2006; Weaver, 2009; Hirayama et al., 1999). MPO enhances inflammatory effects by triggering further neutrophil activation, adhesion, and degranulation. It was suggested that proteases (MPO, elastase) released as a result of neutrophil degranulation oxidize endothelial cell xanthine dehydrogenase to xanthine oxidase and produce reactive oxygen species (ROS) (Thom et al., 2006). MPO and ROS cause changes in myelin basic protein (MBP) structure. ROS and MBP catalyse lipid peroxidation, triggering lymphocyte response and microglia activation (Thom et al., 2006). This mechanism is thought to play a role in late neurological sequelae. In a study conducted in cerebrospinal fluid from patients with CO poisoning who developed late neurological sequelae, increased MBP levels were shown in the 1st month after poisoning compared to those without severe symptoms (Kuroda et al., 2015). These inflammatory effects persist long after initial CO poisoning and are probably independent of COHb levels (Thom et al., 2006; Kuroda et al., 2015). The inflammatory cascade induced by NO and ROS plays an important role in the neurological and cardiac involvement caused by CO poisoning (Thom et al., 2006).

CO can cause ischemic and anoxic brain damage by decreasing oxygen delivery and mitochondrial oxidative phosphorylation, leading to impaired cognitive function in survivors (Geocadin et al., 2008). Ischemia-induced brain damage may result from excitotoxicity, acidosis, ion imbalance and depolarization, oxidative stress, nitrative stress, inflammation, and apoptosis (Doyle et al., 2008). As a result of decreased oxidative phosphorylation and ATP, the Ca ATPase pump in the plasma membrane is inactivated. This results in a large increase in intracellular calcium influx and ultimately increases brain damage (Doyle et al., 2008). Glutamate increases cellular dysfunction and apoptosis by activating N-Methyl-D-aspartate (NMDA) receptors. Decreases in ATP, particularly glutamate, activate intracellular proteases and lipases that cause mitochondrial membrane depolarization, cell death, and neurotransmitter release (Doyle et al., 2008; Kim and Reed, 2008).

Lipid peroxidation occurs in the brain due to the increase in oxidative products. As a result of the products formed after lipid peroxidation (such as malondialdehyde) changing the structure of MBP in the brain and becoming immunogenic, activated microglia cause inflammation (Geocadin et al., 2008; Doyle et al., 2008).

In the pathophysiology of acute CO poisoning, besides CO binding to haemoglobin and causing hypoxemia, inflammatory processes due to CO dissolved in the blood also play an important role. The occurrence of late neurological sequelae after COHb levels fall into the normal range is a result of the inflammatory effect.

Systemic Effects of Carbon Monoxide Poisoning

Carbon monoxide poisoning can easily be missed because it shows non-specific signs and symptoms. The organs most affected by poisoning are organs such as the brain and heart due to high blood flow and high oxygen demand. Patients usually present to the emergency department with complaints of headache, nausea, vomiting, and dizziness. Cardiac ischemic problems, muscle weakness, decreased attention, confusion, convulsion, paralysis, and coma may develop as exposure and severity increase (Jain, 2017) (Table 1).

Table 1. Signs and symptoms at various concentrations of carboxyhemoglobin

CO in atmosphere	Duration of exposure	Saturation of blood	Signs and symptoms
Up to 0.01%	Indefinite	0-10%	None
0.01-0.02%	Indefinite	10-20%	Tightness across the forehead, slight headache, dilatation of cutaneus vessels
0.02-0.03%	5-6 hr	20-30%	Headache, throbbing in temples
0.04-0.06%	4-5 hr	30-40%	Severe headache, weakness, nausea, vomiting, dimness of vision, dizziness, collapse, cherry-red color of lips and skin
0.07-0.10%	3-4 hr	40-50%	As above plus; syncope, increased pulse and respiratory rate
0.11-0.15%	1 1/2 -3 hr	50-60%	Tachycardia, tachypnea, Cheyne-stokes respiration, coma, convulsion
0.16-0.30%	1-1 1/2 hr	60-70%	Coma, convulsion, decreased heart action and respiration, possibly death
0.50-1.00%	1-2 min	70-80%	Weak pulse, depressed respiration, respiratory failure and death

The diagnosis of acute CO poisoning usually depends on 3 factors (Hampson et al., 2012; Hardy and Thom, 1994):

- History of potential exposure to a CO source,
- Symptoms consistent with CO poisoning.

COHb levels above 5% in non-smokers or above 10% in smokers (higher baseline levels have been reported in cigar and hookah smokers) (Dorey et al., 2020).

Measuring COHb and oxyhaemoglobin (O2Hb) by pulse oximetry in a patient with CO poisoning has potential pitfalls. Standard pulse oximetry used in modern medical settings measures the absorption of light at a wavelength of 660 nm. Both O2Hb and COHb have similar absorption characteristics at this wavelength of light, and consequently, the pulse oximeter will report a normal oxygen saturation (Hampson, 1998).

For the purpose of obtaining the HgbCO level, arterial and venous samples are equally reliable and can be used interchangeably. In addition, a fingertip pulse co-oximeter has been available since 2005. Although some investigators have questioned the reliability of these devices, they may be a useful early screening tool until definitive confirmatory laboratory testing is available. COHb above 60% is fatal (Hampson et al., 2012; Weaver et al., 2013).

In patients with a history of cardiovascular disease, myocardial infarction may be triggered as carbon monoxide impairs oxygen transport to the myocardium and increases ischaemia. ST depression may be seen as an ECG change in patients. Arrhythmias, extrasystoles, atrial fibrillation, low voltage, prolongation of the ventricular complex, increased PR interval, conduction defects, and bundle branch block are other ECG findings. In the chronic period, cardiomyopathy, cardiomegaly, hypertension, and atherosclerosis may be observed in patients (Jain, 2017; Raub et al., 2000).

It mostly causes degenerative and demyelinating changes in the nervous system. In the brain, the corpus callosum, hippocampus, and substansia nigra are mostly affected and neuronal damage is observed. In the cerebral cortex, it causes demyelination with perivascular spread. White matter damage is also important in the pathogenesis of parkinsonism. Patients may develop cerebral atrophy in advanced stages, and this is associated with a poor prognosis. Neuropathy may be observed in the peripheral nerves (Jain, 2017; Raub et al., 2000).

In the pulmonary system, it causes pulmonary oedema, interalveolar oedema and has a ground-glass appearance on imaging (Table 2). One of the acute effects is retinal haemorrhages and visual impairment. Due to hypoxia in the cochlear nerve and nuclei in the brainstem, the patient may have central hearing loss with little possibility of recovery. Lactate accumulation in the blood may be observed due to ischemia in the tissues and trigger anaerobic respiration. Intestinal ischemia and infarction have been reported in fatal cases. Late neuropsychiatric sequelae may be more common in the chronic period. These complaints may develop between a few days and about three weeks after exposure. The incidence of late neuropsychiatric sequelae varies between 10% and 40%. Akinetic mutism, apraxia, ataxia, convulsive disorders, cortical blindness, delirium, dementia, depression, mental decline, choreoathetosis, optic neuritis, peripheral neuropathy, psychoses, and multiple sclerosis-like symptoms may be observed in patients. It has been predicted that patients at risk in terms of cognitive sequelae with loss of consciousness in the group not receiving hyperbaric oxygen therapy are those aged 36 years and older and patients with more than 24 hours of exposure (Jain, 2017). Clinical findings and COHb levels are not always compatible. COHb is not directly responsible for toxic effects, as these effects occur as a result of CO dissolved in plasma (Goldbaum, 1975).

In acute carbon monoxide poisoning in pregnant women diagnosed with carbon monoxide poisoning, the maternal mortality rate has been reported as 19-24% and the fetal mortality rate as 36-67%. Toxic effects on the fetus vary according to the degree of exposure, chronicity, and gestational age. As a result of exposure, maternal COHb level increases rapidly in the first 2-3 hours, while fetal COHb level may not show any changes in the first hours. Afterwards, it increases for 24 hours and plateaus at 36-48 hours. Fetal COHb levels rise later than maternal COHb levels, and its elimination is also later than maternal COHb levels even after treatment. Anatomical malformations in the fetus in the early stage of pregnancy and neurological sequelae may develop due to anoxic events in the late stage of pregnancy. Reported fetal morbidities include preterm labor, hypoxic ischemic encephalopathy, hypotonia, cerebral palsy, areflexia, persistent seizures, microcephaly, cardiomegaly, and limb malformations (Friedman et al., 2015).

Table 2. Systemic effects and complications of CO poisoning

System	Clinical findings
Cardiovascular	ECG changes (T wave & ST segment), cardiomegaly, angina pectoris, myocardial infarct, tachycardia, bradycardia, A-V block, atrial fibrillation, prematüre ventricular contraction, ventricular fibrillation, shock
Respiratory	Pneumonia, pulmonary edema, adult respiratory distress syndrome
Genitourinary	Glycosuria, proteinuria, hematuria, myoglobinuria, acute renal failure, abortion, still-birth, menstural disturbance, reduction in weight of testes and in number of spermatozoa
Gastrointestinal	G-I disturbance, G-I bleeding, gastric ulcer, hepatomegaly
Hematological	Leucocytosis, erythrocytosis, anemia, pernicious anemia, thrombotic thrombocytopenic purpura
Metabolic and endocrinological	Hyperglycemia, decreased T_3, acute hyperthyroidism
Dermatological	Bulla, erythema, swelling, ulcer, gangrene, alopecia
Skeletomuscular	Muscle necrosis, Volkman's contracture, osteomyelitis
Ophthalmological	Retinal hemorrhage, papilledema, retinopathy, optic atrophy, amblyopia, scotoma, hemianopsia, blindness
Otologic	Disturbances of cochlear and vestibular functions

Breathing oxygen accelerates the removal of COHb. The half-life of COHb in adults breathing sea-level air is approximately five to six hours but reduced alveolar ventilation will prolong the half-life. The half-life of COHb in adults with normobaric oxygen administration is 74 ± 25 min (mean ± 1 SD) (Weaver et al., 2000). Hyperbaric oxygen accelerates COHb decomposition compared to breathing pure oxygen at sea level pressure (Jasper et al., 2005; Cardellach et al., 2003).

Children may recover uneventfully following poisoning or experience long-term problems (Klees et al., 1985). Based on mathematical modelling from animal experiments, the half-life of fetal COHb is 1.5 times that of adult COHb (Hill et al., 1977). Studies following CO-poisoned patients for a year or more have documented long-term adverse effects on cognitive function, quality of life, and general health (Jasper et al., 2005; Weaver et al., 2008). Therefore, patients with CO poisoning should be followed up after discharge.

The systemic effects and complications of CO poisoning are summarized in Table 2. (Choi, 2001).

Cardiac Effects of Carbon Monoxide Poisoning

Carbon monoxide shows its toxic effects by reducing the delivery of oxygen, which is known to be of vital value, to the tissues, leaving the tissues anoxic. It has arrhythmogenic, haemodynamic and ischemic effects on the cardiovascular system.

Many mechanisms may play a role in myocardial ischemia and cardiac dysfunction in CO poisoning. In animal studies, the decreased systemic oxygen delivery caused by CO poisoning is initially compensated by increased cardiac output and oxygen extraction; when these compensatory mechanisms are insufficient, cardiovascular collapse occurs (Smithline et al., 2003). Decreased oxygen delivery, increased O_2 demand, and increased myocardial contractility resulting from CO poisoning may trigger myocardial infarction in patients with underlying coronary artery disease (Dziewierz et al., 2013).

One of the triple gas signaling molecules, together with nitric oxide and hydrogen sulfide in humans in cell metabolism, tissue or organ systems, CO is also produced endogenously during haemoglobin breakdown (Coburn, 1970; Li et al., 2009). The common feature of all three gases for the vascular system is vasodilatation. Carbon monoxide also plays a critical role in angiogenesis, has anti-inflammatory properties and has been described as a cardiac protective mediator in terms of myocardial damage (Li et al., 2009).

The COHb level formed by endogenous production does not exceed 1% in the body. In haemolytic anaemia or sepsis, the COHb level may increase up to 3-4% (Garg et al., 2018). Ca+2 entry into myocardial cells through a voltage-gated L-type Ca+2 channel is required for the generation of action potentials and the initiation of myocardial contraction with the electrical stimulus. Endogenous CO, a signaling gas molecule, protects myocardial tissue from ischemia and reperfusion damage by inhibiting these channels (Yet et al., 2001). Interruption of the late Na+ current causes prolongation of the plateau phase of the action potential, disruption of myocardial repolarization and consequently arrhythmia. While CO is a strong modulator of cardiac Na+ channels, it has the ability to inhibit peak Na+ current apart from late Na+ current (Elies et al., 2014). These effects of CO on L-type Ca+2 channels and the Na+ current during action potential generation may lead to arrhythmia in the case of toxicity. In addition, perfusion of the cardiac conduction system, which has specialized myocyte cells, is provided by the coronary arteries. Due to CO poisoning, a tendency to coronary thrombosis, a decrease in myocardial O_2 stores and myocardial contractility due to myoglobin-CO (Mb-CO) formation, and a predisposition to arrhythmias will develop as a result of impaired myocardial perfusion secondary to coronary vasoconstriction (Elies et al., 2014).

The reflection of all these processes on the ECG is the prolongation of the QT interval, and the prolongation of the QT interval in acute CO poisoning is associated with cardiac toxicity. The fact that arrhythmia susceptibility is not correlated with serum CO levels highlights the need for close cardiac monitoring for CO poisoning cases (Temrel and Bilge, 2020).

For endogenous CO, which has known functions on the cardiovascular system, porphyrin-iron complex (Haem) related structures are targeted when normal levels are exceeded. Haem-associated proteins include haemoglobin, which is involved in the transport and release of oxygen to tissues, and myoglobin for storage, the cytochrome family that provides ATP production and apoptosis in mitochondria, catalase and peroxidase that protect cells from oxidative damage by reactive oxygen radicals by converting hydrogen peroxide to water and oxygen, and neuronal NO synthetase (nNOS) that centrally regulates blood pressure, endothelial NO synthetase (eNOS), which is a vasodilator and anti-atherogenic/vasoprotective endothelial NO synthetase, inducible NO synthetase (iNOS), which is a multifactorial transmitter in inflammatory cascade activation and platelet aggregation, prostaglandin synthetase, which is involved in the synthesis of prostaglandin and thromboxane, which are regulators of vascular tone and platelet aggregation. CO, which tends to bind to the structure of these proteins, may lead to anaerobic respiration, metabolic acidosis, vascular endothelial damage, thromboembolic processes, and vasoconstriction at the cellular level. High levels of CO compete with and displace NO bound to platelet surface haemoproteins, which may lead to platelet activation (Thom et al., 1994). As with other haem-containing proteins, it activates thromboembolic processes, coronary artery vasoconstriction, and inflammatory cascade in the central nervous system and cardiovascular system. The activated cascade generates free oxygen radicals. This causes neuronal and myocyte damage at the cellular level.

When CO is inhaled into the circulation, it aims to bind to the iron atom in myoglobin (Mb) and haemoglobin (Hb). The affinity of CO for Hb and Mb is higher than that of oxygen (Blumenthal, 2001). In addition to restriction of oxygen delivery to the myocardial tissue by the Hb-CO complex, hypoxia is inevitable for myocardium due to the Mb-CO interaction. Inhaled CO also produces a negative inotropic effect (Lee et al., 2015). The negative inotropic effect on the myocardium decreases the left ventricular ejection fraction and increases the diastolic pressure (Aronow et al., 1974). After reperfusion of the ischemic myocardium, the use of positive inotropic agents is beneficial in the complete reversal of ventricular dysfunction associated with decreased myocardial contractility.

Coronary syndromes with myocardial damage developing at the cellular level when the oxygen required by the myocardium cannot be met in relation to the CO level, arrhythmias with the failure to meet the oxygen demand of the conduction system of the heart, reversible decrease in contractility after myocardial reperfusion independent of myocardial damage or coronary perfusion reduction, hypotension associated with left ventricular dysfunction and with direct CO effect, followed by cardiogenic shock and ultimately death (Garg et al., 2018; Lee et al., 2015).

Although the risk of thromboembolic events in CO poisoning increases in the presence of an underlying cause, carbon monoxide poisoning alone is a risk factor in healthy individuals. Many tests are used in the recognition and evaluation of cardiac involvement in acute carbon monoxide poisoning. Sinus bradycardia, sinus tachycardia (most common), P wave inversion, atrial fibrillation, atrial flutter, first-degree AV block, right and left bundle branch blocks, QRS widening, premature atrial and ventricular complexes, ventricular tachycardia, long QT, ST segment changes, T wave inversion can be observed on electrocardiography in the evaluation of myocardial ischemia

(Garg et al., 2018; Temrel and Bilge, 2020; Ozyurt et al., 2017; Palaniswamy et al., 2013).

There is a negative correlation between BNP and proBNP levels used in the evaluation of left ventricular function in acute CO poisoning cases. Decreases in the ejection fraction are associated with the degree of CO exposure. These changes may occur without myocardial infarction. Changes in ejection fraction typically resolve within 24 hours but may be permanent in some patients (Kalay et al., 2007; Chamberland et al., 2004).

Cardiac troponin, CK, and MB are used as biochemical markers in the evaluation of acute coronary syndrome, but since these markers are also increased in arrhythmias and cerebrovascular events, these parameters cannot completely exclude cardiac toxicity in acute CO poisoning. Therefore, echocardiography, coronary angiography, cardiac scintigraphy, cardiac CT, and MRI should be used in the evaluation of cardiac toxicity. In patients with CO poisoning, elevated cardiac enzymes are associated with an increased five-year mortality rate (Henry et al., 2006). As a means of further investigation, coronary angiography would be the appropriate approach in patients with suspected coronary artery occlusion.

All patients approaching the emergency department with suspicion of carbon monoxide poisoning are firstly evaluated for airway, breathing, and circulation with the ABC approach. In the cases of cardiac arrest, cardiopulmonary resuscitation is initiated. The option of HBO therapy after resuscitation for cardiac arrest cases is controversial due to the time concern for transport to the treatment center (Vanden Hoek et al., 2010). Although extracorporeal membrane oxygenation (ECMO) is available for cardiogenic shock and cardiac arrest cases, the evidence for its usefulness in CO poisoning is still insufficient (Simonsen et al., 2018).

In patients with unstable haemodynamics due to CO poisoning, resuscitative fluid replacement depending on the volume status and the use of positive inotropes will protect myocytes from secondary damage. The treatment approach in all cases of carbon monoxide poisoning is oxygen support to the patient regardless of COHb level. In current practice, response to normal pressure oxygen or hyperbaric oxygen therapy is monitored by COHb levels. Considering that the MbCO bond dissociates later than COHb, it is aimed at using new diagnostic tools and treatments in the follow-up of cases to prevent acute or chronic effects of cardiac toxicity. Solving the molecular dynamics of MbCO with photolysis studies at the molecular level may lead to new treatments to be applied together with protein-based ligands HBO and NBO treatments that can both retain CO and allow its elimination from circulation and tissues (Levantino, et al., 2015; Rose et al., 2018; Azarov et al., 2016).

Neurological Effects of Carbon Monoxide Poisoning

Neurological sequelae are the most common form of morbidity in carbon monoxide poisoning. Neurological morbidity following CO poisoning includes neurological sequelae, brain imaging abnormalities, affective changes, and cognitive disorders (Gorman et al., 2003; Gale et al., 1999). In healthy individuals, cognitive impairments are frequently observed in the acute and late periods following CO poisoning. It is estimated that 15% to 49% of individuals diagnosed with CO poisoning will develop cognitive sequelae (Weaver et al., 2008).

The mechanisms of neural damage resulting from CO poisoning are complex and multifactorial (Weaver, 2009). Although neuropathological damage associated with CO poisoning is mainly related to CO-induced hypoxia, other biochemical mechanisms are also involved. Mechanisms of CO poisoning brain damage include mitochondrial dysfunction, lipid peroxidation resulting in disruption of cellular metabolism, and peroxynitrite accumulation, followed by blood vessel endothelial damage and oxidative stress (Piantadosi et al., 1997). CO-mediated oxidative stress alters the basic protein of myelin, resulting in an immune response and inflammation in the central nervous system (Thom et al., 2004). In accordance with multifactorial neuropathological mechanisms, cognitive, sensory, and neuro behavioral sequelae are seen in the resulting clinical picture.

Survivors of CO poisoning suffer from long-term neurocognitive sequelae related to brain damage. Symptoms include memory impairment, cognitive dysfunction, depression, anxiety and/or vestibular and motor deficits. These deficits become apparent at the sixth week and studies show a greater than 40% incidence of depression, anxiety, and cognitive dysfunction (Hampson et al., 2012; Weaver et al., 2008). Although patients can recover in six months or even up to one year after CO poisoning, studies show that patients still exhibit a 19% incidence of cognitive deficits and a 37% incidence of neurological deficits (Weaver et al., 2008). 33 years after a mining accident involving 156 patients with CO poisoning, 68.6% had mental impairments and 48.7% had neurological symptoms, indicating the irreversible nature of these deficits (Mimura et al., 1999). Risk factors for 6-week cognitive impairment include being 36 years of age or older and a longer duration of CO exposure

(≥24 hours). The severity of initial symptoms is not necessarily associated with the development of long-term neurological problems. Low-level, chronic exposure can also lead to neurological and cognitive deficits that do not improve after removal from the CO source, suggesting neurological damage even at low COHb and environmental CO levels (Penney, 2008; Townsend and Maynard 2002).

The most common neurological symptom of CO toxicity is headache, which is found in approximately 91% of patients. More severely poisoned patients may experience syncope, seizures, altered consciousness (including coma), and altered mental status (Ernst and Zibrak, 1998; Buboltz and Robins, 2023). In surviving patients at initial exposure, a significant proportion may suffer from delayed or persistent neurological symptoms. These symptoms include depression, memory difficulties, ataxia, and motor disorders (Hampson et al., 2012; Weaver et al., 2008).

In the study by Gorman et al., cognitive sequelae lasting one month or longer were observed in 25% of patients with loss of consciousness or carboxyhaemoglobin levels greater than 25% (Gorman et al., 1992). Recent studies using comprehensive standardized neuropsychological tests have found significant cognitive impairment both in the acute phase and several years after recovery from initial CO poisoning symptoms (Gale et al., 1999).

The most frequently reported findings in studies were impaired memory, followed by impaired attention, motor disorders, executive dysfunction, slow mental processing speed, and impaired visuospatial abilities. Similarly, memory impairment was the most common finding in case studies. Memory impairments following CO poisoning include short-term memory loss, anterograde memory loss, retrograde memory loss, recall, and recognition memory impairments. Other cognitive impairments following CO poisoning include visual dysfunction, visual-motor skills, visual-spatial planning, and significant deficits in abstract thinking.

Neurons are the most vulnerable cells in the central nervous system to hypoxic-ischemic insult. Acute or severe CO poisoning can directly lead to diffuse hypoxic-ischemic encephalopathy involving predominantly grey matter (Lo et al., 2007). Acute CO poisoning focally affecting the cerebral cortex has been reported much less frequently (O'Donnell et al., 2000). The temporal lobe and the hippocampus are the most frequently affected areas. Tissue damage may develop due to transient vasogenic oedema or necrosis without any occlusion of the cerebral arteries. Diffusion-weighted MRI examination is useful to distinguish these two conditions (Kavak et al., 2020).

The most common MRI findings are white matter hyperintensities (WMHs) and hippocampal atrophy (Weaver et al., 2015; Parkinson et al., 2002).

The globus pallidus is one of the most commonly affected areas of the brain by CO poisoning. Damage usually occurs immediately. Although the reason why the globus pallidus is affected is unclear, it is thought to be the result of the hypotensive effect of CO poisoning and the inability to supply the tissue with blood flow or the attraction of carbon monoxide to these proteins in this region containing iron-rich proteins (Chu et al., 2004). Globus pallidus necrosis is not always associated with the development of parkinsonism. Because the damage to the nigrostriatal pathway is not complete in all cases (Prockop, 2005). CT usually shows symmetrical hypodensity. On MRI, the medial parts of the globus pallidus appear as bilateral areas of low signal intensity on T1-weighted images and high signal intensity on T2-weighted and FLAIR images. In the acute phase of CO poisoning, contrast-enhanced T1-weighted images may show irregular or peripheral enhancement in necrotic areas (Lo et al., 2007). Diffusion-weighted MRI and apparent diffusion coefficient maps show restriction of fluid diffusion due to cytotoxic oedema resulting from acute tissue necrosis (Kinoshita et al., 2005).

The caudate nucleus, putamen, and thalamus are sometimes affected by CO poisoning, but more rarely than globus pallidus. The lesions are usually seen as asymmetric hyperintense foci in T2-weighted and FLAIR MRI sequences. Involvement of the brainstem and cerebellum may be a reflection of more severe poisoning because posterior structures are more resistant to hypoxia (O'Donnell et al., 2000).

Delayed posthypoxic leukoencephalopathy (DPHL) can develop within days to weeks after prolonged cardiac arrest or severe haemorrhagic shock. In the case of CO poisoning, DPHL is thought to result from direct myelinotoxicity resulting from impaired cellular respiration, again secondary to inhibition of aerobic respiration by CO binding to COX. MRI findings of DPHL are seen on T2-weighted images, especially in the central semiovale, showing diffuse cerebral and CO intoxication (Shprecher and Mehta, 2010).

After carboxyhaemoglobin levels decrease, mitochondrial function recovers and energy production is restored, but transient changes can cause neuronal necrosis and apoptotic death leading to brain atrophy. CT and MRI show enlargement of the brain ventricles and an increased ventricle-to-brain ratio. They found that within six months after CO exposure, 80% of the cases had marked atrophic changes and half of the patients developed cognitive impairment. However, the atrophic change did not correlate well with cognitive impairment (Gorman et al., 2003).

Demyelination of cerebral white matter is usually not specific to acute CO poisoning. The most commonly involved areas are periventricular white matter and centrum semioval (O'Donnell et al., 2000). However, in severe cases, demyelination may involve subcortical white matter, corpus callosum, external and internal capsules. CT usually shows diffuse and confluent hypodensity in these areas. Hyperintensity on T1-weighted images and hyperintensity on T2-weighted and FLAIR images indicate demyelination. White matter demyelination is believed to be responsible for the delayed neuropsychiatric syndrome (Kim et al., 2003; Murata et al., 2001). In a small proportion of patients who regain consciousness after acute CO poisoning, the initial neurological deficit does not appear to persist, but delayed neuropsychiatric involvement may occur after the lucid interval (O'Donnell et al., 2000). The most common symptoms of the delayed neuropsychiatric syndrome are mental impairment (amnesia, cognitive dysfunction), emotional disturbance (depression, anxiety, mutism), urinary and fecal incontinence, and motor impairment (Kim et al., 2003).

In animal studies, it has been predicted that hyperbaric oxygen therapy may prevent the development of delayed neuropsychiatric pathologies by preventing the lipid peroxidation process (Gorman et al., 2003).

Late Neuropsychiatric Sequelae

The two centers in our body where oxygen is consumed the most are the heart and the brain; therefore, the pathophysiological mechanisms caused by carbon monoxide (CO) most frequently lead to cardiovascular and neuropsychiatric symptoms (Keith, 2000). It has been observed that neuropsychiatric sequelae develop in most long-term and/or severe exposures. The most common neuropsychiatric findings are disorders including anterograde and retrograde amnesia accompanying confabulation. Apart from these, psychiatrically, decreased cognitive functions, emotional lability, and impaired judgement may be seen. Neurologically, apraxia, agnosia, tic disorders, rigidity, hearing and vestibular dysfunction, gait and movement disorders, stupor, and even coma may be seen. Studies have shown that coma is an indicator of severe CO exposure (Penney, 2008; Weaver et al., 2007).

Mental status changes and nutritional intolerance in infancy and headache and vomiting complaints in older children are the most frequently detected symptoms (Yarar et al., 2008; Kurt et al., 2013).

The clinical findings and the time of onset of the clinical findings due to carbon monoxide poisoning vary from person to person. Symptoms and signs may manifest themselves acutely or may occur after days or even months. In addition, these clinical symptomatologies may manifest themselves in monophasic or biphasic forms. In monophasic form, survival varies between days and years, and at the end of this process, it may recover with or without sequelae. In the biphasic form, there is a period of normality called the Lucid interval, which follows the coma period and lasts between a week and a month (Choi, 2001).

Due to these complex reasons, the diagnosis of CO poisoning can be very difficult. In fact, the possibility of misdiagnosis increases in cases of late anoxic encephalopathy due to the asymptomatic period following acute poisoning (Werner et al., 1985; Wood and Murray, 1999). In a study following 86 patients who developed late neuropsychiatric sequelae after CO intoxication, it was reported that 35 patients were first taken to a psychiatrist by their families because of psychiatric symptoms and three of these patients were diagnosed with acute functional psychosis and two of these patients were diagnosed with schizophrenia (Min, 1986).

The late anoxic encephalopathy symptom triad was defined to clarify these diagnostically difficult processes. Late anoxic encephalopathy symptom triad includes deterioration in mental status, urinary and/or fecal incontinence and gait disturbance (Choi, 1983). Myoclonus, ballismus, tremor, parkinsonism, apraxia, peripheral neuropathy, neurological deficits caused by neurological deficits due to spinal cord damage and various gait disturbances can be observed (Şenoğlu et al., 2005; Choi, 1983). The reason why there are many different psychiatric findings in CO poisoning is related to the affected brain region. For example, when the white matter, prefrontal cortex and basal ganglia are affected, symptoms such as periodic depression, major depression, social withdrawal, personality changes, apathy, perception disorders, obsessive-compulsive disorder, catatonia, and even psychosis are observed. It has also been observed to cause exacerbations of the disease after intoxication in patients with a previous history of mania (Ku et al., 2006). Pallidal lesions lead to decreased intellectual capacity and behavioral activity, as well as stereotypic behaviors and amnesia (Starkstein et al., 1989).

The prognosis of delayed encephalopathy due to CO intoxication is relatively good. In a clinical study, 75% of patients recovered within 1 year.

However, some findings such as mild memory impairment and parkinsonism may remain as sequelae (Weaver, 2009). Information on the treatment of hypoxic encephalopathy that occurs in the late period due to CO poisoning is limited. It is seen that psychopharmacological treatments are preferred considering the symptoms and findings of the patients in the studies, most of which were prepared as case reports (Borras et al., 2009; Kwon et al., 2004; Gürlek et al., 2007).

Conclusion

CO poisoning still remains important because of its mortal course and the fact that it occurs in different people in different ways and at different times, causing difficulties for physicians in the diagnostic process. Although the current technological possibilities are advanced, the suspicion that occurs in the minds of doctors after a good anamnesis is more important than all other methods. The fact that the clinical course of the diagnosed patients is good in the acute process should not mislead the physicians; it should be kept in mind that late neurological, cardiac, and neuropsychiatric findings may occur in patients and patients should be followed up regularly.

References

Agency for Toxic Substances and Disease Registry (ATSDR). *Toxicological Profile of Carbon Monoxide* (2012). Available at: https://www.atsdr.cdc.gov/ToxProfiles/tp201.pdf. Accessed April 1,2023.

Aronow, W. S., Cassidy, J., Vangrow, J. S., March, H., Kern, J. C., Goldsmith, J. R., Khemka, M., Pagano, J., & Vawter, M. (1974). Effect of cigarette smoking and breathing carbon monoxide on cardiovascular hemodynamics in anginal patients. *Circulation*, *50*(2), 340–347. https://doi.org/10.1161/01.cir.50.2.340

Azarov, I., Wang, L., Rose, J. J., Xu, Q., Huang, X. N., Belanger, A., Wang, Y., Guo, L., Liu, C., Ucer, K. B., McTiernan, C. F., O'Donnell, C. P., Shiva, S., Tejero, J., Kim-Shapiro, D. B., & Gladwin, M. T. (2016). Five-coordinate H64Q neuroglobin as a ligand-trap antidote for carbon monoxide poisoning. *Science translational medicine*, *8*(368), 368ra173. https://doi.org/10.1126/scitranslmed.aah6571

Bernard, C. (1857). Leçons sur les effets des substances toxiques et médicamenteuses [*Lessons on the effects of toxic and drug substances*]. JB Baillière.

Blumenthal I. (2001). Carbon monoxide poisoning. *Journal of the Royal Society of Medicine*, *94*(6), 270–272. https://doi.org/10.1177/014107680109400604

Boehning, D., Moon, C., Sharma, S., Hurt, K. J., Hester, L. D., Ronnett, G. V., Shugar, D., & Snyder, S. H. (2003). Carbon monoxide neurotransmission activated by CK2 phosphorylation of heme oxygenase-2. *Neuron, 40*(1), 129–137. https://doi.org/10.1016/s0896-6273(03)00596-8

Borras, L., Constant, E., De Timary, P., Huguelet, P., & Khazaal, Y. (2009). Intoxication au monoxyde de carbone: quelles séquelles neuropsychiatriques? À propos d'un cas clinique et revue de la littérature. [Long-term psychiatric consequences of carbon monoxide poisoning: A case report and literature review] *La Revue de médecine interne*, *30*(1), 43-48. https://doi.org/10.1016/j.revmed.2008.04.014

Brown, S. D., & Piantadosi, C. A. (1990). In vivo binding of carbon monoxide to cytochrome c oxidase in rat brain. *Journal of applied physiology (Bethesda, Md.: 1985)*, *68*(2), 604–610. https://doi.org/10.1152/jappl.1990.68.2.604

Brown, S. D., & Piantadosi, C. A. (1992). Recovery of energy metabolism in rat brain after carbon monoxide hypoxia. *The Journal of clinical investigation, 89*(2), 666–672. https://doi.org/10.1172/JCI115633

Buboltz, J. B., & Robins, M. (2023). Hyperbaric Treatment Of Carbon Monoxide Toxicity. In *StatPearls*. StatPearls Publishing.

Buckley, N. A., Juurlink, D. N., Isbister, G., Bennett, M. H., & Lavonas, E. J. (2011). Hyperbaric oxygen for carbon monoxide poisoning. *Cochrane database of systematic reviews*, (4). https://doi.org/10.1002/14651858.CD002041.pub3

Cardellach F, Miro O, Casademont J. (2003 Feb). Hyperbaric oxygen for acute carbon monoxide poisoning. *N Engl J Med.* 6;348(6):557-560; author reply 557-560.

Chamberland, D. L., Wilson, B. D., & Weaver, L. K. (2004). Transient cardiac dysfunction in acute carbon monoxide poisoning. *The American journal of medicine*, *117*(8), 623–625. https://doi.org/10.1016/j.amjmed.2004.04.025

Chenoweth, J. A., Albertson, T. E., & Greer, M. R. (2021). Carbon monoxide poisoning. *Critical care clinics*, *37*(3), 657-672. https://doi.org/10.1016/j.ccc.2021.03.010

Choi, S. (1983). Delayed neurologic sequelae in carbon monoxide intoxication. *Archives of Neurology*, *40*(7), 433-435. https://doi.org/10.1001/archneur.1983.04050070063016

Choi, I. S. (2001). Carbon monoxide poisoning: systemic manifestations and complications. *Journal of Korean medical science*, *16*(3), 253-261. https://doi.org/10.3346/jkms.2001.16.3.253

Choi, A. M., & Otterbein, L. E. (2002). Emerging role of carbon monoxide in physiologic and pathophysiologic states. *Antioxidants and Redox Signaling*, *4*(2), 227-228. https://doi.org/10.1089/15230860275366271

Chu, K., Jung, K. H., Kim, H. J., Jeong, S. W., Kang, D. W., & Roh, J. K. (2004). Diffusion-weighted MRI and 99mTc-HMPAO SPECT in delayed relapsing type of carbon monoxide poisoning: evidence of delayed cytotoxic edema. *European neurology*, *51*(2), 98–103. https://doi.org/10.1159/000076536

Churchill-Davidson, I. (1966). Therapeutic uses of hyperbaric oxygen. *Annals of the Royal College of Surgeons of England*, *39*(3), 164.

Clemens, J. B. (1926). Carbon monoxide poisoning. *Bulletin of the New York Academy of Medicine*, *2*(8), 402.

Coburn R. F. (1970). Endogenous carbon monoxide production. *The New England journal of medicine*, *282*(4), 207–209. https://doi.org/10.1056/NEJM197001222820407

Coburn, R. F., & Mayers, L. B. (1971). Myoglobin O2 tension determined from measurement of carboxymyoglobin in skeletal muscle. *American Journal of Physiology-Legacy Content*, *220*(1), 66-74. https://doi.org/10.1152/ajplegacy.1971.220.1.66

Cooper, A. G. (1966). Carbon Monoxide, A Bibliography with Abstracts. Superintendent of Documents, U.S. Government Printing Office, Washington, D.C.

Danesh-Sani, S. A., Shariati-Sarabi, Z., & Feiz, M. R. (2012). Comprehensive review of hyperbaric oxygen therapy. *The Journal of craniofacial surgery*, *23*(5), e483–e491. https://doi.org/10.1097/SCS.0b013e3182668777

Dillehay, T. D., Ocampo, C., Saavedra, J., Sawakuchi, A. O., Vega, R. M., Pino, M., Collins, M. B., Scott Cummings, L., Arregui, I., Villagran, X. S., Hartmann, G. A., Mella, M., González, A., & Dix, G. (2015). New archaeological evidence for an early human presence at Monte Verde, Chile. *PloS one*, *10*(11), e0141923. https://doi.org/10.1371/journal.pone.0141923

Dorey, A., Scheerlinck, P., Nguyen, H., & Albertson, T. (2020). Acute and Chronic Carbon Monoxide Toxicity from Tobacco Smoking. *Military medicine*, *185*(1-2), e61–e67. https://doi.org/10.1093/milmed/usz280

Doyle, K. P., Simon, R. P., & Stenzel-Poore, M. P. (2008). Mechanisms of ischemic brain damage. *Neuropharmacology*, *55*(3), 310–318. https://doi.org/10.1016/j.neuropharm.2008.01.005

Drinker, Cecil K. (1938). Carbon Monoxide Asphyxia, Founders of the Harvard School of Public Health,: With biographical notes, 1909-1946, Family Portrait.

Dziewierz, A., Ciszowski, K., Gawlikowski, T., Rakowski, T., Kleczyński, P., Surdacki, A., & Dudek, D. (2013). Primary angioplasty in patient with ST-segment elevation myocardial infarction in the setting of intentional carbon monoxide poisoning. *The Journal of emergency medicine*, *45*(6), 831–834. https://doi.org/10.1016/j.jemermed.2013.05.061

Elies, J., Dallas, M. L., Boyle, J. P., Scragg, J. L., Duke, A., Steele, D. S., & Peers, C. (2014). Inhibition of the cardiac Na^+ channel Nav1.5 by carbon monoxide. *The Journal of biological chemistry*, *289*(23), 16421–16429. https://doi.org/10.1074/jbc.M114.569996

Ernst, A., & Zibrak, J. D. (1998). Carbon monoxide poisoning. *The New England journal of medicine*, *339*(22), 1603–1608. https://doi.org/10.1056/NEJM199811263392206

Friedman, P., Guo, X. M., Stiller, R. J., & Laifer, S. A. (2015). Carbon monoxide exposure during pregnancy. *Obstetrical & Gynecological Survey*, *70*(11), 705-712. https://doi.org/10.1097/OGX.0000000000000238

Gale, S. D., Hopkins, R. O., Weaver, L. K., Bigler, E. D., Booth, E. J., & Blatter, D. D. (1999). MRI, quantitative MRI, SPECT, and neuropsychological findings following carbon monoxide poisoning. *Brain injury*, *13*(4), 229–243. https://doi.org/10.1080/026990599121601

Garg, J., Krishnamoorthy, P., Palaniswamy, C., Khera, S., Ahmad, H., Jain, D., Aronow, W. S., & Frishman, W. H. (2018). Cardiovascular Abnormalities in Carbon Monoxide Poisoning. *American journal of therapeutics*, *25*(3), e339–e348. https://doi.org/10.1097/MJT.0000000000000016

Garland, H., & Pearce, J. (1967). Neurological complications of carbon monoxide poisoning. *The Quarterly journal of medicine*, *36*(144), 445–455.

Geocadin, R. G., Koenig, M. A., Jia, X., Stevens, R. D., & Peberdy, M. A. (2008). Management of brain injury after resuscitation from cardiac arrest. *Neurologic clinics*, *26*(2), 487–ix. https://doi.org/10.1016/j.ncl.2008.03.015

Gnaiger, E., Lassnig, B., Kuznetsov, A., Rieger, G., & Margreiter, R. (1998). Mitochondrial oxygen affinity, respiratory flux control and excess capacity of cytochrome c oxidase. *The Journal of experimental biology*, *201*(Pt 8), 1129–1139. https://doi.org/10.1242/jeb.201.8.1129

Goldbaum, L. R., Ramirez, R. G., & Absalon, K. B. (1975). What is the mechanism of carbon monoxide toxicity?. *Aviation, space, and environmental medicine*, *46*(10), 1289-1291.

Goldbaum, L. R., Orellano, T., & Dergal, E. (1976). Mechanism of the toxic action of carbon monoxide. *Annals of clinical and laboratory science*, *6*(4), 372–376.

Goren-Inbar, N., Alperson, N., Kislev, M. E., Simchoni, O., Melamed, Y., Ben-Nun, A., & Werker, E. (2004). Evidence of hominin control of fire at Gesher Benot Yaaqov, Israel. *Science*, *304*(5671), 725-727. https://doi.org/10.1126/science.1095443

Gorman, D. F., Clayton, D., Gilligan, J. E., & Webb, R. K. (1992). A longitudinal study of 100 consecutive admissions for carbon monoxide poisoning to the Royal Adelaide Hospital. *Anaesthesia and intensive care*, *20*(3), 311–316. https://doi.org/10.1177/0310057X9202000306

Gorman, D., Drewry, A., Huang, Y. L., & Sames, C. (2003). The clinical toxicology of carbon monoxide. *Toxicology*, *187*(1), 25–38. https://doi.org/10.1016/s0300-483x(03)00005-2

Grace, A. M. (2014). *Carbon monoxide exposure to emergency medical services personnel and firefighters* (Doctoral dissertation). University of Central Missouri Warrensburg, Missouri.

Grieb, G., Simons, D., Schmitz, L., Piatkowski, A., Grottke, O., & Pallua, N. (2011). Glasgow Coma Scale and laboratory markers are superior to COHb in predicting CO intoxication severity. *Burns : journal of the International Society for Burn Injuries*, *37*(4), 610–615. https://doi.org/10.1016/j.burns.2010.03.007

Gürlek Yüksel E, Taşkin EO, Yilmaz Ovali G, Karaçam M, Esen Danaci A. Olgu Sunumu: Case report: kleptomania and other psychiatric symptoms after carbon monoxide intoxication. *Turk Psikiyatri Derg* 2007;18:80-86.

Haldane, J. (1895). The relation of the action of carbonic oxide to oxygen tension. *The Journal of Physiology*, *18*(3), 201. https://doi.org/10.1113/jphysiol.1895.sp000562

Haldane J. (1895). The Action of Carbonic Oxide on Man. *The Journal of physiology*, *18*(5-6), 430–462. https://doi.org/10.1113/jphysiol.1895.sp000578

Hampson N. B. (1998). Pulse oximetry in severe carbon monoxide poisoning. *Chest*, *114*(4), 1036–1041. https://doi.org/10.1378/chest.114.4.1036

Hampson, N. B., & Weaver, L. K. (2007). Carbon monoxide poisoning: a new incidence for an old disease. *Undersea & hyperbaric medicine : journal of the Undersea and Hyperbaric Medical Society, Inc*, *34*(3), 163–168.

Hampson, N. B., Piantadosi, C. A., Thom, S. R., & Weaver, L. K. (2012). Practice recommendations in the diagnosis, management, and prevention of carbon monoxide poisoning. *American journal of respiratory and critical care medicine*, *186*(11), 1095–1101. https://doi.org/10.1164/rccm.201207-1284CI

Hardy, K. R., & Thom, S. R. (1994). Pathophysiology and treatment of carbon monoxide poisoning. *Journal of toxicology. Clinical toxicology*, *32*(6), 613–629. https://doi.org/10.3109/15563659409017973

Henry, C. R., Satran, D., Lindgren, B., Adkinson, C., Nicholson, C. I., & Henry, T. D. (2006). Myocardial injury and long-term mortality following moderate to severe carbon monoxide poisoning. *JAMA*, *295*(4), 398–402. https://doi.org/10.1001/jama.295.4.398

Hill, E. P., Hill, J. R., Power, G. G., & Longo, L. D. (1977). Carbon monoxide exchanges between the human fetus and mother: a mathematical model. *American Journal of Physiology-Heart and Circulatory Physiology*, *232*(3), H311-H323. https://doi.org/10.1152/ajpheart.1977.232.3.H311

Hirayama, A., Noronha-Dutra, A. A., Gordge, M. P., Neild, G. H., & Hothersall, J. S. (1999). S-nitrosothiols are stored by platelets and released during platelet–neutrophil interactions. *Nitric Oxide*, *3*(2), 95-104. https://doi.org/10.1006/niox.1999.0208

Hopper, C. P., Zambrana, P. N., Goebel, U., & Wollborn, J. (2021). A brief history of carbon monoxide and its therapeutic origins. *Nitric oxide: biology and chemistry*, *111-112*, 45–63. https://doi.org/10.1016/j.niox.2021.04.001

Houston, G. W. (1989). *The state of the art: current work in the technology of Ancient Rome.*

Jain, K. K. (2017). Carbon Monoxide and Other Tissue Poisons. In Jain KK (ed.) *Textbook of Hyperbaric Medicine.* (6th ed., pp. 131-154) Basel: Springer International Publishing. https://doi.org/10.1007/978-3-319-47140-2_13

Janík, M., Ublová, M., Kučerová, Š., & Hejna, P. (2017). Carbon monoxide-related fatalities: A 60-year single institution experience. *Journal of forensic and legal medicine*, *48*, 23–29. https://doi.org/10.1016/j.jflm.2017.04.002

Jasper, B. W., Hopkins, R. O., Van Duker, H., & Weaver, L. K. (2005). Affective outcome following carbon monoxide poisoning: a prospective longitudinal study. *Cognitive and behavioral neurology*, *18*(2), 127-134. https://doi.org/10.1097/01.wnn.0000160820.07836.cf

Kalay, N., Ozdogru, I., Cetinkaya, Y., Eryol, N. K., Dogan, A., Gul, I., Inanc, T., Ikizceli, I., Oguzhan, A., & Abaci, A. (2007). Cardiovascular effects of carbon monoxide poisoning. *The American journal of cardiology*, *99*(3), 322–324. https://doi.org/10.1016/j.amjcard.2006.08.030

Kavak, N., Doğan, B., Sultanoğlu, H., Kavak, R. P., & Özdemir, M. (2020). Clinical and Magnetic Resonance Imaging Findings of Patients with Acute Carbon Monoxide Poisoning. *Konuralp Medical Journal*, *12*(3), 443-450. https://doi.org/10.18521/ktd.735274

Keith, W. (2000). Van Meter. *Carbon monoxide Poisoning. Emergency Medicine A Comprehensive Study Guide*, New York: McGraw-Hill, 1302-06.

Kim, J. H., Chang, K. H., Song, I. C., Kim, K. H., Kwon, B. J., Kim, H. C., Kim, J. H., & Han, M. H. (2003). Delayed encephalopathy of acute carbon monoxide intoxication: diffusivity of cerebral white matter lesions. *AJNR. American journal of neuroradiology*, *24*(8), 1592–1597.

Kim, I., Xu, W., & Reed, J. C. (2008). Cell death and endoplasmic reticulum stress: disease relevance and therapeutic opportunities. *Nature reviews. Drug discovery*, *7*(12), 1013–1030. https://doi.org/10.1038/nrd2755

Kinoshita, T., Sugihara, S., Matsusue, E., Fujii, S., Ametani, M., & Ogawa, T. (2005). Pallidoreticular damage in acute carbon monoxide poisoning: diffusion-weighted MR imaging findings. *AJNR. American journal of neuroradiology*, *26*(7), 1845–1848.

Klees, M., Heremans, M., & Dougan, S. (1985). Psychological sequelae to carbon monoxide intoxication in the child. *Science of the total environment*, *44*(2), 165-176. https://doi.org/10.1016/0048-9697(85)90120-2

Ku, B. D., Shin, H. Y., Kim, E. J., Park, K. C., Seo, S. W., & Na, D. L. (2006). Secondary mania in a patient with delayed anoxic encephalopathy after carbon monoxide intoxication. *Journal of clinical neuroscience*, *13*(8), 860-862. https://doi.org/10.1016/j.jocn.2005.10.013

Kuroda, H., Fujihara, K., Kushimoto, S., & Aoki, M. (2015). Novel clinical grading of delayed neurologic sequelae after carbon monoxide poisoning and factors associated with outcome. *Neurotoxicology*, *48*, 35–43. https://doi.org/10.1016/j.neuro.2015.03.002

Kurt, F., Bektas, Ö., Kalkan, G., Öncel, M. Y., Yakut, H. I., & Kocabas, C. N. (2013). Does age affect presenting symptoms in children with carbon monoxide poisoning?. *Pediatric emergency care*, *29*(8), 916-921. https://doi.org/10.1097/PEC.0b013e31829ec22b

Kwon, O. Y., Chung, S. P., Ha, Y. R., Yoo, I. S., & Kim, S. W. (2004). Delayed postanoxic encephalopathy after carbon monoxide poisoning. *Emergency Medicine Journal*, *21*(2), 250-251. https://doi.org/10.1136/emj.2002.002014

Levantino, M., Lemke, H. T., Schirò, G., Glownia, M., Cupane, A., & Cammarata, M. (2015). Observing heme doming in myoglobin with femtosecond X-ray absorption spectroscopy. *Structural dynamics (Melville, N.Y.)*, *2*(4), 041713. https://doi.org/10.1063/1.4921907

Lee, F. Y., Chen, W. K., Lin, C. L., & Kao, C. H. (2015). Carbon monoxide poisoning and subsequent cardiovascular disease risk: a nationwide population-based cohort study. *Medicine*, *94*(10), e624. https://doi.org/10.1097/MD.0000000000000624

Li, L., Hsu, A., & Moore, P. K. (2009). Actions and interactions of nitric oxide, carbon monoxide and hydrogen sulphide in the cardiovascular system and in inflammation--a tale of three gases! *Pharmacology & therapeutics*, *123*(3), 386–400. https://doi.org/10.1016/j.pharmthera.2009.05.005

Lo, C. P., Chen, S. Y., Lee, K. W., Chen, W. L., Chen, C. Y., Hsueh, C. J., & Huang, G. S. (2007). Brain injury after acute carbon monoxide poisoning: early and late complications. *AJR. American journal of roentgenology*, *189*(4), W205–W211. https://doi.org/10.2214/AJR.07.2425

Lo Iacono, L., Boczkowski, J., Zini, R., Salouage, I., Berdeaux, A., Motterlini, R., & Morin, D. (2011). A carbon monoxide-releasing molecule (CORM-3) uncouples mitochondrial respiration and modulates the production of reactive oxygen species. *Free radical biology & medicine*, *50*(11), 1556–1564. https://doi.org/10.1016/j.freeradbiomed.2011.02.033

Mannaioni, P. F., Vannacci, A., & Masini, E. (2006). Carbon monoxide: the bad and the good side of the coin, from neuronal death to anti-inflammatory activity. *Inflammation research: official journal of the European Histamine Research Society 55*(7), 261–273. https://doi.org/10.1007/s00011-006-0084-y

Megas, I. F., Beier, J. P., & Grieb, G. (2021). The History of Carbon Monoxide Intoxication. *Medicina (Kaunas, Lithuania)*, *57*(5), 400. https://doi.org/10.3390/medicina57050400

Mimura, K., Harada, M., Sumiyoshi, S., Tohya, G., Takagi, M., Fujita, E., Takata, A., & Tatetsu, S. (1999). *Seishin shinkeigaku zasshi = Psychiatria et neurologia Japonica*, *101*(7), 592–618.

Min, S. K. (1986). A brain syndrome associated with delayed neuropsychiatric sequelae following acute carbon monoxide intoxication. *Acta Psychiatrica Scandinavica*, *73*(1), 80-86. https://doi.org/10.1111/j.1600-0447.1986.tb02671.x

Murata, T., Kimura, H., Kado, H., Omori, M., Onizuka, J., Takahashi, T., Itoh, H., & Wada, Y. (2001). Neuronal damage in the interval form of CO poisoning determined by serial diffusion weighted magnetic resonance imaging plus 1H-magnetic resonance spectroscopy. *Journal of neurology, neurosurgery, and psychiatry*, *71*(2), 250–253. https://doi.org/10.1136/jnnp.71.2.250

O'Donnell, P., Buxton, P. J., Pitkin, A., & Jarvis, L. J. (2000). The magnetic resonance imaging appearances of the brain in acute carbon monoxide poisoning. *Clinical radiology*, *55*(4), 273–280. https://doi.org/10.1053/crad.1999.0369

Ozyurt, A., Karpuz, D., Yucel, A., Tosun, M. D., Kibar, A. E., & Hallioglu, O. (2017). Effects of Acute Carbon Monoxide Poisoning on ECG and Echocardiographic Parameters in Children. *Cardiovascular toxicology*, *17*(3), 326–334. https://doi.org/10.1007/s12012-016-9389-4

Palaniswamy, C., Aronow, W. S., Sugunaraj, J. P., Kang, J. J., Kar, K., & Kalra, A. (2013). Brugada electrocardiographic pattern in carbon monoxide poisoning. *Archives of medical science: AMS*, *9*(2), 377–380. https://doi.org/10.5114/aoms.2013.34538

Pankow, D. (2000). History of carbon monoxide toxicology. *Carbon Monoxide Toxicology*, 1-19.

Parkinson, R. B., Hopkins, R. O., Cleavinger, H. B., Weaver, L. K., Victoroff, J., Foley, J. F., & Bigler, E. D. (2002). White matter hyperintensities and neuropsychological outcome following carbon monoxide poisoning. *Neurology*, *58*(10), 1525–1532. https://doi.org/10.1212/wnl.58.10.1525

Prockop L. D. (2005). Carbon monoxide brain toxicity: clinical, magnetic resonance imaging, magnetic resonance spectroscopy, and neuropsychological effects in 9 people. *Journal of neuroimaging: official journal of the American Society of Neuroimaging*, *15*(2), 144–149. https://doi.org/10.1177/1051228404273819

Penney, D. G. (2008). Chronic carbon monoxide poisoning: a case series. In *Carbon Monoxide Poisoning* (pp. 577-594). CRC Press.

Piantadosi, C. A., Zhang, J., Levin, E. D., Folz, R. J., & Schmechel, D. E. (1997). Apoptosis and delayed neuronal damage after carbon monoxide poisoning in the rat. *Experimental neurology*, *147*(1), 103–114. https://doi.org/10.1006/exnr.1997.6584

Piantadosi C. A. (2002). Biological chemistry of carbon monoxide. *Antioxidants & redox signaling*, *4*(2), 259–270. https://doi.org/10.1089/15230860275366316

Raphael, J. C., Elkharrat, D., Jars-Guincestre, M. C., Chastang, C., Vercken, J. B., Chasles, V., & Gajdos, P. (1989). Trial of normobaric and hyperbaric oxygen for acute carbon monoxide intoxication. *The Lancet*, *334*(8660), 414-419. https://doi.org/10.1016/s0140-6736(89)90592-8

Raub, J. A., Mathieu-Nolf, M., Hampson, N. B., & Thom, S. R. (2000). Carbon monoxide poisoning a public health perspective. *Toxicology*, *145*(1), 1-14. https://doi.org/10.1016/s0300-483x(99)00217-6

Robbins, R. C., Cavanagh, L. A., Salas, L. J., & Robinson, E. (1973). Analysis of ancient atmospheres. *Journal of Geophysical Research*, *78*(24), 5341-5344. https://doi.org/10.1029/JC078i024p05341

Roughton, F. J. W., & Darling, R. C. (1944). The effect of carbon monoxide on the oxyhemoglobin dissociation curve. *American Journal of Physiology-Legacy Content*, *141*(1), 17-31. https://doi.org/10.1152/ajplegacy.1944.141.1.17

Rose, J. J., Xu, Q., Bachman, T. N., Hu, J., Azarov, I., Huang, X. N., Wang L., Corey, C.G., Guimarães, D., Mc Tiernan, C.F., O'Donnel, C.P., & Gladwin, M. T. (2018). Reversal of Carbon Monoxide (CO) Mediated Mitochondrial Dysfunction and Cardiovascular Collapse with Molecularly Engineered Neuroglobin-Based CO Scavenger. In *A70. Environmental Stressors, Gases, And Host Responses* (pp. A2277-A2277). American Thoracic Society.

Sayers, R. R., & Davenport, S. J. (1937). *Review of Carbon Monoxide Poisoning: 1936*. US Government Printing Office.

Schofield, R. (2005). Joseph Priestley, natural philosopher. *Bull. Hist. Chem*, *30*(2), 57-62. https://doi.org/10.1179/amb.1967.14.1.1

Sinkovič, A., Smolle-Juettner, F. M., Krunic, B., & Marinšekz, M. (2006). Severe carbon monoxide poisoning treated by hyperbaric oxygen therapy—A case report. *Inhalation toxicology*, *18*(3), 211-214. https://doi.org/10.1080/08958370500434289

Schallner, N., & Otterbein, L. E. (2015). Friend or foe? Carbon monoxide and the mitochondria. *Frontiers in Physiology*, *6*, 17. https://doi.org/10.3389/fphys.2015.00017

Shprecher, D., & Mehta, L. (2010). The syndrome of delayed post-hypoxic leukoencephalopathy. *NeuroRehabilitation*, *26*(1), 65–72. https://doi.org/10.3233/NRE-2010-0536

Shiva, S., Huang, Z., Grubina, R., Sun, J., Ringwood, L. A., MacArthur, P. H., Xu, X., Murphy, E., Darley-Usmar, V. M., & Gladwin, M. T. (2007). Deoxymyoglobin is a nitrite reductase that generates nitric oxide and regulates mitochondrial respiration. *Circulation research*, *100*(5), 654–661. https://doi.org/10.1161/01.RES.0000260171.52224.6b

Simonsen, C., Magnusdottir, S. O., Andreasen, J. J., Rohde, M. C., & Kjærgaard, B. (2018). ECMO improves survival following cardiogenic shock due to carbon monoxide poisoning - an experimental porcine model. *Scandinavian journal of trauma, resuscitation and emergency medicine*, *26*(1), 103. https://doi.org/10.1186/s13049-018-0570-6

Smithline, H. A., Ward, K. R., Chiulli, D. A., Blake, H. C., & Rivers, E. P. (2003). Whole body oxygen consumption and critical oxygen delivery in response to prolonged and severe carbon monoxide poisoning. *Resuscitation*, *56*(1), 97–104. https://doi.org/10.1016/s0300-9572(02)00272-1

Starkstein, S. E., Berthier, M. L., & Leiguarda, R. (1990). Psychic akinesia following bilateral pallidal lesions. *The International Journal of Psychiatry in Medicine*, *19*(2), 155-164. https://doi.org/10.2190/ae1q-qy7b-lu2f-gjhf

Stoller, K. P. (2007). Hyperbaric oxygen and carbon monoxide poisoning: a critical review. *Neurological Research*, *29*(2), 146-155. https://doi.org/10.1179/016164107X181770

Suliman, H. B., Carraway, M. S., Tatro, L. G., & Piantadosi, C. A. (2007). A new activating role for CO in cardiac mitochondrial biogenesis. *Journal of cell science*, *120*(Pt 2), 299–308. https://doi.org/10.1242/jcs.03318

Sykes, O. T., & Walker, E. (2016). The neurotoxicology of carbon monoxide–Historical perspective and review. *Cortex*, *74*, 440-448. https://doi.org/10.1016/j.cortex.2015.07.033

Şenoğlu, N., Öksüz, H., Zencirci, B., Ezberci, M., & Tuncer, D. (2005). Parkinsonism after carbon monoxide intoxication: Case Report. *Journal of neurological sciences (Turkish)*, *22*(3), 292-296.

Temrel, T. A., & Bilge, S. (2020). Myocardial Repolarization Parameters and Neutrophil-to-Lymphocyte Ratio are Associated with Cardiotoxicity in Carbon Monoxide Poisoning. *Cardiovascular toxicology*, *20*(2), 190–196. https://doi.org/10.1007/s12012-019-09560-7

Thom, S. R., Ohnishi, S. T., & Ischiropoulos, H. (1994). Nitric oxide released by platelets inhibits neutrophil B2 integrin function following acute carbon monoxide poisoning. *Toxicology and applied pharmacology*, *128*(1), 105–110. https://doi.org/10.1006/taap.1994.1186

Thom, S. R., Bhopale, V. M., Fisher, D., Zhang, J., & Gimotty, P. (2004). Delayed neuropathology after carbon monoxide poisoning is immune-mediated. *Proceedings of the National Academy of Sciences of the United States of America*, *101*(37), 13660–13665. https://doi.org/10.1073/pnas.0405642101

Thom, S. R., Bhopale, V. M., & Fisher, D. (2006). Hyperbaric oxygen reduces delayed immune-mediated neuropathology in experimental carbon monoxide toxicity. *Toxicology and applied pharmacology*, *213*(2), 152–159. https://doi.org/10.1016/j.taap.2005.10.006

Thom, S. R., Bhopale, V. M., Han, S. T., Clark, J. M., & Hardy, K. R. (2006). Intravascular neutrophil activation due to carbon monoxide poisoning. *American journal of respiratory and critical care medicine*, *174*(11), 1239–1248. https://doi.org/10.1164/rccm.200604-557OC

Townsend, C. L., & Maynard, R. L. (2002). Effects on health of prolonged exposure to low concentrations of carbon monoxide. *Occupational and environmental medicine*, *59*(10), 708–711. https://doi.org/10.1136/oem.59.10.708

Turner, M., Hamilton-Farrell, M. R., & Clark, R. J. (1999). Carbon monoxide poisoning: an update. *Journal of accident & emergency medicine*, *16*(2), 92–96. https://doi.org/10.1136/emj.16.2.92

Vreman, H. J., Wong, R. J., & Stevenson, D. K. (2000). Carbon monoxide in breath, blood, and other tissues. *Carbon monoxide toxicity*, *1*, 19-60.

Wald, G., & Allen, D. W. (1957). The equilibrium between cytochrome oxidase and carbon monoxide. *The Journal of general physiology*, *40*(4), 593–608. https://doi.org/10.1085/jgp.40.4.593

Watt, S., Prado, C. E., & Crowe, S. F. (2018). Immediate and delayed neuropsychological effects of carbon monoxide poisoning: a meta-analysis. *Journal of the International Neuropsychological Society*, *24*(4), 405-415. https://doi.org/10.1017/S1355617717001035

Weaver, L. K., Howe, S., Hopkins, R., & Chan, K. J. (2000). Carboxyhemoglobin half-life in carbon monoxide-poisoned patients treated with 100% oxygen at atmospheric pressure. *Chest*, *117*(3), 801-808. https://doi.org/10.1378/chest.117.3.801

Weaver, L. K., Valentine, K. J., & Hopkins, R. O. (2007). Carbon monoxide poisoning: risk factors for cognitive sequelae and the role of hyperbaric oxygen. *American journal of respiratory and critical care medicine*, *176*(5), 491-497. https://doi.org/10.1164/rccm.200701-026OC

Weaver, L. K., Hopkins, R. O., Churchill, S. K., & Deru, K. (2008). Neurological outcomes 6 years after acute carbon monoxide poisoning. *Undersea Hyperb Med*, *35*(4), 241-323.

Weaver, L. K. (2009). Carbon monoxide poisoning. *New England Journal of Medicine*, *360*(12), 1217-1225. https://doi.org/10.1056/NEJMcp0808891

Weaver, L. K., Churchill, S. K., Deru, K., & Cooney, D. (2013). False positive rate of carbon monoxide saturation by pulse oximetry of emergency department patients. *Respiratory care*, *58*(2), 232–240. https://doi.org/10.4187/respcare.01744

Weaver, L. K., Orrison, W. W., Deru, K., & McIntosh, J. (2015). Brain imaging abnormalities in carbon monoxide-poisoned patients with ongoing symptoms at least 6 months after poisoning. *Undersea Hyperb Med. Soc*, *100*, 39.

Weaver L. K. (2020). Carbon monoxide poisoning. *Undersea & hyperbaric medicine: journal of the Undersea and Hyperbaric Medical Society, Inc*, *47*(1), 151–169. https://doi.org/10.22462/01.03.2020.17

Werner, B., Bäck, W., Åkerblom, H., & Barr, F. O. (1985). Two cases of acute carbon monoxide poisoning with delayed neurological sequelae after a "free" interval. *Journal of Toxicology: Clinical Toxicology*, *23*(4-6), 249-265. https://doi.org/10.3109/15563658508990633

Wilbur, S., Williams, M., Williams, R., Scinicariello, F., Klotzbach, J. M., Diamond, G. L., & Citra, M. (2012). *Toxicological Profile for Carbon Monoxide*. Agency for Toxic Substances and Disease Registry (US).

Wood, P. S., & Murray, G. B. (1999). Neuropsychiatric Aspects of Carbon Monoxide Poisoning: A Review and Single Case Report Suggesting a Role for Amphetamines. *Annals of clinical psychiatry*, *11*(1), 21-27. https://doi.org/10.1023/a:1022856015103

World Health Organization. (2010). *WHO guidelines for indoor air quality: selected pollutants*. World Health Organization. Regional Office for Europe.

Vanden Hoek, T. L., Morrison, L. J., Shuster, M., Donnino, M., Sinz, E., Lavonas, E. J., Jeejeebhoy, F. M., & Gabrielli, A. (2010). Part 12: cardiac arrest in special situations: 2010 American Heart Association Guidelines for Cardiopulmonary Resuscitation and Emergency Cardiovascular Care. *Circulation*, *122*(18 Suppl 3), S829–S861. https://doi.org/10.1161/CIRCULATIONAHA.110.971069

Yarar, C., Yakut, A., Akin, A., Yildiz, B., & Dinleyici, E. C. (2008). Analysis of the features of acute carbon monoxide poisoning and hyperbaric oxygen therapy in children. *The Turkish Journal of Pediatrics*, *50*(3), 235.

Yet, S. F., Tian, R., Layne, M. D., Wang, Z. Y., Maemura, K., Solovyeva, M., Ith, B., Melo, L. G., Zhang, L., Ingwall, J. S., Dzau, V. J., Lee, M. E., & Perrella, M. A. (2001). Cardiac-specific expression of heme oxygenase-1 protects against ischemia and reperfusion injury in transgenic mice. *Circulation research*, *89*(2), 168–173. https://doi.org/10.1161/hh1401.093314

Chapter 6

Diagnostic Methods for Carbon Monoxide Poisoning

Murat Daş*, MD
Okhan Akdur, MD
and Gökhan Akdur, MD
Department of Emergency Medicine, Çanakkale Onsekiz Mart University,
Çanakkale, Turkey

Abstract

The diagnosis of Carbon Monoxide (CO) poisoning consists of three elements: symptoms associated with carbon monoxide poisoning, exposure to CO, and an increase in COHb levels. The most common symptoms in people exposed to CO are non-specific complaints such as headache, nausea, vomiting, and dizziness. The most common environments that produce CO are counted as stoves or ovens using wood or coal as fuel, heaters using propane fuel, and building or forest fires. The COHb level is performed most accurately by co-oximetry blood gas analysis devices with samples obtained from arterial or venous blood samples. There is no correlation between Dechb level and clinical status. In victims with normal COHb levels, the diagnosis should be managed according to the complaints of exposure to CO and admission.

Keywords: carbon monoxide poisoning, co-oximetry, carboxyhemoglobin level, pulse co-oximetry

---

* Corresponding Author's Email: muratdas58@gmail.com.

In: Carbon Monoxide Poisoning
Editors: Seda Özkan and Afsin Ipekci
ISBN: 979-8-89113-217-7

Introduction

The diagnosis of carbon monoxide (CO) poisoning is largely based on clinical suspicion. History is the first step in uncovering exposure to CO. It is important to know the exogenous sources that may cause CO poisoning to create suspicion of poisoning in clinicians. Fires, geyser, or stove leaks have the potential to create CO poisoning. However, the exhaust fumes of motor vehicles, fuels used in industry, and barbecues can form exogenous CO gas. In the detailed history taken by the clinician, it can be revealed whether there is exposure.

Complaints of patients experiencing CO poisoning may have mild symptoms such as headache, weakness, nausea, and dizziness, or may also manifest themselves with serious conditions such as hypotension, arrhythmia, seizure, coma, and death. This varies depending on the amount of CO exposed and the duration of exposure.

The most accurate diagnostic method in patients with suspected poisoning is to determine the carboxyhemoglobin (COHb) concentration by CO-oximetry. The CO-oximeter measures the concentrations of oxygenated hemoglobin (oxyHb), deoxygenated hemoglobin (deoxyHb or reduced Hb), carboxyhemoglobin (COHb) and methemoglobin (MetHb) as a percentage of the total hemoglobin concentration in a blood sample.

It is not reliable to diagnose CO poisoning by standard pulse oximetry. Because the measurements of COHb wavelengths and oxyhemoglobin wavelengths are very close to each other.

Diagnostic Approaches for Carbon Monoxide Poisoning

There is a clinical trial in the diagnosis of carbon monoxide poisoning, which consists of symptoms associated with carbon monoxide poisoning, exposure to CO, and an increase in COHb levels (Rose et al., 2017).

Symptoms and Clinical Features

The clinic of carbon monoxide poisoning can be confused with many clinical tables that can lead to an incorrect diagnosis. Poisoning victims may complain of flu-like symptoms, such as a simple headache and weakness. In severely affected victims, it is possible to experience cardiac arrest with a level of consciousness changing from confusion to coma or cardiac dysrhythmias. In addition to the personal characteristics of the victims, the intensity of the exposed CO gas and the duration of exposure also play an important role in the formation of these different clinical tables.

A study conducted in the United States (USA) between 2005 and 2018 using data from the national poison information system found that the most common symptoms of Dec poisoning victims were headache (58%), nausea (33%), dizziness (29%), and drowsiness- weakness (14%) (Shin et al., 2023). In a study conducted in the pediatric age group, it was found that the most common symptoms were nausea and vomiting (53.6%), headache (39.5%), dizziness (21.1%), and weakness (20.7%) (Kandis et al., 2009).

In CO poisoning, symptoms may differ depending on the COHb level. In mild poisoning (COHb level 5%-20%), headache, nausea, vomiting, blurred vision, tachycardia, and dizziness may be observed. In moderate intoxication (COHb level 20%-50%); syncope chest pain, shortness of breath, changes in consciousness, and coordination disorders can be detected. In patients with severe or life-threatening COHb levels (COHb level >50%): cardiac dysrhythmias, signs of cardiac ischemia, cerebral infarction, severe metabolic acidosis, seizures, pulmonary edema, coma, and hemodynamic deterioration may be found (Kandis et al., 2009). As a result, for health professionals working in a center where the COHb level cannot be obtained, this information can be used to predict whether it is necessary to transfer the patient to a center where he can be managed at an advanced level.

If there is no accompanying trauma or burn condition in CO poisoning, there may be a change in consciousness that can range from tachypnea, tachycardia, or confusion to coma. Neurological, metabolic, and cardiac findings are at the forefront in severely affected victims. Neurological signs such as seizures, syncope, temporary loss of consciousness, or coma may be observed. Metabolic conditions such as cellular hypoxia or lactic acidosis caused by cytochrome oxidase inhibition can be detected. Cardiac conditions such as acute myocardial ischemia or infarction, ventricular dysrhythmias, and pulmonary edema may be found (Harper & Croft-Baker, 2004).

Exposure to CO Gas

The sources that can produce carbon monoxide gas must be known by clinical and pre-hospital health professionals to reveal the exposure to CO. Especially during the winter months, the most common sources that can produce CO are stoves or ovens that burn wood or coal, heaters using propane fuel, and building or forest fires (Hampson, 2016). Heaters burned using natural gas, methylene chloride used in decking agents, and paint removers can also be considered among the sources that can produce CO gas (Chang et al., 1999). Victims who indicate in the story that they were affected or came into contact with such sources should be evaluated for CO poisoning. It is necessary to look for clues that the victim has been in contact with such resources at the scene by pre-hospital health professionals or that he has been exposed. However, the smell of smoke and signs that may be soot stains or inhalation burns may be an important clue in people who are not able to take an unconscious history.

Determination of COHb Level

The most accurate diagnosis of CO poisoning is to show that the COHb level has exceeded the threshold level that can cause poisoning. For this reason, the most important diagnostic tool used is the blood oximeter blood gas analyzer (Hampson, 2016; Touger et al., 1995). In addition, pulse co-oximetry devices can also measure COHb levels by spectrophotometric method. The detection of CO gas in the air expelled by the respiratory tract can also be considered as another method. However, no information about the use of this method in patients with CO poisoning has been found in a clinical study (Hampson, 2016; Touger et al., 1995).

Co-Oximeter Measurement in a Blood Sample

A co-oximeter device calculates the concentrations of oxyHb, deoxyHb, COHb, and MetHb as a percentage of total hemoglobin in a blood sample by spectrophotometric method. The use of co-oximetry is indicated in cases where hypoxia persists despite oxygen administration in the history of toxin exposure, there is a discrepancy between partial O2 (PaO2) measured in blood gas and oxygen saturation measured by pulse oximetry, and the clinician suspects other Dechemoglobinemia, such as methemoglobinemia or carboxyhemoglobinemia.

Pulse oximetry measures the oxygen saturation of hemoglobin (SaO2) in arterial blood, or the average amount of oxygen bound to each hemoglobin molecule. Blood gas analyzers calculate the oxygen saturation from PO2 and pH parameters measured based on standard oxygen dissociation curves. However, a standard pulse o Decimeter, a non-invasive procedure, does not distinguish between different types of hemoglobin. For this reason, the SaO2 measured by pulse oximetry results in artificially high (Wolf et al., 2017). For example, in the case of methemoglobinemia, pulse oximetry can read 88%, but desaturation can be indicated by co-oxymetry, which records 70% oxyHb and 30% MetHb.

Each of the dishemoglobins has a unique absorption spectrum. The concentration can be calculated by Beer-Lambert's law by measuring the absorption at four specific wavelengths. The reference ranges of the percentage of normal hemoglobin ranges measured by co-oximetry are shown in Table 1. It has been shown in (Mack, 2007). Total hemoglobin levels are age-dependent in children.

Oxygen saturation deficiency is defined as the difference of more than 5% between the saturation calculated from a standard arterial blood gas analyzer and the saturation measured by a co-oximeter. The presence of a deficit in oxygen saturation is compatible with the presence of dishemoglobins.

Correct blood collection techniques are necessary for the proper interpretation of co-oxymetry. Co-oximeter gases require a minimum of 0.3 mL of blood (venous or arterial). Blood should be collected in an airless, heparinized injector, thoroughly mixed, air bubbles should be removed, and placed on ice. Whether the blood sample taken is arterial or venous, the effect on COHb measurement is negligible (Mack, 2007).

Table 1. Reference ranges based on hemoglobin levels (Mack, 2007)

Type of hemoglobin	Reference Range
Oxy-hemoglobin	45%-70%
Deoxy-hemoglobin	0%-5% Arterial 15%-40% venous
CO-hemoglobin	0%-2.5% (in non-smokers) 5%-10% (in smokers)
Methemoglbin	0%-1,5%

Measurement of COHb Level with Pulse Co-Oximeter

The latest technology in hemoglobin measurement is pulse co-oximety devices capable of measuring dishemoglobin such as COHb and MetHb. Although pulse co-oximety and standard pulse oximetry devices have a similar working principle, pulse co-oximety has the ability to measure different wavelengths of dishemoglobins such as COHb (Ruckman, 2012). The standard pulse oximeter does not have the ability to distinguish the wavelengths of oxyHb and COHb. As a result, in carbon monoxide poisoning, oxygen saturation obtained by standard pulse oximetry may be artificially high (Yurtseven et al., 2016).

In a study comparing the co-oximetry measurements made from blood samples with pulse co-oximetry in CO poisoning, it was found that the COHb levels examined by both methods were similar (Hampson, 2012). As a result, it can be used as a screening tool in patients with suspected carbon monoxide poisoning in emergency triage areas. However, patients with high COHb levels measured by pulse co-oximetry should be confirmed with COHb levels of arterial or venous blood samples in a laboratory setting. Because there are a limited number of studies comparing the results obtained by measuring COHb levels by pulse co-oximetry and blood samples in laboratory environment in CO poisoning, more research is needed on this issue.

Interpretation of COHb Level

The level of COHb is not an absolute indicator of clinical severity. When interpreting COHb levels, it is necessary to take into account the time and duration of exposure, the time from exposure to admission, and treatments such as high-current oxygen given on the way (Radford, & Drizd, 1982). It can be argued that there is a serious impact on a victim with a COHb level of 50% or more. A COHb level of 10% in a victim with symptoms a few hours before admission should also be considered CO poisoning.

According to a study of CO poisoning with 163-series of Yurtseven et al., they found that in 49 of the cases (about 30%), they had normal COHb levels (0-5%) at the time of admission (Yurtseven et al., 2016). Therefore, even in the absence of a high COHb level, the diagnosis should still be made with a history of exposure and compatible symptoms and signs.

In fires, cyanide gas can also occur together with CO gas. It has been reported that COHb levels of patients who were treated with hydroxycobalamin during the pre-hospital period were incorrectly high (Livshits et al., 2012; Lee et al., 2007; Pace et al., 2014). However, this information should not deter clinicians from treating CO poisoning.

Other Diagnostic Tests

In all patients with moderate to severe CO poisoning, the heart and central nervous system (CNS), which are highly susceptible to hypoxia, should be examined for involvement. A blood gas evaluation should also be performed to diagnose hypoxia and other metabolic disorders. Investigations of the liver, kidneys, and musculoskeletal system, which are likely to be affected by poisoning, should also be ordered.

Laboratory Investigations

Acute CO poisoning causes electrical, functional, and morphological changes in the heart (Koga et al., 2021). However, there is no specific ECG finding for CO poisoning. Patients may present with a completely normal ECG or an ST elevation myocardial infarction (STEMI) ECG (Cha et al., 2016). ST-T changes indicating myocardial ischemia may be seen. The most common ECG changes are sinus tachycardia, ischemic ST-T changes, and non-specific ST changes (Satran et al., 2005).

Another diagnostic tool for demonstrating cardiac involvement in CO poisoning is ECHO (Park et al., 2016). It should be evaluated especially in patients with chest pain and moderate to severe cardiac involvement. In addition to ECHO findings such as left ventricular systolic dysfunction, global hypokinesia, ejection fraction less than 50% in patients with CO poisoning, and high sensitive troponin levels, some patients showed findings similar to Takotsubo cardiomyopathy (Cha et al., 2016). Therefore, the evaluation of myocardial function is important in patients with moderate to severe intoxication, with a history of cardiac disease, and at risk of cardiac diseases (Wolf et al., 2017).

Cardiac biomarkers are another diagnostic test to be ordered in cardiac involvement due to CO poisoning. Currently, the recommended diagnostic test for this purpose is the high sensitivity troponin T assay to demonstrate myocardial damage (Collet et al., 2021). Increased blood troponin levels can be seen in acute and severe CO poisoning (Abdel Aziz et al., 2021; Coşkun et al., 2019). Troponin-positive results were statistically more common in males, in patients with neuro psychosis and in those with the mortal outcome (Coşkun et al., 2019).

Both COHb levels and metabolic status can be evaluated by blood gas analysis. In CO poisoning, the anaerobic metabolism pathway is activated due to the decrease in oxygenated respiration at the cellular level. The resulting increase in lactate in the blood is reflected in the blood gas as metabolic acidosis. The development of metabolic acidosis is associated with the duration of exposure and severe clinical and neurological sequelae (Kao & Nañagas, 2004). However, elevated blood lactate levels also indicate the severity and prognosis of the disease (Sokal & Kralkowska, 1985).

Severe metabolic acidosis is associated with high short-term mortality in CO-poisoned patients, and if the CO source is a house fire, it is probably due to concomitant cyanide poisoning. This study demonstrated short-term mortality in 30-50% of patients whose initial pH did not exceed 7.20, regardless of COHb levels (Hampson & Hauff, 2008). If arterial blood gas analysis shows a pH of less than 7.20 (Hampson & Hauff 2008) or a plasma lactate level of 10 mmol/L or more (Baud, 2007), cyanide poisoning should also be considered in this severe metabolic acidosis if the source of CO is a house fire. The specific antidote is hydroxocobalamin, which has few side effects in smoke-inhaled individuals (Baud, 2007; Lawson-Smith et al., 2011).

Imaging Methods

Chest X-Ray does not give a specific finding in CO poisoning. However, images such as ground glass, perihilar fullness, and intra-alveolar edema indicate a poor prognosis. In severe poisoning, in the presence of pulmonary symptoms, in patients with signs of hypoxia, and in patients receiving hyperbaric oxygen therapy, a chest X-Ray should be obtained for differential diagnosis or exclusion of other accompanying pathologies (Medscape, 2023).

In severe carbon monoxide poisoning or changes in the state of consciousness that do not improve rapidly despite treatment, screening with computed brain tomography (CT) should be performed. Serial CT scanning should be performed especially in patients with deteriorating mental status (So et al., 1997) Cerebral edema and low-density (hypodense) lesions, most of which are characteristically seen in the basal ganglia, can be seen on CT. The presence of positive findings on CT scans usually predicts neurologic complications. In one study, neurological sequelae were found in all hospitalized patients with CT findings, whereas neurological sequelae were found in only 11% of those without CT findings (Jones et al., 1994).

Magnetic resonance imaging (MRI) provides better images than CT in detecting focal lesions and demyelination in the white matter (Inagaki et al., 1997). The introduction of diffusion-weighted imaging (DWI) and diffusion tensor imaging (DTI) after conventional MRI has allowed for more sensitive detection of damage that may occur in CO poisoning. DTI allows the detection of pathological changes in the early stage of CO toxicity, allowing the prediction of chronic disorders (Beppu, 2014).

Conclusion

The diagnosis of CO poisoning is made with three main elements. The first is the finding of symptoms associated with CO poisoning. The most common symptoms are nonspecific signs such as headache, nausea, vomiting, and dizziness. Neurological, metabolic, and cardiac effects are observed in victims with serious clinics. The second point is the exposure to CO gas. Heaters and fires can produce significant levels of CO gas. Therefore, the exposure to CO gas should be questioned in the story. The third point in the diagnosis is confirmed by COHb level. Measurements made by looking at the blood give the most accurate result. However, the fact that the COHb level is within normal limits does not mean that there is no CO poisoning. In such cases, clinicians should conduct management according to the symptoms associated with poisoning and exposure to CO gas, if in doubt.

References

Abdel Aziz, M. H., El Dine, F. M. M. B., Hussein, H. A. S. M., Abdelazeem, A. M., & Sanad, I. M. (2021). Prediction of troponin I and N-terminal pro-brain natriuretic peptide levels in acute carbon monoxide poisoning using advanced electrocardiogram analysis, Alexandria, Egypt. *Environmental science and pollution research international, 28*(35), 48754–48766. https://doi.org/10.1007/s11356-021-14171-3.

Baud, F. J. (2007). Cyanide: critical issues in diagnosis and treatment. *Human & experimental toxicology, 26*(3), 191–201. https://doi.org/10.1177/0960327107070566.

Beppu, T. (2014). The role of MR imaging in assessment of brain damage from carbon monoxide poisoning: a review of the literature. AJNR. *American journal of neuroradiology, 35*(4), 625–631. https://doi.org/10.3174/ajnr.A3489.

Cha, Y. S., Kim, H., Hwang, S. O., Kim, J. Y., Kim, Y. K., Choi, E. H., Kim, O. H., Kim, H. I., Cha, K. C., & Lee, K. H. (2016). Incidence and patterns of cardiomyopathy in carbon monoxide-poisoned patients with myocardial injury. *Clinical toxicology (Philadelphia, Pa.), 54*(6), 481–487. https://doi.org/10.3109/15563650.2016.1162310.

Chang, Y. L., Yang, C. C., Deng, J. F., Ger, J., Tsai, W. J., Wu, M. L., Liaw, H. C., & Liaw, S. J. (1999). Diverse manifestations of oral methylene chloride poisoning: report of 6 cases. *Journal of toxicology: Clinical toxicology*, 37(4), 497–504. https://doi.org/10.1081/clt-100102442.

Collet, J. P., Thiele, H., Barbato, E., Barthélémy, O., Bauersachs, J., Bhatt, D. L., Dendale, P., Dorobantu, M., Edvardsen, T., Folliguet, T., Gale, C. P., Gilard, M., Jobs, A., Jüni, P., Lambrinou, E., Lewis, B. S., Mehilli, J., Meliga, E., Merkely, B., Mueller, C., Roffi, M., Rutten, F. H, Sibbing, D., Siontis, G. C. M, & ESC Scientific Document Group (2021). 2020 ESC Guidelines for the management of acute coronary syndromes in patients presenting without persistent ST-segment elevation. *European heart journal, 42*(14), 1289–1367. https://doi.org/10.1093/eurheartj/ehaa575.

Coşkun, A., Eren, F. A., Eren, Ş. H., & Korkmaz, İ. (2019). Predicting of neuropsychosis in carbon monoxide poisoning according to the plasma troponin, COHb, RDW and MPV levels: Neuropsychoses in carbon monoxide poisoning. *The American journal of emergency medicine, 37*(7), 1254–1259. https://doi.org/10.1016/j.ajem.2018.09.017.

Hampson, N. B. (2012). Noninvasive pulse CO-oximetry expedites evaluation and management of patients with carbon monoxide poisoning. *The American journal of emergency medicine*, 30(9), 2021–2024. https://doi.org/10.1016/j.ajem.2012.03.026

Hampson, N. B. (2016). Myth busting in carbon monoxide poisoning. *The American journal of emergency medicine*, 34(2), 295–297. https://doi.org/10.1016/j.ajem.2015.10.051.

Hampson, N. B. (2016). U.S. Mortality Due to Carbon Monoxide Poisoning, 1999-2014. Accidental and Intentional Deaths. *Annals of the American Thoracic Society*, 13(10), 1768–1774. https://doi.org/10.1513/AnnalsATS.201604-318OC.

Harper, A., & Croft-Baker, J. (2004). Carbon monoxide poisoning: undetected by both patients and their doctors. *Age and ageing, 33*(2), 105–109. https://doi.org/10.1093/ageing/afh038.

Inagaki, T., Ishino, H., Seno, H., Umegae, N., & Aoyama, T. (1997). A long-term follow-up study of serial magnetic resonance images in patients with delayed encephalopathy after acute carbon monoxide poisoning. *Psychiatry and clinical neurosciences, 51*(6), 421–423. https://doi.org/10.1111/j.1440-1819.1997.tb02611.x.

Jones, J. S., Lagasse, J., & Zimmerman, G. (1994). Computed tomographic findings after acute carbon monoxide poisoning. *The American journal of emergency medicine, 12*(4), 448–451. https://doi.org/10.1016/0735-6757(94)90059-0.

Kandis, H., Katırcı, Y., & Karapolat, B. S. (2009). Kabonmonoksit zehirlenmesi [Carbonmonoxide Poisoning]. *Düzce Medical Journal*, 11, 54-60.

Kao, L. W., & Nañagas, K. A. (2004). Carbon monoxide poisoning. *Emergency medicine clinics of North America, 22*(4), 985–1018. https://doi.org/10.1016/j.emc.2004.05.003.

Koga, H., Tashiro, H., Mukasa, K., Inoue, T., Okamoto, A., Urabe, S., Sagara, S., Yano, K., Onitsuka, K., & Yamashita, H. (2021). Can indicators of myocardial damage predict carbon monoxide poisoning outcomes?. *BMC emergency medicine, 21*(1), 7. https://doi.org/10.1186/s12873-021-00405-7.

Lawson-Smith, P., Jansen, E. C., & Hyldegaard, O. (2011). Cyanide intoxication as part of smoke inhalation--a review on diagnosis and treatment from the emergency perspective. *Scandinavian journal of trauma, resuscitation and emergency medicine, 19*, 14. https://doi.org/10.1186/1757-7241-19-14.

Lee, J., Mukai, D., Kreuter, K., Mahon, S., Tromberg, B., & Brenner, M. (2007). Potential interference by hydroxocobalamin on cooximetry hemoglobin measurements during cyanide and smoke inhalation treatments. *Annals of emergency medicine*, 49(6), 802–805. https://doi.org/10.1016/j.annemergmed.2006.11.016.

Livshits, Z., Lugassy, D. M., Shawn, L. K., & Hoffman, R. S. (2012). Falsely low carboxyhemoglobin level after hydroxocobalamin therapy. *The New England journal of medicine*, 367(13), 1270–1271. https://doi.org/10.1056/NEJMc1114820.

Mack E. (2007). Focus on diagnosis: co-oximetry. *Pediatrics in review*, 28(2), 73–74. https://doi.org/10.1542/pir.28-2-73.

Medscape (2023) *Carbon Monoxide Toxicity Workup*. Retrieved from https://emedicine.medscape.com/article/819987-workup#c6.

Pace, R., Bon Homme, M., Hoffman, R. S., & Lugassy, D. (2014). Effects of hydroxocobalamin on carboxyhemoglobin measured under physiologic and pathologic conditions. *Clinical toxicology (Philadelphia, Pa.)*, 52(7), 647–650. https://doi.org/10.3109/15563650.2014.939659.

Park, J. S., Seo, K. W., Choi, B. J., Choi, S. Y., Yoon, M. H., Hwang, G. S., Tahk, S. J., Choi, S. C., Min, Y. G., & Shin, J. H. (2016). Various Echocardiographic Patterns of Left Ventricular Systolic Dysfunction Induced by Carbon Monoxide Intoxication. *Cardiovascular toxicology, 16*(4), 361–369. https://doi.org/10.1007/s120 12-015-9347-6.

Radford, E. P., & Drizd, T. A. (1982). Blood carbon monoxide levels in persons 3-74 years of age: United States, 1976-80. *Advance data*, (76), 1–24.

Rose, J. J., Wang, L., Xu, Q., McTiernan, C. F., Shiva, S., Tejero, J., & Gladwin, M. T. (2017). Carbon Monoxide Poisoning: Pathogenesis, Management, and Future Directions of Therapy. *American journal of respiratory and critical care medicine*, 195(5), 596–606. https://doi.org/10.1164/rccm.201606-1275CI.

Ruckman J. S. (2012). CO-oximeters. *Biomedical instrumentation & technology*, 46(1), 61–63. https://doi.org/10.2345/0899-8205-46.1.61.

Satran, D., Henry, C. R., Adkinson, C., Nicholson, C. I., Bracha, Y., & Henry, T. D. (2005). Cardiovascular manifestations of moderate to severe carbon monoxide poisoning. *Journal of the American College of Cardiology, 45*(9), 1513–1516. https://doi.org/10.1016/j.jacc.2005.01.044.

Shin, M., Bronstein, A. C., Glidden, E., Malone, M., Chang, A., Law, R., Boehmer, T. K., Strosnider, H., & Yip, F. (2023). Morbidity and Mortality of Unintentional Carbon Monoxide Poisoning: United States 2005 to 2018. *Annals of emergency medicine*, 81(3), 309–317. https://doi.org/10.1016/j.annemergmed.2022.10.011.

So, G. M., Kosofsky, B. E., & Southern, J. F. (1997). Acute hydrocephalus following carbon monoxide poisoning. *Pediatric neurology, 17*(3), 270–273. https://doi.org/10.1016/s0887-8994(97)00097-0.

Sokal, J. A., & Kralkowska, E. (1985). The relationship between exposure duration, carboxyhemoglobin, blood glucose, pyruvate and lactate and the severity of intoxication in 39 cases of acute carbon monoxide poisoning in man. *Archives of toxicology, 57*(3), 196–199. https://doi.org/10.1007/BF00290887.

Touger, M., Gallagher, E. J., & Tyrell, J. (1995). Relationship between venous and arterial carboxyhemoglobin levels in patients with suspected carbon monoxide poisoning. *Annals of emergency medicine,* 25(4), 481–483. https://doi.org/10.1016/s0196-0644(95)70262-8.

Wolf, S. J., Maloney, G. E., Shih, R. D., Shy, B. D., Brown, M. D. & American College of Emergency Physicians Clinical Policies Subcommittee (Writing Committee) on Carbon Monoxide Poisoning, (2017). Clinical Policy: Critical Issues in the Evaluation and Management of Adult Patients Presenting to the Emergency Department with Acute Carbon Monoxide Poisoning. *Annals of emergency medicine*, 69(1), 98–107.e6. https://doi.org/10.1016/j.annemergmed.2016.11.003.

Yurtseven, S., Arslan, A., Eryigit, U., Gunaydin, M., Tatli, O., Ozsahin, F., Karaca, Y., Aksut, N., Aygun, A., & Gunduz, A. (2016). Analysis of patients presenting to the emergency department with carbon monoxide intoxication. *Turkish journal of emergency medicine*, 15(4), 159–162. https://doi.org/10.1016/j.tjem.2015.05.001.

Chapter 7

Biomarkers Used in the Diagnosis and Prognosis of Carbon Monoxide Poisoning

Gökcan Aman[1,*], MD
and Türker Demirtakan[2], MD
[1]Department of Emergency Medicine, Sultan 1. Murat State Hospital, Edirne, Turkey
[2]Department of Emergency Medicine, University of Health Sciences,
Kanuni Sultan Süleyman Research and Training Hospital, Istanbul, Turkey

Abstract

Carbon monoxide (CO) poisoning is a significant public health concern worldwide, with millions of cases and thousands of deaths each year. The diagnosis and management of CO poisoning can be challenging, as its symptoms are non-specific and can mimic other conditions. Therefore, identifying reliable biomarkers to diagnose and monitor the progression of CO poisoning is crucial.

This chapter reviews current research on biomarkers that can be used to diagnose and diagnose CO poisoning. The main focus is on the role of carboxyhemoglobin (COHb) levels as a biomarker, as they are widely used in clinical practice. However, other potential biomarkers, including lactate, neuron-specific biomarkers, and cytokines, are also discussed.

The chapter provides an overview of the diagnostic and prognostic value of these biomarkers and their limitations.

Overall, this chapter highlights the potential of biomarkers in improving the diagnosis and prognosis of CO poisoning and provides insight into their use in clinical practice.

* Corresponding Author's Email: gokcan.aman@hotmail.com.

In: Carbon Monoxide Poisoning
Editors: Seda Özkan and Afsin Ipekci
ISBN: 979-8-89113-217-7

Keywords: carboxyhemoglobin, cardiac biomarkers, inflammatory biomarkers

Introduction

Carbon monoxide (CO) poisoning is a major public health problem worldwide, associated with high rates of morbidity and mortality. Diagnosis and management of CO poisoning is based mainly on clinical features, history, and laboratory investigations, such as carboxyhemoglobin (COHb) levels. However, the clinical presentation of CO poisoning can be non-specific, and COHb levels may not correlate well with the severity of the poisoning. In recent years, there has been growing interest in identifying new biomarkers that can help with the diagnosis and prognosis of CO poisoning. Biomarkers, such as cytokines, oxidative stress markers, and cardiac enzymes, have been studied in various settings to evaluate their potential utility in CO poisoning. This chapter will provide an overview of the current understanding of biomarkers in CO poisoning and their potential use in diagnosis and prognosis.

Elevated Biomarkers in Acute CO Poisoning

Carboxyhemoglobin

Carboxyhemoglobin is a protein that carries carbon monoxide in the blood, but before describing its structure and functions, we must know about hemoglobin, heme, and globin protein.

Globular Proteins

Globular proteins (sometimes called spheroproteins) are proteins that are spherical (globe-like) in shape. They are one of the more common types of proteins with fibrous, disordered, and membrane proteins. Unlike fibrous or membrane proteins, globular proteins tend to form colloids in aqueous environments due to their possession of hydrophilic amino acids on their surface on the outside (Andreeva et al., 2014). To further stabilize the spherical nature of the protein structure, hydrophobic non-polar amino acids face the interior parts.

Globular proteins can act as enzymes (catalyzing reactions in the body), messenger proteins (to regulate biological processes), amino acid stocks, other regulatory roles, structural proteins (such as tubulin and actin), and transporters.

Hemoglobin is the most known member of this protein family and the most important for our chapter. Other than hemoglobin, there is alpha, beta, and gamma globulin. Many signal proteins and most enzymes with primary metabolic functions have spherical shapes. Another globular protein is albumin, but unlike some water-soluble members, it is completely soluble in aqueous environments (Hassan et al., 1997).

Heme Structure

Heme is a planar structure, and it is a precursor to hemoglobin. It is biologically synthesized in the marrow of the bone and the liver (Bloomer, 1998). The system comprises a porphyrin ring and a ferrous iron (Fe^{2+}) coordinated in the center of the ring by bonds to four nitrogens, leaving two free bonds to Fe^{2+} heme along the two sides of the planar structure (Abali et al., 2021).

Globular Hemeproteins

Globular hemeproteins are a family of proteins that contain a heme group, a complex organic molecule that contains iron, which is responsible for their characteristic red color. The three-dimensional build of the protein dictates the function of the heme group. Hemeproteins involve many biological processes, including oxygen transport, electron transfer, and catalysis (Lehninger et al., 2000; Chelikani et al., 2004).

In electron transfer in mitochondria, the structure of the cytochrome protein makes way for reversible and fast oxidation-reduction electron transfer of heme-coordinated iron. This redox function is reversible between the ferrous (Fe^{2+}) and ferric (Fe^{3+}) states of iron (Lehninger et al., 2000). In catalysis, the heme is at the active site of the catalase, which helps the breakdown of hydrogen peroxide (Chelikani et al., 2004).

The structure of the hemoglobin protein can affect the alignment of ferrous iron with respect to the heme group. The changes in this alignment affect the binding capacity oxygen molecules and the transportation of the protein around the lungs and tissues (Lehninger et al., 2000).

Hemoglobin

Organisms require oxygen to support metabolic processes and generate energy. However, oxygen diffusion from the atmosphere into the body tissues of an organism is limited by its solubility in water-based fluids, such as blood.

Larger organisms have evolved circulatory systems to transport oxygen more efficiently throughout their bodies to overcome this limitation. However, oxygen transport remains challenging even with a circulatory system because it is only slightly soluble in blood. Organisms have developed transport molecules such as hemoglobin to address this issue (Hardison, 2012).

Hemoglobin (Hb) is the metalloprotein that is found exclusively in red blood cells (erythrocytes and RBCs) and contains iron. Its main functionality is the transportation of oxygen molecules from the lungs to the capillaries of tissues. The major hemoglobin variant in adults is Hemoglobin A (HbA), composed of two alpha (α) and two beta (β) polypeptide chains. Non-covalent interactions hold together those four chains (Farid et al., 2022).

Hemoglobin can carry four oxygen molecules from the lungs to cells and can take protons (H+) and carbon dioxide (CO2) from cells to the lungs (Hsia, 1998). Allosteric effector interactions regulate the oxygen-binding abilities of hemoglobin (Kneipp et al., 2006).

Quaternary structure: Components of the hemoglobin tetramer composed of two identical dimers, αβ1, and αβ2 (Perutz, 1987). The two polypeptide chains are tightly arranged within each dimer, primarily by hydrophobic interactions. On the contrary, the two dimers are mainly held together by polar bonds. Weaker interactions between dimers allow them to move relative to each other. This action causes the two dimers to occupy different relative positions in the oxyhemoglobin versus deoxyhemoglobin.

T and R forms: While the deoxy form of hemoglobin is named the "T" form, the taut form, the oxy form, is called the relaxed "R" form. While the oxygen affinity for the R form is higher, the oxygen affinity for the T form is low. In the T conformation, the interaction of two αβ dimers through ionic and hydrogen bonds limits the movement of the chains, and iron (Fe2+) is pulled out from the planar structure of the heme. The binding of O2 to hemoglobin results in the rupture of some of the bonds between two dimers and allows the movement of the Fe^{2+} toward the planar heme structure (Abali et al., 2021).

The oxygenation of hemoglobin as a function of the oxygen concentration can be shown as a sigmoid curve with two characteristics. First, the shape of the sigmoid curve is because of cooperativity, which increases the affinity of the empty hemes for oxygen when the hemoglobin is partially saturated with oxygen (Chou, 1989; Mihailescu & Russu, 2001). The second characteristic is that the oxygen affinity of hemoglobin can be shifted right or left, modified by external factors.

The completely deoxygenated hemoglobin is slow to bind with an oxygen molecule, but the oxygenation process accelerates as it reacts with oxygen.

With four hemes saturated with the oxygen molecule, T to R transformation occurs, and the oxygen affinity markedly increases (Monod et al., 1965).

The P50 designates oxygen affinity, meaning that the partial pressure of oxygen at the hemoglobin protein is 50% saturated. The modulators of oxygen affinity are pH, CO_2, 2,3-bisphosphoglycerate (2,3-BPG), and temperature (Benner et al., 2023).

The right and left shift of the hemoglobin-oxygen association/dissociation curve happens when these modulators change. A shift to the right means that a larger P50 is required to saturate hemoglobin; on the other hand, the left shift means that a decreased P50 can saturate hemoglobin at the level of the lungs (Benner et al., 2023).

The affinity of hemoglobin for oxygen molecules increases as a function of pH in the range of 6.0 to 8.5. This is known as the Bohr effect (Benner et al., 2023). Hemoglobin that is deoxygenated binds protons stronger than oxyhemoglobin. When deoxyhemoglobin becomes oxyhemoglobin, salt bonds are broken, and protons are released. Because of this Bohr effect, oxygen molecules are released easier at the capillary level. The carbon dioxide (CO_2) tension is higher, and the pH is lower at the tissue level. On the contrary, oxygen is taken up at the lung level with a higher pH.

The alpha and beta chains have free amino groups at the N termini, and CO_2 can react with these to form carbimino complexes. At any given pH level, CO_2 lowers oxygen affinity because deoxyhemoglobin forms these complexes easier than oxy forms (Perutz, 1987).

Another modulator of the hemoglobin oxygen affinity is 2,3-BPG; it is available in RBCs and is synthesized with the bisphosphoglycerate mutase (BPGM) enzyme of 1,3-BPG (Pritlove et al., 2006). 2,3-BPG binds strongly to deoxyhemoglobin but weakly to oxyhemoglobin. The reaction is as follows:

$$\text{Hb-BPG} + 4O_2 \Leftrightarrow \text{Hb}(O_2)_4 + \text{BPG}$$

Increased 2,3-BPG levels decrease oxygen affinity, corresponding to a right shift on the hemoglobin-oxygen curve. A variation in BPGM can reduce 2,3-BPG levels, and a left shift will occur, leading to decreased tissue oxygenation of at the tissue level (Petousi et al., 2014).

When body temperature is elevated, oxygen affinity decreases to oxygenate tissues when oxygen needs are higher than usual.

Normal hemoglobin levels for males are between 14 and 18 g/dl, while for females, the range is between 12 and 16 g/dl (Billet, 1990).

Carboxyhemoglobin

Carboxyhemoglobin (COHb) is a stable complex that binds carbon monoxide and hemoglobin in red blood cells. While non-smokers typically have a systemic carboxyhemoglobin level under 3%, smokers can approach 10% (Ernst & Zibrak, 1998; Hopper et al., 2021). Toxicity occurs consistently at levels exceeding 15% COHb, which the FDA has previously set as a threshold of 14% COHb in specific clinical trials involving carbon monoxide as a potential therapy (Motterlini & Foresti, 2017; Yang et al., 2020).

Despite its low solubility in water and high bond enthalpy, carbon monoxide has a high affinity for the iron core site in hemoglobin (also shared by oxygen). It binds to it with affinity greater than of oxygen. This binding is what causes the toxicity of carbon monoxide.

Under normal physiological conditions, the affinity of carbon monoxide for hemoglobin is approximately 240 times greater than that of oxygen (Berg et al., 2011; Hopper et al., 2021). However, in humans with the Hb-Kirklareli (α H58L) mutation, the affinity for carbon monoxide is even more significant, resulting in a sustained level of 16% COHb in the bloodstream (Bissé et al., 2017; Motterlini & Foresti, 2017). When two carbon monoxide molecules bind to hemoglobin, the molecule shifts to a relaxed state, which can be dangerous for those exposed to carbon monoxide. The two globin chains that can still bind to oxygen will remain in their high-affinity conformation, making it more difficult for the remaining oxygen binding sites to deliver oxygen to tissues. This phenomenon is called the Darling-Roughton effect and increases hemoglobin's oxygen affinity as carbon monoxide levels increase (Darling & Roughton, 1942).

Carbon monoxide can be present in the bloodstream without environmental exposure. Adults typically have around 1-2% carboxyhemoglobin (COHb) from endogenously produced CO, which comes from the degradation of heme by the heme oxygenase-cytochrome P450 complex (SJÖSTRAND, 1949). The levels of endogenous CO can vary due to factors such as genetics, caloric restriction, dehydration, and certain medical conditions. Exogenous sources of CO include atmospheric CO from incomplete combustion and oxidation of hydrocarbons, as well as natural sources. High-altitude polycythemia and hypoxemia can also contribute to increased COHb levels, exacerbating the already decreased tissue oxygen delivery associated with high altitude. It is important to note that endogenous CO production can have physiological consequences, and exogenous CO exposure can be toxic (Marks et al., 1991; McGrath, 1992).

Carbon monoxide poisoning is diagnosed by measuring carboxyhemoglobin levels in the blood using co-oximetry in patients with known or suspected CO exposure. Venous blood samples are commonly used in hemodynamically stable patients, with levels above 3% for non-smokers and 10% for smokers, indicating CO poisoning (Lopez et al., 2000; Touger et al., 1995). However, COHb levels do not always indicate the extent of poisoning, as they may not accurately reflect the severity of symptoms if significant time has passed since exposure due to CO removal from the body. Therefore, the management of CO poisoning is based on symptoms and signs of the patient rather than just COHb levels. Any abnormally high level of COHb associated with severe symptoms such as cardiac ischemia or altered mental state should indicate severe poisoning (Piantadosi, 1999).

Lactate Levels in Acute CO Poisoning

In acute CO poisoning, body tissues can become oxygen-deprived due to the displacement of oxygen by carbon monoxide, leading to anaerobic metabolism and the accumulation of lactic acid. Lactic acidosis can occur and lactate levels in the blood can be used as a marker of tissue hypoxia and the severity of CO poisoning. Elevated lactate levels in CO poisoning may indicate tissue hypoxia and a poor prognosis. As a result, the body switches to anaerobic metabolism, producing lactate (Henry et al., 2006; Weaver et al., 2007). Higher levels of lactate can indicate more severe tissue hypoxia and a poorer prognosis in cases of CO poisoning. Lactate levels may be used to monitor the response to treatment and guide decisions regarding the need for further interventions. It is important to note that elevated lactate levels can be a valuable marker of tissue hypoxia. However, they can also be elevated in conditions such as sepsis, shock, and liver failure (Buehler et al., 1975; Weaver et al., 2007).

RDW Levels in Acute CO Poisoning

RDW, a measure of red blood cell size variability, has been associated with adverse events in various clinical conditions, including heart-related diseases. Elevated levels of RDW have been observed in CO poisoning patients compared to control subjects.

While RDW is commonly used in the diagnosis and monitoring of hematologic diseases, recent studies have explored its relationship with cardiovascular conditions. Elevated levels of RDW have been associated with morbidity and mortality in acute coronary syndrome, coronary artery disease (CAD), pulmonary thromboembolism, and heart failure. RDW is associated with the presence and severity of CAD, and in individuals with asymptomatic atherosclerosis, inflammation, and oxidative stress can disrupt erythropoiesis and lead to the release of immature RBCs into the circulation, resulting in higher levels of RDW levels. In the context of CO poisoning, the mechanisms underlying the relationship between RDW, and the condition are multifactorial. Patients with elevated RDW may have a higher incidence of CAD, which could exacerbate the severity of CO poisoning. Additionally, the acute effects of carboxyhemoglobin (COHb) molecules, formed by binding of CO to erythrocyte heme instead of oxygen, can cause structural changes and anisocytosis, contributing to elevated RDW. Furthermore, chronic CO exposure prior to the index event, possibly due to living or working conditions, could stimulate erythropoiesis through hypoxia. Studies on long-term outcomes of CO poisoning are scarce and have predominantly focused on moderate to severe cases. Some studies have indicated that myocardial injury and troponin elevation are predictors of long-term mortality from CO poisoning. In the present study, with more than half of the patients having mild to moderate CO poisoning, the long-term mortality rate was 5.8%. Although the majority of deaths occurred in the first year, the mortality rate remained elevated after the first year in patients with high RDW values (Sunman et al., 2018).

Neuron-Specific Biomarkers Acute CO Poisoning

Severe CO poisoning can lead to prominent central nervous system (CNS) symptoms, with neuropsychiatric symptoms in about 67% of cases. Brain injury can occur to varying degrees depending on the severity of the poisoning, and the diagnosis and prognosis of patients with CO poisoning remain a topic of debate. Several studies have investigated the use of brain injury markers, including S100B, neuron-specific enolase (NSE), and glial fibrillary acidic protein (GFAP), to determine the prognosis following brain injury in cases of poisoning (Akdemir et al., 2014).

S100-Beta

S100-Beta is a protein that belongs to the S100 family of proteins. It is a dimeric protein that consists of two identical subunits, each containing 92 amino acids. The primary structure of S100-Beta includes six alpha helices and several beta strands arranged in a compact globular shape. The protein has a high content of acidic amino acid residues, particularly glutamic and aspartic acids, which contribute to its acidic nature and ability to bind calcium ions. The secondary and tertiary structures of S100-Beta are stabilized by the formation of disulfide bonds between cysteine residues in each subunit and by interactions between hydrophobic amino acid residues (Donato, 2001).

S100-Beta is a calcium-binding protein and can bind up to two calcium ions per subunit. Calcium binding induces conformational changes in the protein, which can regulate its interaction with target proteins. The biological function of S100-Beta is still being studied. However, it is known to be involved in various cellular processes, including regulating cell growth and differentiation, intracellular signaling, and calcium homeostasis. S100-Beta is also used as a biomarker to diagnose and monitor neurological disorders, including traumatic brain injury, stroke, and Alzheimer's disease (Réty et al., 1999; H. Y. Zhang et al., 2012).

Neuron-specific Enolase

Neuron-specific enolase (NSE) is a type of glycolytic enzyme that is expressed primarily in neurons and neuroendocrine cells. It exists in several isoforms, with the gamma and alpha/gamma isoforms being the most abundant in the nervous system. The primary structure of NSE consists of two identical subunits, each containing 434 amino acids. The protein has a molecular weight of approximately 78 kDa. Secondary and tertiary structures of NSE are stabilized by forming multiple intramolecular disulfide bonds between cysteine residues and interactions between hydrophobic and hydrophilic amino acid residues (Burté et al., 2015; Kornblatt & Klugerman, 1989).

In addition to its role in energy metabolism, NSE has been shown to have other functions in the nervous system, such as promoting neurite outgrowth and regulating synaptic plasticity. It is also used as a biomarker to diagnose and monitor several neurological and neoplastic disorders, including brain injury, stroke, and small-cell lung cancer (Goyal et al., 2013; Isgrò et al., 2015).

Glial Fibrillary Acidic Protein

Glial fibrillary acidic protein (GFAP) is a type of intermediate filament protein that is expressed primarily in astrocytes, a type of glial cell in the central nervous system. GFAP plays an essential role in providing structural support to astrocytes and regulating astrocyte function in response to various stimuli (Akdemir et al., 2014; L. Zhang et al., 2021).

The primary structure of GFAP consists of a single polypeptide chain that contains approximately 432 amino acids. The protein has a molecular weight of about 50 kDa. The GFAP monomer consists of a central rod domain flanked by a globular N-terminal head domain and a globular C-terminal tail domain. GFAP monomers form dimers that can be assembled into tetramers, which can be assembled into intermediate filaments. The assembly of GFAP filaments is regulated by the phosphorylation and dephosphorylation of specific serine and threonine residues within the protein. The degree of phosphorylation is thought to influence the properties of GFAP filaments, such as their stability and ability to interact with other proteins (Akdemir et al., 2014; L. Zhang et al., 2021).

In addition to its role in providing structural support to astrocytes, GFAP has been implicated in a variety of neurological disorders, including Alzheimer's disease, Parkinson's disease, and multiple sclerosis. GFAP is also used as a biomarker for certain neurological conditions, such as brain injury and certain types of brain tumors (Akdemir et al., 2014; L. Zhang et al., 2021).

Determining Clinical Severity

The normal range of S100 beta in plasma can vary depending on the laboratory that performs the test, but it is generally less than 0.1 ng/mL. It is important to note that S100 beta levels should be interpreted in conjunction with other clinical findings and diagnostic tests. Elevated levels of S100 beta may suggest the presence of brain damage, such as traumatic brain injury, stroke, or carbon monoxide poisoning. However, an elevated level alone is not diagnostic and should be correlated with other clinical and laboratory findings (Liu et al., 2015; E. Park et al., 2012).

In the case of carbon monoxide poisoning, some studies suggest that an initial S100 beta level greater than 0.3 ng/mL can indicate the likelihood of delayed neurological sequelae. On the contrary, levels above 1.0 ng/mL can indicate a worse prognosis and a higher risk of neurological sequelae.

However, more research is needed to confirm these findings and determine the optimal cut-off levels for S100 beta in the diagnosis and prognosis of CO poisoning. Elevated levels of S100 beta can contribute to the development of brain edema, impaired cognitive function, and other neurologic complications (Brvar et al., 2004).

The average plasma level of neuron-specific enolase (NSE) varies depending on the laboratory reference ranges, but it is typically less than or equal to 17 ng/mL in adults. In acute carbon monoxide (CO) poisoning, elevated levels of NSE can indicate neuronal damage and may be a predictor of a poor prognosis. NSE levels may begin to increase within hours of CO exposure and peak within 48 to 72 hours. However, it is essential to note that NSE levels may also be elevated in other conditions, such as stroke, traumatic brain injury, and some cancers. Therefore, NSE levels should be interpreted in the context of the patient's overall clinical presentation and medical history (Böttiger et al., 2001; Cha et al., 2018; Feng, 2022; Kao & Nañagas, 2005).

The normal plasma level of glial fibrillary acidic protein (GFAP) is generally considered to be less than 0.07 ng/mL. Elevated GFAP levels have been observed in patients with acute carbon monoxide poisoning, particularly those with neurological symptoms. GFAP levels may be helpful as a biomarker for detecting and monitoring brain injury in these patients. However, the interpretation of GFAP levels should be made in conjunction with other clinical and diagnostic findings. It is important to note that GFAP is not specific to carbon monoxide poisoning and may also be elevated in other types of brain injury or neurological conditions. Therefore, GFAP levels should be interpreted in the context of the overall clinical presentation and medical history of the patient (L. Zhang et al., 2021).

Copeptin in Acute CO Poisoning

Plasma copeptin levels have been observed to increase during the early stages of acute developing diseases. Copeptin, a stress hormone synthesized alongside vasopressin, has emerged as a novel diagnostic biomarker for patients presenting with acute illnesses. This biomarker consists of a 39-amino acid sequence of the glycoprotein and holds promise in aiding the identification of individuals with acute diseases. The secretion of copeptin from the hypothalamus increases in response to stress. Consequently, copeptin may provide vital information for risk stratification in a variety of clinical scenarios. Notably, there is a significant disparity between the serum copeptin levels of healthy individuals and those poisoned, highlighting the diagnostic potential of copeptin for acute carbon monoxide (CO) poisoning. These findings underscore the preferential use of copeptin in diagnosing such cases, thus enhancing patient management and outcomes (Ozkan et al., 2020).

Cardiac Biomarkers in Acute CO Poisoning

High-sensitive Troponin I (hs-TnI) is a cardiac biomarker that is used to evaluate acute myocardial injury. The biochemical structure of hs-TnI is a protein complex consisting of three subunits, TnI, TnT, and TnC. TnI is the inhibitory subunit that blocks the interaction of actin and myosin, while TnT and TnC are the regulatory subunits responsible for Ca^{2+} binding. In acute carbon monoxide poisoning, hs-TnI can be elevated due to the presence of a myocardial injury. Carbon monoxide poisoning can cause hypoxia and subsequent tissue damage, including damage to heart muscles. Elevated levels of hs-TnI can indicate the presence of cardiac injury and may be helpful in the diagnosis and prognosis of carbon monoxide poisoning. It is worth noting that elevated hs-TnI levels can also be seen in other conditions, such as myocardial infarction, heart failure, and pulmonary embolism, so further evaluation and differential diagnosis are necessary to determine the underlying cause (Geng et al., 2020; Huysal et al., 2016; J. S. Kim et al., 2020; J. H. Park et al., 2020).

The fatty acid binding protein (FABP) is a small cytoplasmic protein involved in the transport and metabolism of fatty acids in cells. In acute CO poisoning, elevated levels of FABP have been reported in studies as a potential biomarker of myocardial injury. FABP has a beta-barrel structure consisting of 10 antiparallel beta-strands and two alpha-helices. It contains a fatty acid binding pocket where fatty acids can bind, and it is involved in the transport of fatty acids from the cell membrane to the mitochondria for β-oxidation (Erenler et al., 2013).

In cases of acute CO poisoning, FABP may be released from damaged myocardial cells and can be detected in the blood as a marker of myocardial injury. Elevated levels of FABP have been associated with an increased risk of adverse cardiovascular events and mortality in patients with CO poisoning (J.-S. Kim et al., 2020).

Creatine phosphokinase (CPK), also known as creatine kinase (CK), is an enzyme found primarily in the heart, brain, and skeletal muscle. It is composed of two subunits, M (muscle) and B (brain), which combine to form three isoenzymes: CK-MM, CK-MB, and CK-BB. In acute CO poisoning, elevated levels of CK-MB and CK-MM have been reported, indicating potential cardiac and skeletal muscle damage. However, these markers are less specific to CO poisoning and can also be elevated in other conditions, such as myocardial infarction and rhabdomyolysis. Therefore, their interpretation in the context of CO poisoning requires careful consideration of other clinical and laboratory findings (Rhodes et al., 2009).

Inflammatory Biomarkers in Acute CO Poisoning

Inflammatory biomarkers have been studied as potential predictors of the severity and outcomes of acute carbon monoxide (CO) poisoning. CO poisoning can cause damage to various organs, including the brain, heart, and lungs, leading to inflammation in these tissues. Elevated levels of inflammatory biomarkers, such as C-reactive protein (CRP), interleukin-6 (IL-6), and tumor necrosis factor-alpha (TNF-α), have been reported in patients with severe CO poisoning.

Akcali et al. suggested that elevated levels of CRP and IL-6 are associated with the severity of CO poisoning and may be useful in determining the clinical severity of the condition. The study showed that patients with severe CO poisoning had significantly higher levels of CRP and IL-6 compared to those with mild or moderate CO poisoning (Akcali et al., 2018).

IL-6 (Interleukin-6) is a proinflammatory cytokine that plays a crucial role in the immune response and inflammation. In cases of acute carbon monoxide poisoning, IL-6 levels have been found to be elevated and may be used as a marker for the severity of the poisoning. The normal range of IL-6 levels can vary depending on the laboratory and the test used for the measurement. Generally, the normal range for IL-6 levels in healthy individuals is less than 10 pg/mL (H. Kim et al., 2018; Pepe et al., 2011).

In acute CO poisoning, the interpretation of IL-6 levels can depend on the severity of the poisoning. Some studies have shown that IL-6 levels are significantly elevated in patients with severe CO poisoning compared to those with mild or moderate poisoning and that IL-6 levels may be a valuable biomarker to predict the severity of CO poisoning and the risk of developing complications such as acute respiratory distress syndrome (ARDS) and delayed neuropsychiatric sequelae (Akcali et al., 2018; H. Kim et al., 2018).

Tumor necrosis factor alpha (TNF-α) is an important cytokine involved in the regulation of the immune response. It is produced by a variety of cells, including macrophages, monocytes, T-cells, and natural killer cells, and plays a crucial role in host defense against infections and in the development of inflammation. TNF-α has many functions in the immune system, including inducing fever, activating neutrophils and other immune cells, and promoting the production of other inflammatory cytokines. It is also involved in the regulation of cell proliferation, differentiation, and apoptosis (Angus & van der Poll, 2013; Cohen, 2002).

The normal level of TNF-alpha in the blood can vary depending on the laboratory reference range used, but it is general less than 10 pg/mL. In acute carbon monoxide poisoning, TNF-alpha levels have been found to increase significantly, and their levels can be used as a marker of the severity and prognosis of the poisoning (Thom et al., 2010). However, it is important to note that TNF-alpha is not specific to CO poisoning and can also be elevated in other inflammatory conditions. Overproduction of TNF-α can lead to chronic inflammation and tissue damage and has been implicated in the pathogenesis of a variety of inflammatory and autoimmune diseases, including rheumatoid arthritis, Crohn's disease sepsis, and psoriasis. As a result, TNF-α inhibitors are widely used as therapeutic agents for these conditions (Hack & Zeerleder, 2001; Opal & Esmon, 2002).

Conclusion

In conclusion, the diagnosis and management of carbon monoxide poisoning can be challenging due to the non-specific nature of its symptoms. The use of biomarkers can provide valuable information on the diagnosis and prognosis of this condition. Measuring carboxyhemoglobin levels is the most widely used biomarker for the diagnosis of carbon monoxide poisoning. However, other biomarkers such as lactate, S100B, and interleukins have also shown promising results in predicting the severity of the poisoning and its clinical outcome.

The availability and feasibility of these biomarkers in clinical practice need further evaluation to improve the management and outcome of carbon monoxide poisoning. Biomarkers can also help identify patients who would benefit from hyperbaric oxygen therapy, which is the recommended treatment for severe cases of carbon monoxide poisoning. Further research in this area is needed to standardize the use of biomarkers in clinical practice and develop more sensitive and specific biomarkers for the diagnosis and prognosis of carbon monoxide poisoning.

References

Abali, E. E., Cline, S. D., Franklin, D. S., & Viselli, S. M. (2021). Chapter 3: Globular Proteins. In *Lippincott Illustrated Reviews: Biochemistry* (Eighth). Lippincott Williams & Wilkins.

Akcali, G., Uzun, G., Arziman, I., Aydin, I., & Yildiz, S. (2018). The relationship between intoxication severity and blood interleukin 6, interleukin 10 and CRP levels in carbon monoxide-poisoned patients. *Undersea and Hyperbaric Medicine*, *45*(6), 645–652. https://doi.org/10.22462/11.12.2018.4.

Akdemir, H. U., Yardan, T., Kati, C., Duran, L., Alacam, H., Yavuz, Y., & Okuyucu, A. (2014). The role of S100B protein, neuron-specific enolase, and glial fibrillary acidic protein in the evaluation of hypoxic brain injury in acute carbon monoxide poisoning. *Human & Experimental Toxicology*, *33*(11), 1113–1120. https://doi.org/10.1177/0960327114521049.

Andreeva, A., Howorth, D., Chothia, C., Kulesha, E., & Murzin, A. G. (2014). SCOP2 prototype: a new approach to protein structure mining. *Nucleic Acids Research*, *42*(Database issue), D310-4. https://doi.org/10.1093/nar/gkt1242.

Angus, D. C., & van der Poll, T. (2013). Severe Sepsis and Septic Shock. *New England Journal of Medicine*, *369*(9), 840–851. https://doi.org/10.1056/NEJMra1208623.

Benner, A., Patel, A. K., Singh, K., & Dua, A. (2023). *Physiology, Bohr Effect*.

Berg, J., Tymoczko, J., & Stryer, L. (2011). *Biochemistry* (Seventh). Palgrave MacMillan.

Billet, H. (1990). Hemoglobin and Hematocrit. In H. Walker, W. Hall, & J. Hurst (Eds.), *Clinical Methods: The History, Physical, and Laboratory Examinations.* (Third). Buttersworths.

Bissé, E., Schaeffer-Reiss, C., Van Dorsselaer, A., Alayi, T. D., Epting, T., Winkler, K., Benitez Cardenas, A. S., Soman, J., Birukou, I., Samuel, P. P., & Olson, J. S. (2017). Hemoglobin Kirklareli (α H58L), a New Variant Associated with Iron Deficiency and Increased CO Binding. *Journal of Biological Chemistry*, *292*(6), 2542–2555. https://doi.org/10.1074/jbc.M116.764274.

Bloomer, J. R. (1998). Liver metabolism of porphyrins and haem. *Journal of Gastroenterology and Hepatology*, *13*(3), 324–329. https://doi.org/10.1111/j.1440-1746.1998.01548.x.

Böttiger, B. W., Möbes, S., Glätzer, R., Bauer, H., Gries, A., Bärtsch, P., Motsch, J., & Martin, E. (2001). Astroglial Protein S-100 Is an Early and Sensitive Marker of Hypoxic Brain Damage and Outcome After Cardiac Arrest in Humans. *Circulation*, *103*(22), 2694–2698. https://doi.org/10.1161/01.CIR.103.22.2694.

Brvar, M., Mozina, H., Osredkar, J., Mozina, M., Noc, M., Brucan, A., & Bunc, M. (2004). S100B protein in carbon monoxide poisoning: a pilot study. *Resuscitation*, *61*(3), 357–360. https://doi.org/10.1016/j.resuscitation.2004.01.009.

Buehler, J. H., Berns, A. S., Webster, J. R., Addington, W. W., & Cugell, D. W. (1975). Lactic acidosis from carboxyhemoglobinemia after smoke inhalation. *Annals of Internal Medicine*, *82*(6), 803–805. https://doi.org/10.7326/0003-4819-82-6-803.

Burté, F., Carelli, V., Chinnery, P. F., & Yu-Wai-Man, P. (2015). Disturbed mitochondrial dynamics and neurodegenerative disorders. *Nature Reviews. Neurology*, *11*(1), 11–24. https://doi.org/10.1038/nrneurol.2014.228.

Cha, Y., Kim, H., Do, H., Kim, H., Kim, O., Cha, K. C., Lee, K., & Hwang, S. (2018). Serum neuron-specific enolase as an early predictor of delayed neuropsychiatric sequelae in patients with acute carbon monoxide poisoning. *Human & Experimental Toxicology*, *37*(3), 240–246. https://doi.org/10.1177/0960327117698544.

Chelikani, P., Fita, I., & Loewen, P. C. (2004). Diversity of structures and properties among catalases. *Cellular and Molecular Life Sciences: CMLS*, *61*(2), 192–208. https://doi.org/10.1007/s00018-003-3206-5.

Chou, K. C. (1989). Low-frequency resonance and cooperativity of hemoglobin. *Trends in Biochemical Sciences*, *14*(6), 212–213. https://doi.org/10.1016/0968-0004(89)90026-1.

Cohen, J. (2002). The immunopathogenesis of sepsis. *Nature*, *420*(6917), 885–891. https://doi.org/10.1038/nature01326.

Darling, R. C., & Roughton, F. J. W. (1942). The Effect of Methemoglobın on The Equılıbrıum Between Oxygen and Hemoglobın. *American Journal of Physiology-Legacy Content*, *137*(1), 56–68. https://doi.org/10.1152/ajplegacy.1942.137.1.56.

Donato, R. (2001). S100: a multigenic family of calcium-modulated proteins of the EF-hand type with intracellular and extracellular functional roles. *The International Journal of Biochemistry & Cell Biology*, *33*(7), 637–668. https://doi.org/10.1016/s1357-2725(01)00046-2.

Erenler, A. K., Yardan, T., Baydin, A., Gunay, M., & Amanvermez, R. (2013). Heart-type fatty acid-binding protein as a potential biomarker of acute carbon monoxide poisoning. *The American Journal of Emergency Medicine*, *31*(8), 1165–1169. https://doi.org/10.1016/j.ajem.2013.04.005.

Ernst, A., & Zibrak, J. D. (1998). Carbon monoxide poisoning. *The New England Journal of Medicine*, *339*(22), 1603–1608. https://doi.org/10.1056/NEJM199811263392206.

Farid, Y., Bowman, N. S., & Lecat, P. (2022). *Biochemistry, Hemoglobin Synthesis*. StatPearls Publishing.

Feng, S. Y. (2022). Magnetic resonance imaging for predicting delayed neurologic sequelae caused by carbon monoxide poisoning: A systematic review and meta-analysis. *Medicine*, *101*(47), e31981. https://doi.org/10.1097/MD.0000000000031981.

Geng, S., Hao, X., Xu, H., Yao, J., He, D., Xin, H., Gong, X., & Zhang, R. (2020). Cardiac injury after acute carbon monoxide poisoning and its clinical treatment scheme. *Experimental and Therapeutic Medicine*, *20*(2), 1098–1104. https://doi.org/10.3892/etm.2020.8801.

Goyal, A., Failla, M. D., Niyonkuru, C., Amin, K., Fabio, A., Berger, R. P., & Wagner, A. K. (2013). S100b as a Prognostic Biomarker in Outcome Prediction for Patients with Severe Traumatic Brain Injury. *Journal of Neurotrauma*, *30*(11), 946–957. https://doi.org/10.1089/neu.2012.2579.

Hack, C. E., & Zeerleder, S. (2001). The endothelium in sepsis: source of and a target for inflammation. *Critical Care Medicine*, *29*(7 Suppl), S21-7. https://doi.org/10.1097/00003246-200107001-00011.

Hardison, R. C. (2012). Evolution of Hemoglobin and Its Genes. *Cold Spring Harbor Perspectives in Medicine*, *2*(12), a011627–a011627. https://doi.org/10.1101/cshperspect.a011627.

Hassan, M., Azzazy, E., & Christenson, R. H. (1997). All About Albumin: Biochemistry, Genetics, and Medical Applications. *Clinical Chemistry*, *43*(10), 2014a–2015. https://doi.org/10.1093/clinchem/43.10.2014a.

Henry, C. R., Satran, D., Lindgren, B., Adkinson, C., Nicholson, C. I., & Henry, T. D. (2006). Myocardial injury and long-term mortality following moderate to severe carbon monoxide poisoning. *JAMA*, *295*(4), 398–402. https://doi.org/10.1001/jama.295.4.398.

Hopper, C. P., Zambrana, P. N., Goebel, U., & Wollborn, J. (2021). A brief history of carbon monoxide and its therapeutic origins. *Nitric Oxide*, *111–112*, 45–63. https://doi.org/10.1016/j.niox.2021.04.001.

Hsia, C. C. (1998). Respiratory function of hemoglobin. *The New England Journal of Medicine*, *338*(4), 239–247. https://doi.org/10.1056/NEJM199801223380407.

Huysal, K., Ustundag Budak, Y., Aydin, U., Demirci, H., Turk, T., & Karadag, M. (2016). COHb Level and High-Sensitivity Cardiac Troponin T in 2012 in Bursa, Turkey: A Retrospective Single-Center Study. *Iranian Red Crescent Medical Journal*, *18*(5). https://doi.org/10.5812/ircmj.27061.

Isgrò, M. A., Bottoni, P., & Scatena, R. (2015). Neuron-Specific Enolase as a Biomarker: Biochemical and Clinical Aspects. *Advances in Experimental Medicine and Biology*, *867*, 125–143. https://doi.org/10.1007/978-94-017-7215-0_9.

Kao, L. W., & Nañagas, K. A. (2005). Carbon Monoxide Poisoning. *Medical Clinics of North America*, *89*(6), 1161–1194. https://doi.org/10.1016/j.mcna.2005.06.007.

Kim, H., Choi, S., Park, E., Yoon, E., Min, Y., & Lampotang, S. (2018). Serum markers and development of delayed neuropsychological sequelae after acute carbon monoxide poisoning: anion gap, lactate, osmolarity, S100B protein, and interleukin-6. *Clinical and Experimental Emergency Medicine*, *5*(3), 185–191. https://doi.org/10.15441/ceem.17.217.

Kim, J. S., Ko, B. S., Sohn, C. H., Kim, Y. J., & Kim, W. Y. (2020). High-Sensitivity Troponin I and Creatinine Kinase-Myocardial Band in Screening for Myocardial Injury in Patients with Carbon Monoxide Poisoning. *Diagnostics (Basel, Switzerland)*, *10*(4). https://doi.org/10.3390/diagnostics10040242.

Kneipp, J., Balakrishnan, G., Chen, R., Shen, T. J., Sahu, S. C., Ho, N. T., Giovannelli, J. L., Simplaceanu, V., Ho, C., & Spiro, T. G. (2006). Dynamics of allostery in hemoglobin: roles of the penultimate tyrosine H bonds. *Journal of Molecular Biology*, *356*(2), 335–353. https://doi.org/10.1016/j.jmb.2005.11.006.

Kornblatt, M. J., & Klugerman, A. (1989). Characterization of the enolase isozymes of rabbit brain: kinetic differences between mammalian and yeast enolases. *Biochemistry and Cell Biology = Biochimie et Biologie Cellulaire*, *67*(2–3), 103–107. https://doi.org/10.1139/o89-016.

Lehninger, A., Nelson, D., & Cox, M. (2000). *Lehninger Principle of Biochemistry* (Third). Worth Publishers.

Liu, H., Zhang, Y., Ren, Y. B., Kang, J., Xing, J., Qi, Q. H., Gao, D. N., Ma, T., Liu, X. W., & Liu, Z. (2015). Serum S100B level may be correlated with carbon monoxide poisoning. *International Immunopharmacology*, *27*(1), 69–75. https://doi.org/10.1016/j.intimp.2015.04.027.

Lopez, D. M., Weingarten-Arams, J. S., Singer, L. P., & Conway, E. E. (2000). Relationship between arterial, mixed venous, and internal jugular carboxyhemoglobin concentrations at low, medium, and high concentrations in a piglet model of carbon monoxide toxicity. *Critical Care Medicine*, *28*(6), 1998–2001. https://doi.org/10.1097/00003246-200006000-00053.

Marks, G. S., Brien, J. F., Nakatsu, K., & McLaughlin, B. E. (1991). Does carbon monoxide have a physiological function? *Trends in Pharmacological Sciences*, *12*, 185–188. https://doi.org/10.1016/0165-6147(91)90544-3.

McGrath, J. J. (1992). Effects of altitude on endogenous carboxyhemoglobin levels. *Journal of Toxicology and Environmental Health*, *35*(2), 127–133. https://doi.org/10.1080/15287399209531601.

Mihailescu, M. R., & Russu, I. M. (2001). A signature of the T → R transition in human hemoglobin. *Proceedings of the National Academy of Sciences*, *98*(7), 3773–3777. https://doi.org/10.1073/pnas.071493598.

Monod, J., Wyman, J., & Changeux, J.-P. (1965). On the nature of allosteric transitions: A plausible model. *Journal of Molecular Biology*, *12*(1), 88–118. https://doi.org/10.1016/S0022-2836(65)80285-6.

Motterlini, R., & Foresti, R. (2017). Biological signaling by carbon monoxide and carbon monoxide-releasing molecules. *American Journal of Physiology-Cell Physiology*, *312*(3), C302–C313. https://doi.org/10.1152/ajpcell.00360.2016.

Opal, S. M., & Esmon, C. T. (2002). Bench-to-bedside review: Functional relationships between coagulation and the innate immune response and their respective roles in the pathogenesis of sepsis. *Critical Care*, *7*(1), 23. https://doi.org/10.1186/cc1854.

Ozkan, S., Salt, O., Durukan, P., Sen, A., Bulbul, E., Duman, A., & Kavalci, C. (2020). The relationship among plasma copeptin, carboxyhemoglobin, and lactate levels in carbon monoxide poisoning. *Human & experimental toxicology*, 39(3), 311–318. https://doi.org/10.1177/0960327119886063.

Park, E., Ahn, J., Min, Y. G., Jung, Y. S., Kim, K., Lee, J., & Choi, S. C. (2012). The usefulness of the serum s100b protein for predicting delayed neurological sequelae in acute carbon monoxide poisoning. *Clinical Toxicology*, *50*(3), 183–188. https://doi.org/10.3109/15563650.2012.658918.

Park, J. H., Heo, R., Kang, H., Oh, J., Lim, T. H., & Ko, B. S. (2020). Diagnostic performance and optimal cut-off values of cardiac biomarkers for predicting cardiac injury in carbon monoxide poisoning. *Clinical and Experimental Emergency Medicine*, *7*(3), 183–189. https://doi.org/10.15441/ceem.19.072.

Pepe, G., Castelli, M., Nazerian, P., Vanni, S., Del Panta, M., Gambassi, F., Botti, P., Missanelli, A., & Grifoni, S. (2011). Delayed neuropsychological sequelae after carbon monoxide poisoning: predictive risk factors in the Emergency Department. A retrospective study. *Scandinavian Journal of Trauma, Resuscitation and Emergency Medicine*, *19*(1), 16. https://doi.org/10.1186/1757-7241-19-16.

Perutz, M. (1987). Molecular anatomy, physiology, and pathology of hemoglobin. In G. Stamatoyannopoulos & A. Nienhuis (Eds.), *The Molecular Basis of Blood Disorders* (p. 127). WB Saunders.

Petousi, N., Copley, R. R., Lappin, T. R. J., Haggan, S. E., Bento, C. M., Cario, H., Percy, M. J., WGS Consortium, Ratcliffe, P. J., Robbins, P. A., & McMullin, M. F. (2014).

Erythrocytosis associated with a novel missense mutation in the BPGM gene. *Haematologica*, *99*(10), e201-4. https://doi.org/10.3324/haematol.2014.109306

Piantadosi, C. A. (1999). Diagnosis and treatment of carbon monoxide poisoning. *Respiratory Care Clinics of North America*, *5*(2), 183–202.

Pritlove, D., Gu, M., Boyd, C., Randeva, H., & Vatısh, M. (2006). Novel Placental Expression of 2,3-Bisphosphoglycerate Mutase. *Placenta*, *27*(8), 924–927. https://doi.org/10.1016/j.placenta.2005.08.010

Réty, S., Sopkova, J., Renouard, M., Osterloh, D., Gerke, V., Tabaries, S., Russo-Marie, F., & Lewit-Bentley, A. (1999). The crystal structure of a complex of p11 with the annexin II N-terminal peptide. *Nature Structural Biology*, *6*(1), 89–95. https://doi.org/10.1038/4965.

Rhodes, M. A., Carraway, M. S., Piantadosi, C. A., Reynolds, C. M., Cherry, A. D., Wester, T. E., Natoli, M. J., Massey, E. W., Moon, R. E., & Suliman, H. B. (2009). Carbon monoxide, skeletal muscle oxidative stress, and mitochondrial biogenesis in humans. *American Journal of Physiology. Heart and Circulatory Physiology*, *297*(1), H392-9. https://doi.org/10.1152/ajpheart.00164.2009.

Sjöstrand, T. (1949). Endogenous Formation of Carbon Monoxide in Man. *Nature*, *164*(4170), 580–581. https://doi.org/10.1038/164580a0.

Sunman, H., Çimen, T., Erat, M., Yayla, K. G., Efe, T. H., Özkan, S., Arslan, E. D., & Açıkel, S. (2018). Red blood cell distribution width as a predictor of long-term mortality in patients with carbon monoxide poisoning. *Turkish journal of emergency medicine*, 18(4), 158–161. https://doi.org/10.1016/j.tjem.2018.05.003.

Thom, S. R., Bhopale, V. M., Milovanova, T. M., Hardy, K. R., Logue, C. J., Lambert, D. S., Troxel, A. B., Ballard, K., & Eisinger, D. (2010). Plasma biomarkers in carbon monoxide poisoning. *Clinical Toxicology (Philadelphia, Pa.)*, *48*(1), 47–56. https://doi.org/10.3109/15563650903468209.

Touger, M., Gallagher, E. J., & Tyrell, J. (1995). Relationship between venous and arterial carboxyhemoglobin levels in patients with suspected carbon monoxide poisoning. *Annals of Emergency Medicine*, *25*(4), 481–483. https://doi.org/10.1016/s0196-0644(95)70262-8.

Weaver, L. K., Valentine, K. J., & Hopkins, R. O. (2007). Carbon monoxide poisoning: risk factors for cognitive sequelae and the role of hyperbaric oxygen. *American Journal of Respiratory and Critical Care Medicine*, *176*(5), 491–497. https://doi.org/10.1164/rccm.200701-026OC.

Yang, X., Caestecker, M., Otterbein, L. E., & Wang, B. (2020). Carbon monoxide: An emerging therapy for acute kidney injury. *Medicinal Research Reviews*, *40*(4), 1147–1177. https://doi.org/10.1002/med.21650.

Zhang, H. Y., Zheng, X. Z., Wang, X. H., Xuan, X. Y., Wang, F., & Li, S. S. (2012). S100A4 mediated cell invasion and metastasis of esophageal squamous cell carcinoma via the regulation of MMP-2 and E-cadherin activity. *Molecular Biology Reports*, *39*(1), 199–208. https://doi.org/10.1007/s11033-011-0726-1.

Zhang, L., Zhao, J., Hao, Q., Xu, X., Han, H., & Li, J. (2021). Serum NSE and S100B protein levels for evaluating the impaired consciousness in patients with acute carbon monoxide poisoning. *Medicine*, *100*(25), e26458. https://doi.org/10.1097/MD.0000000000026458.

Chapter 8

Imaging Methods and Findings in Carbon Monoxide Poisoning

Turkan Ikizceli[1,*]
and Ibrahim Ikizceli[2]
[1]Department of Radiology, University of Health Sciences,
Istanbul Haseki Training and Research Hospital, Istanbul, Turkey
[2]Department of Emergency Medicine,
Istanbul University-Cerrahpasa, Istanbul, Turkey

Abstract

Carbon monoxide (CO) is the most common poisonous gas known, which is a colorless, odorless gas produced by the combustion of organic materials. Symptoms of CO poisoning spread over a large scale. Imaging plays an important role in the diagnosis of CO poisoning with the onset of symptoms. There may be acute or chronic poisoning, and the imaging findings vary accordingly. In addition, imaging methods can objectively and quantitatively evaluate nervous system damage after CO poisoning, evaluate the prognosis of the disease, and evaluate the delayed onset of encephalopathy. Imaging studies, particularly cerebral magnetic resonance imaging (MRI), have high sensitivity but low specificity for detecting brain abnormalities after CO poisoning. Involvement of both the globus pallidus in both the modalities of Computed Tomography (CT) and MRI is typical. In addition, deep white cell involvement is a more suggestive indicator. In the presence of pulmonary symptoms, the first examination is a chest X-ray. In a poor prognosis, a Thorax CT scan is required to demonstrate the damage and spread of the disease in the lungs. Nevertheless, a correlation of imaging studies with clinical history

* Corresponding Author's Email: turkan.ikizceli@sbu.edu.tr.

In: Carbon Monoxide Poisoning
Editors: Seda Özkan and Afsin Ipekci
ISBN: 979-8-89113-217-7

and laboratory data is crucial to perform the correct diagnosis. The importance of imaging in CO poisoning and its findings are summarized.

Keywords: computed tomography, diagnostic imaging, imaging modalities, magnetic resonance imaging

Introduction

Carbon monoxide (CO) is a colorless, odorless, and highly toxic gas produced by the combustion of organic materials (Chenoweth et al., 2021). CO binds to hemoglobin and other heme molecules in the blood, causing tissue hypoxia (Rose et al., 2017). Carboxyhemoglobin (COHb) binds CO to hemoglobin with a 230-270 times greater affinity than oxygen, resulting in tissue hypoxia, reducing the oxygen-carrying capacity and oxygen release to tissues (Varrassi et al., 2017; Bleecker 2015). At low levels of COHb (1-5%), blood flow increases by intrinsic compensatory physiological mechanisms and prevents CO hypoxia through increased oxygen extraction. At a COHb of less than 20%, changes in brain oxygen consumption are negligible, and therefore, brain function is generally unaffected. A 10% reduction in brain oxygen consumption does not occur until a COHb level of 27% is reached (Benignus et al., 1990). In CO poisoning, loss of consciousness with cerebral hypotension occurs, with the possibility of developing delayed neurological sequelae (DNS). DNS may develop after a lucid interval duration of approximately 2-40 days after the acute event; meanwhile, a loss of myelin occurs in the brain, accompanied by a variety of signs and symptoms that are reversible in most patients (Roderique et al., 2015).

Symptoms of CO poisoning spread over a larger scale. Although all organs are affected by CO poisoning, symptoms related to organs with high O2 consumption, especially the brain and heart, are seen in the foreground. Symptoms may appear early or weeks later (Keith et al., 2000). In acute carbon monoxide poisoning, obvious damage occurs mainly in the central nervous system. There are different neuroimaging changes that are relatively specific at different stages of the disease (Liu et al., 2023).

Imaging plays an important role in the diagnosis of CO poisoning with the onset of symptoms. There may be acute or chronic poisoning and imaging findings vary accordingly. In addition, imaging methods can objectively and quantitatively evaluate nervous system damage after CO poisoning, evaluate the prognosis of the disease, and evaluate the delayed onset of encephalopathy

(Liu et al., 2023; Hao et al., 2017). When exposed to CO poisoning, it is a situation that needs urgent treatment.

The severity of symptoms is a more significant indicator to determine the severity of poisoning. The findings of the disease and whether it is acute or chronic determine the first imaging method. In particular, the possibility of delayed sequela may be related to exposure time and blood CO (Kandis et al., 2009).

The pathophysiology can be two-fold:

1. CO strongly binds to hemoglobin and the resulting carboxyhemoglobin in the bloodstream can cause profound hypoxic/anoxic ischemia. Neuronal necrosis or apoptotic cell death may develop with an increase in the level of carboxyhemoglobin (COHb) in the blood. Brain hypoxia that occurs in CO poisoning damages the cerebral cortex through increased excitatory amino acids, as well as oxidative stress, apoptosis, cellular necrosis, and inflammation. This process is probably responsible for the initial neurological abnormalities.
2. CO is also a toxin that interferes with mitochondrial oxidative phosphorylation and activates polymorphonuclear leukocytes, which undergo diapedesis and cause brain lipid peroxidation; this results in the delayed effects of CO poisoning.

Patients can present with acute symptoms of headache, dizziness, different levels of consciousness, seizures, shortness of breath, and angina. Cardiac arrest may occur. In addition to acute symptoms, urinary and fecal incontinence, features of Parkinsonism, gradual psychiatric symptoms, and cognitive dysfunction may develop in chronic poisonings (Lo et al., 2007).

Imaging

Imaging methods according to the clinics of the patients (Table 1).

Chest X-rays (CXR)

Chest X-ray (CXR) is an imaging modality that is easily accessible, inexpensive and takes a short time. CO poisoning may result in hypoxia as a direct result of CO inhalation or cardiac ischemia due to non-cardiogenic pulmonary edema. CXR is the first imaging method to evaluate pulmonary edema in patients with pulmonary symptoms such as dyspnea and hypoxia and is generally normal (Lim et al., 2014). Perihilar fullness, peribronchial findings, or intra-alveolar edema findings may be seen and show a poor prognosis. In this situation, serial chest radiographs reveal progressively worsening changes in acute respiratory distress syndrome (ARDS). In addition, patients should be treated with hyperbaric oxygen (HBO). In pediatric patients, CXR should be performed to see any congenital lung abnormalities that may cause pneumothorax (Baran et al., 2020).

Table 1. Overview of the routinely used imaging modalities, their advantages, and disadvantages for the imaging modality in CO poisoning

Imaging Methods	Advantages	Disadvantages
CXR	Fast imaging	Low specificity
	Low costs	Low sensitivity
	Easily accessible	Not anatomical information
	Low dose radiation	
	Follow-up	
	Pediatric patients	
Ultrasound	High resolution	User dependence
	Not X-ray	Not appropriate for the whole body
	Easily accessible	
	Fast imaging	
	Low costs	
	Real-time imaging	
CT	High resolution	Radiation exposure
	Fast imaging	Low specificity
	Low costs	
MRI	High resolution	High costs
	High sensitivity	Low specificity
	Excellent soft tissue contrast	Time-consuming
PET	Very high sensitivity	Low resolution
	Quantitative analyses	Low specificity
		Radiation exposure

CXR: Chest X-rays, CT: Computed Tomography, MRI: Magnetic Resonance Imaging, PET: Positron Emission Tomography.

Ultrasound

Although ultrasound is a modality that is in real-time, fast imaging, and easily accessible, ultrasound has no place in acute CO toxicity. However, it can be used in the follow-up of chronic organ failure in chronic poisoning and pregnant patients (Delomenie et al., 2015). In addition, cranial ultrasound is useful in the follow-up of neonatal cranial changes after CO poisoning in pediatric patients (Ginsberg et al., 1976). User dependency is its main disadvantage.

Computed Tomography (CT)

Acute CO poisoning occurs as neuronal damage in both the basal ganglia and white matter in the brain of patients. On CT, it is most widely seen as hypodense areas in the deep white matter and low density in both globus pallidus (Figure 1). While the findings increase with the duration and depth of the patient's confusion, they can also be seen in patients with mild mental changes. The presence of low densities in the white matter rather than in globus pallidus is an indicator that determines the prognosis (Silver et al., 1996; Choi et al., 1993). Additionally, cerebral cortical lesions, cerebral edema, hippocampal lesions, and complete loss of gray-white differentiation may be seen on CT imaging. According to studies, age, duration of CO exposure, and time between CO exposure and treatment do not appear to be significantly associated with clinical outcomes, although blood carboxyhemoglobin levels correlate with clinical prognosis (Pracyk et al., 1995).

Thorax CT should be performed to define lung injury and to determine whether CXR is normal in the presence of severe pulmonary symptoms. The appearance of ground glass, the fullness of the perihilar, the findings of the peribronchial or intra-alveolar edema can be seen and show a poor prognosis (Figure 2) (Baran et al., 2020).

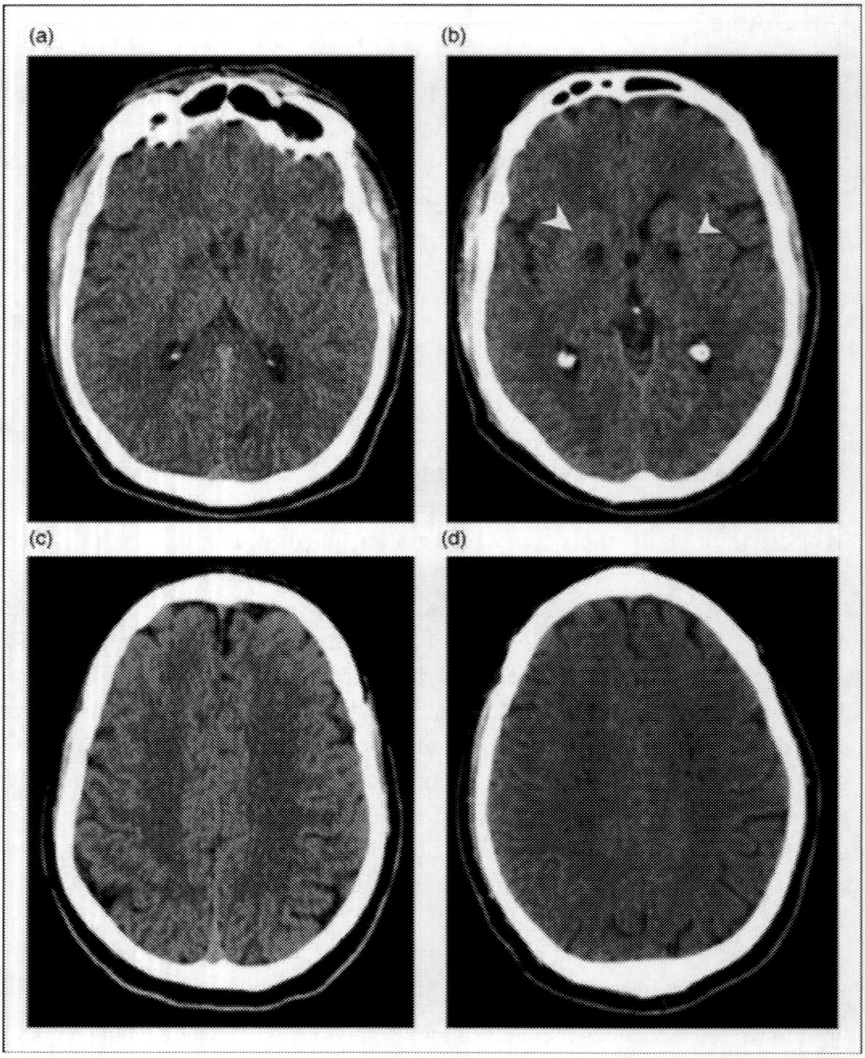

Figure 1. (a) and (c): mildly hypodense areas in bilaterally globus pallidus (yellow aroowheads); no relevant findings in the centrum semiovale. (b) and (d): Six weeks follow-up showing malacic evolution of the bilateral and symmetrical hypodensities in the globus pallidus. The appearance of micro lacunar lesions bilaterally involving centrum semiovale (red arrowhead) (Varrassi et al., 2017).

Magnetic Resonance Imaging (MRI)

Several studies have shown that neuroimaging, especially MRI, has superiority in diagnosing acute damage and neuropathological changes in CO toxicity in the brain. MRI is more sensitive and has higher penetration into soft tissue than CT scanning and is a preferred imaging method in this regard (Saji et al., 2022; Jasne et al., 2019; Kanaya et al., 1992). In acute CO poisoning, a brain MRI should be obtained after the patient is stable in order to show the affected areas and the rate of involvement. The areas of the brain affected by MRI often show greater variation, although in areas similar to CT. The extent of damage seen in MRI is related to clinical outcome, and therefore MRI is not only an imaging modality but also aids in treatment and prognosis (O'Donnell, 2000). Commonly, globus pallidus and white matter involvement are seen with conventional MRI of the brain because poor oxygenation and the hypotension-hypoxia process cause damage (Figure 3a).

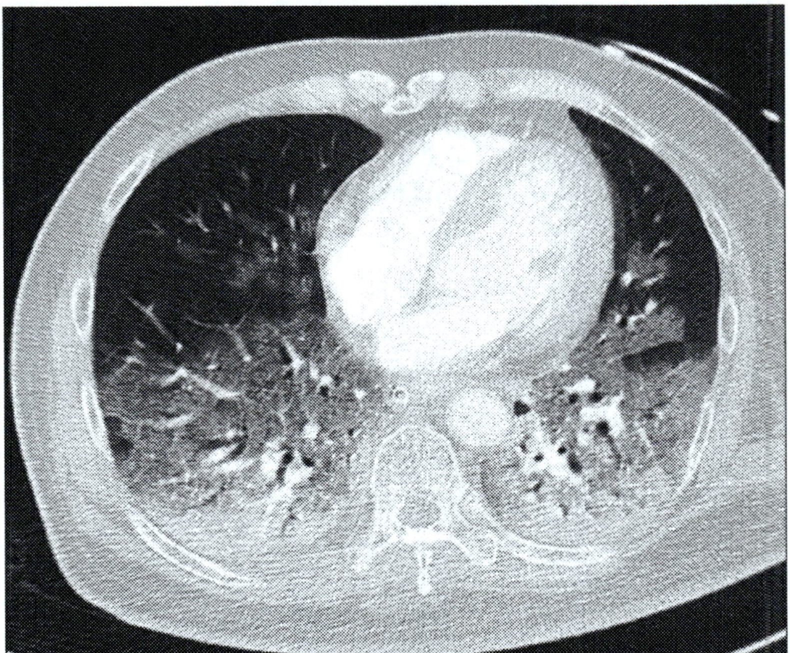

Figure 2. CT image shows compact parenchymal opacification in the dependent lung and non-dependent ground-glass opacification, consistent with acute respiratory distress syndrome (Lim et al., 2014).

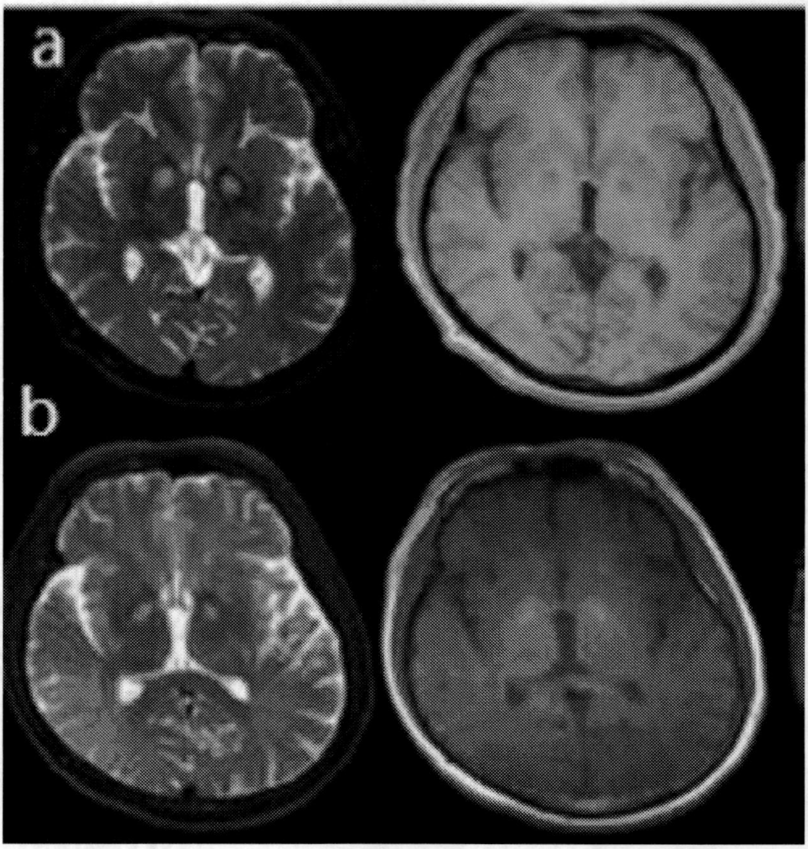

Figure 3a. Brain MRIs in the acute (a) and subacute (b) CO intoxication stages. T2WI shows high signal intensities in the bilateral globus pallidus (red arrowheads), also visualized as subtle low signal intensities on T1WI. (b) Follow-up brain MRIs 26 days after CO exposure reveal slightly high signal changes of the globus pallidus on T2WI and T1WI (Bae et al., 2012).

The area's most commonly affected are those of the brain with higher iron levels. Because of that, these regions are the highest binding target areas for carboxyhemoglobin (Hopkins et al., 2006). Normal iron transport is crucial for brain functions. Iron accumulates gradually over the years in certain regions of the normal brain and especially in the basal ganglia. Histologically, the most iron-rich structures are the globus pallidus and substantia nigra, followed by putamen, caudate nucleus, dentate nucleus, and subthalamic nucleus (Lehéricy et al., 2020). In some hereditary neurodegenerative diseases, this is the reason for iron accumulation in the globus pallidus and other basal ganglia. The reason for the hypointensity of the basal ganglia on MRI as a result of iron accumulation in these diseases is that ferritin shortens the T2 relaxation time on MRI. Using T2-weighted images at 1.5T on MRI, iron deposition is first seen in the globus pallidus, then in the red nucleus and substantia nigra, and then in the dentate nucleus (Aoki et al., 1989).

Signal characteristics include:

- *T1:* usually low signal (affected areas), high signal (hemorrhagic areas)
- *T2/FLAIR:* high signal (affected areas)
- *T1 C+ (Gd):* patchy peripheral enhancement
- *DWI:* increased diffusion signal (affected areas), in the acute phase

Diffusion-weighted imaging (DWI) is an MRI technique based on both qualitative and quantitative measurements of the Brownian movement of water molecules. In cerebral white matter, water molecules tend to be freely distributed along the direction of the axonal fascicles. The DWI should be taken at values of b=1000 s/mm^2. (Lo et al., 2007b). In the acute phase of carbon monoxide poisoning, DWI obtained at b=1000 s/mm^2 shows high-signal-intensity lesions consistent with limited diffusion in the white matter (Figure 3b). It has been reported that lesions may decrease in follow-up MRI. This suggests that white matter may be more sensitive to ischemia than gray matter (Sener, 2003; Durak et al., 2005).

The bilateral globus pallidus with restricted diffusion could be a characteristic MRI finding in patients with acute CO poisoning. However, the relationship between carboxyhemoglobin levels and the variety or severity of MRI findings is unclear (Kim et al., 2016).

Diffusion tensor imaging (DTI) is an MRI technique that uses anisotropic diffusion to estimate the axonal (white matter) microstructures, the location, orientation, and anisotropy of the white matter tracts of the brain (Jellison et al., 2004). Traditionally, in diffusion-weighted imaging (DWI), a three-direction gradient is generally applied. This is sufficient to estimate the trace, or 'average diffusivity' of the diffusion tensor. Clinically, it is considered that trace-weighted images will be useful in the diagnosis of vascular strokes in the brain, for the initial detection (within a few minutes) of hypoxic edema. Further expansion is achieved by the diffusion tensor imaging (DTI) scanning, where at least 6 gradient directions must be scanned to calculate the diffusion tensor. The fractional anisotropy can be calculated. Moreover, the essential aspect of the diffusion tensor can be used to understand the brain's white-matter connections (e.g., tractography; trying to see how parts of the brain relate to others). DTI is capable of sensitively reflecting the damage to gray matter nuclei caused by acute carbon monoxide intoxication and quantifying the degree of hypoxic brain damage to a certain extent and may be related to cognitive impairment (Jiang et al., 2019). DTI can quantitatively reveal white matter microstructure damage and has been correlated with cognitive functions (Hou et al., 2013; Wang et al., 2014).

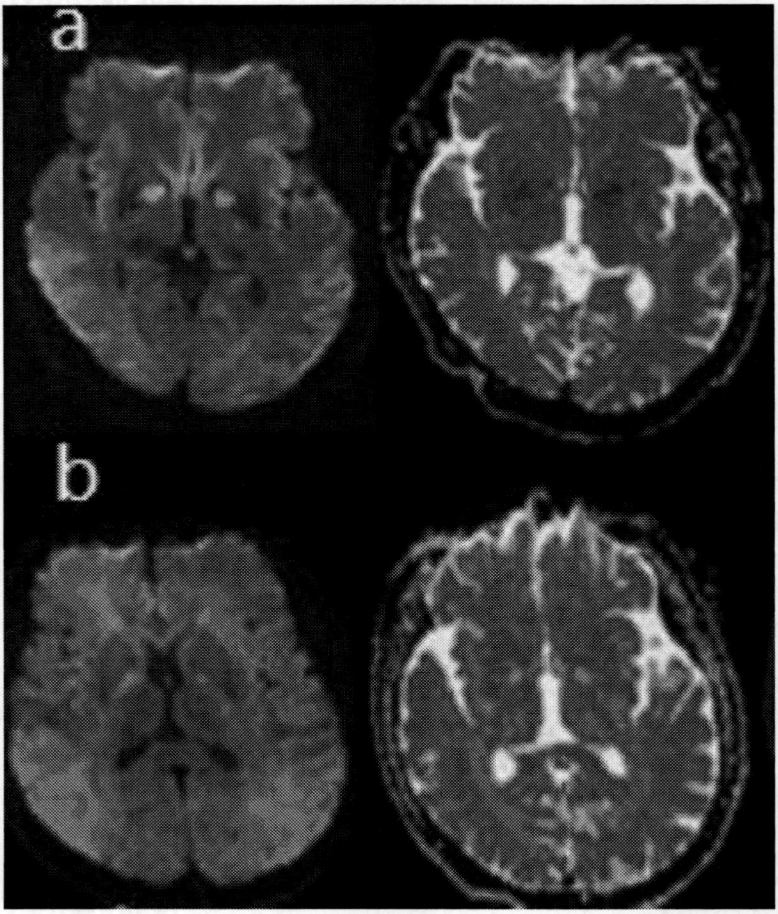

Figure 3b. DWI shows high signal intensities in the bilateral globus pallidus and subtle low signal intensities on ADC. (b) Follow-up brain MRIs 26 days after CO exposure reveal slightly high signal changes of the globus pallidus on DWI, and ADC map (Bae et al., 2012).

Recently developed Susceptibility-weighted imaging (SWI) is more sensitive than other sequences in detecting accumulated hemosiderin and iron secondary to cerebral hemorrhage. Following petechial hemorrhages secondary to acute hypoxic injury during acute and subacute CO poisoning, a low signal on SWI in the globus pallidus, which represents iron or calcium deposition secondary to hypoxic damage in the basal ganglia, especially in the late period, suggests that SWI may be a useful MRI technique to show brain damage in delayed CO poisoning (Figure 3c) (Bae et al., 2012).

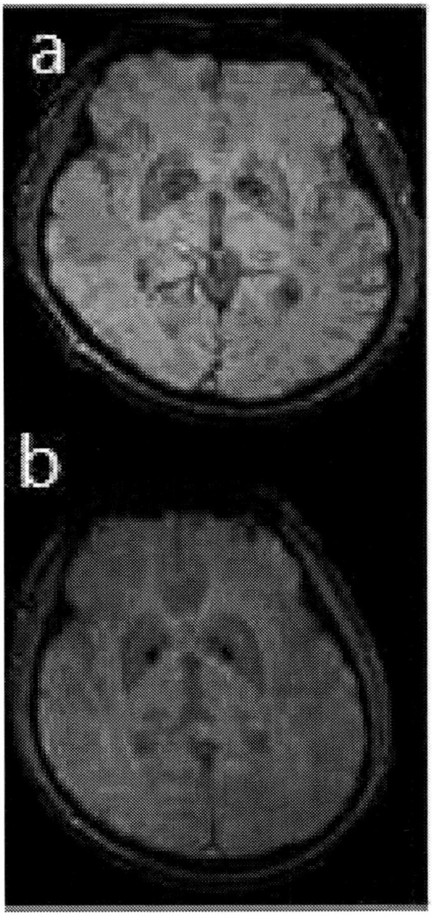

Figure 3c. Brain SWI MRIs in the acute (a) and subacute (b) CO intoxication stages. SWI shows subtle low signal intensities (a) and definite lower signal in the subacute stage (b) (Bae et al., 2012).

The magnetic resonance spectroscopy technique (MRS), one of the most advanced MRI techniques, allows the presence and concentration of various metabolites within the brain tissue to be demonstrated (Al-Okaili et al., 2006). The basic principle of MR spectroscopy (MRS) is that the distribution of electrons within an atom causes nuclei in different molecules to experience a different magnetic field. This results in slightly different resonant frequencies, which return a slightly different signal. The technique is the same as nuclear magnetic resonance (NMR) used in analytical chemistry, but the community often refers to in vivo NMR as MRS to avoid confusion (Mabray & Cha, 2016). Thus, MRS can provide insight into the pathophysiology of CO poisoning by monitoring neurochemical changes, but to date only limited data is available regarding the use of this sequence in detecting the neurological effects of CO poisoning (Kondziella et al., 2009).

According to studies, when white matter and globus pallidus hyperintensities are revealed in MRI, decreased choline (Cho) and N-acetyl aspartate (NAA) creatinine (Cr) ratios can be demonstrated in MRS. MRS may show that ongoing biochemical changes persist despite MRI scanning showing normalization of morphological changes. Generally, MRS is normal in patients with chronic low-dose CO exposure, whereas patients with high-dose exposure show abnormal gray and white matter NAA/Cr, Cho/Cr, and lactate levels in MRS. However, it needs to be confirmed in larger future studies (Kamada et al., 1994; Beppu et al., 2011).

Nuclear Medicine

Positron emission tomography (PET) is a nuclear medicine method that has been used for years and gives a 3D view of physiological processes in the body. Combining the PET device with CT provides anatomical and physiological information to be obtained in a single session and increases the accuracy of the examination (Townsend et al., 2004). PET is a part of neuroimage. The first studies on acute CO poisoning were conducted with single-photon emission computed tomography (SPECT), and regional cerebral perfusion abnormalities were detected in the early period of toxicity (Denays et al., 1994; Lu et al., 2012). Cerebral perfusion failures were observed in 17 (85%) patients, mainly in the frontal, parietal cortex, and basal ganglia. 99mTc-HmPAO scintigraphy appears to be useful in demonstrating early cerebral dysfunction and predicting the extent to which perfusion abnormalities affect brain damage (Figure 4) (Pach et al., 2004; Ozyurt et al., 2008).

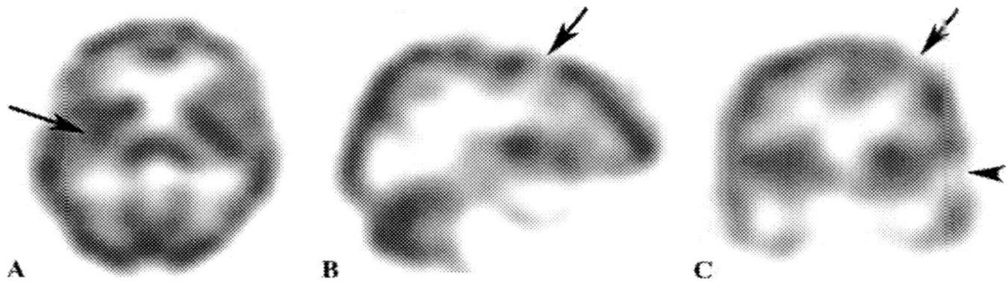

Figure 4. Patients with acute CO intoxication had HMPAO perfusion abnormalities (a) in the basal ganglia (SPECT, transaxial section), (b) frontal lobe (SPECT, sagittal section), (c) temporal lobe and frontal lobe (SPECT, coronal section), respectively (Lu et al., 2012).

On the other hand, in 18 fluoro-deoxyglucose positron emission tomography (18FDG-PET) studies, decreased glucose uptake is observed in the regional areas of cerebral abnormalities in the late period of poisoning (Tengvar et al., 2001). According to case study studies, the presence of hypometabolic activity areas in PET in very late sequelae with symptoms even though there is no finding in MRI shows that PET is a more sensitive imaging tool (Rissanen et al., 2010). In addition, the hypometabolic areas seen in the perivascular areas on PET examination show that the "watershed" areas secondary to hypoxia are not affected (Pinkston et al., 2000).

Further studies are needed to evaluate rCBF for poisoning severity scoring.

Conclusion

As a result, imaging of CO poisoning is widely used in acute and chronic periods and the follow-up of treatment. Although CT and MRI show similar areas of involvement, MRI also provides more detailed findings with advanced techniques (DWI, Spectroscopy, DTI, and SWI). Although nuclear medicine techniques provide more metabolic information, more studies are needed.

References

Al-Okaili, R. N., Krejza, J., Wang, S., Woo, J. H., & Melhem, E. R. (2006). Advanced MR imaging techniques in the diagnosis of intraaxial brain tumors in adults. *Radiographics,* 26, 173-189. https://doi.org/10.1148/rg.26si065513

Aoki, S., Okada, Y., Nishimura, K., Barkovich, A. J., Kjos, B. O., Brasch, R. C., & Norman, D. (1989). Normal deposition of brain iron in childhood and adolescence: MR imaging at 1.5 T. *Radiology*, 172(2), 381-385. https://doi.org/10.1148/radiology.172.2.2748819.

Bae, J. W., Cha, S. Y., Kang, T. H., Lee, J. H., Kim, H. J., Jung, D. S., & Kim, E. J. (2012). Susceptibility-weighted imaging findings of subacute delayed carbon monoxide intoxication: a report of five cases. *Journal of the Neurological Sciences,* 15, 312(1-2), 13-17. https://doi.org/10.1016/j.jns.2011.08.033.

Baran, D. A., Stelling, K., McQueen, D., Pearson, M., & Shah, V. (2020). Pediatric veno-veno extracorporeal membrane oxygenation rescue from carbon monoxide poisoning. *Pediatric Emergency Care,* 36(10), 592-594. https://doi.org/10.1097/PEC.0000000000001486.

Benignus, V. A., Muller, K. E., & Malott, C. M. (1990). Dose-effects functions for carboxyhemoglobin and behavior. *Neurotoxicology and Teratology,* 12(2), 111-118. https://doi.org/10.1016/0892-0362(90)90121-r.

Beppu, T., Nishimoto, H., Fujiwara, S., Kudo, K., Sanjo, K., Narumi, S., Oikawa, H., Onodera, M., Ogasawara, K., & Sasaki, M. (2011). 1H-magnetic resonance spectroscopy indicates damage to cerebral white matter in the subacute phase after CO poisoning. *Journal of Neurology, Neurosurgery, and Psychiatry,* 82(8), 869-875. https://doi.org/10.1136/jnnp.2010.222422.

Bleecker, M. L. (2015). *Carbon monoxide intoxication.* Handbook of Clinical Neurology, 131, 191-203. https://doi.org/10.1016/B978-0-444-62627-1.00024-X.

Chenoweth, J. A., Albertson, T. E., & Greer, M. R. (2021). Carbon monoxide poisoning. *Critical Care Clinics*. 37(3), 657-672. https://doi.org/10.1016/j.ccc.2021.03.010.

Choi, I. S., Kim, S. K., Choi, Y. C., Lee, S. S., & Lee, M. S. (1993). Evaluation of outcome after acute carbon monoxide poisoning by brain CT. *Journal of Korean Medical Science,* 8(1), 78-83. https://doi.org/10.3346/jkms.1993.8.1.78 .

Delomenie, M., Schneider, F., Beaudet, J., Gabriel, R., Bednarek, N., & Graesslin, O. (2015). Carbon monoxide poisoning during pregnancy: presentation of a rare severe case with fetal bladder complications. *Case Reports in Obstetrics and Gynecology,* 2015, 687975. https://doi.org/10.1155/2015/687975.

Denays, R., Makhoul, E., Dachy, B., Tondeur, M., Noel, P., Ham, H. R., & Mols, P. (1994). Electroencephalographic mapping and 99mTc HMPAO single-photon emission computed tomography in carbon monoxide poisoning. *Annals of Emergency Medicine,* 24(5), 947-952. https://doi.org/10.1016/s0196-0644(94)70212-8.

Durak, A. C., Coskun, A., Yikilmaz, A., Erdogan, F., Mavili, E., & Guven, M. (2005). Magnetic resonance imaging findings in chronic carbon monoxide intoxication. *Acta Radiology,* 46(3), 322-327. https://doi.org/10.1080/02841850510021085.

Ginsberg M. D., & Myers R. E. (1976). Fetal brain injury after maternal carbon monoxide intoxication. Clinical and neuropathologic aspects. *Neurology,* 26(1), 15–23. https://doi.org/0.1212/wnl.26.1.15.

Hao, N. N., Tian, C., Lian, K. X., Han, T., & Jin, S. (2017). Imaging diagnosis of 95 cases of moderate and severe acute carbon monoxide poisoning. *Chinese Journal of Industrial Hygiene and Occupational Diseases,* 35(6), 463-467. https://doi.org/10.3760/cma.j.issn.1001-9391.2017.06.016.

Hopkins, R. O., Fearing, M. A., Weaver, L. K., & Foley, J. F. (2006). Basal ganglia lesions following carbon monoxide poisoning. *Brain Injury,* 20(3), 273-281. https://doi.org/10.1080/02699050500488181.

Hou, X., Ma, L., Wu, L., Zhang, Y., Ge, H., Li, Z., Gao, Y., Zhou, Y., & Gao, C. (2013). Diffusion tensor imaging for predicting the clinical outcome of delayed encephalopathy of acute carbon monoxide poisoning. *European Journal of Neurology,* 69(5), 275-280. https://doi.org/10.1159/000346117.

Jasne, A. S., Alsherbini, K. H., Smith, M. S., Pandhi, A., Vagal, A., & Kanter, D. (2019). cerebellar hippocampal and basal nuclei transient edema with restricted diffusion (CHANTER) syndrome. *Neurocritical Care,* 31(2), 288-296. https://doi.org/10.1007/s12028-018-00666-4.

Jellison, B. J., Field, A. S., Medow, J., Lazar, M., Salamat, M. S., & Alexander, A. L. (2004). Diffusion tensor imaging of cerebral white matter: a pictorial review of physics, fiber tract anatomy, and tumor imaging patterns. *American Journal of Roentgenology,* 25(3), 356-369.

Jiang, W., Wu, Q., Zhou, C., Zhao, Z., & Tan, Y. (2020). Gray matter nuclei damage in acute carbon monoxide intoxication assessed in vivo using diffusion tensor MR imaging. *La Radiologia Medica,* 125(1), 80-86. https://doi.org/10.1007/s11547-019-01078-w.

Kamada, K., Houkin, K., Aoki, T., Koiwa, M., Kashiwaba, T., Iwasaki, Y., & Abe, H. (1994). Cerebral metabolic changes in delayed carbon monoxide sequelae studied by proton MR spectroscopy. *Neuroradiology,* 36(2), 104-106. https://doi.org/10.1007/BF00588070.

Kanaya, N., Imaizumi, H., Nakayama, M., Nagai, H., Yamaya, K., & Namiki, A. (1992). The utility of MRI in acute stage of carbon monoxide poisoning. *Intensive Care Medicine,* 18(6), 371-372. https://doi.org/10.1007/BF01694368.

Kandis, H., Katırcı, Y. & Karapolat, B. S. (2009). Karbonmonoksit zehirlenmesi [Carbon Monoxide Poisoning]. *Duzce Medical Journal,* 11 (3), 54-60.

Keith, W., & Van, Meter. (2000). Carbon monoxide poisoning. In Tintinalli, J. E., Kelen, G. D., & Stapczynski, J. S. (Eds). *Emergency Medicine A Comprehensive Study Guide,* (pp: 1302-1306). New York: McGraw-Hill.

Kim, D. M., Lee, I. H., Park, J. Y., Hwang, S. B., Yoo, D. S., & Song, C. J. (2017). Acute carbon monoxide poisoning: MR imaging findings with clinical correlation. *Diagnostic and Interventional Imaging,* 98(4), 299-306. https://doi.org/10.1016/j.diii.2016.10.004.

Kondziella, D., Danielsen, E. R., Hansen, K., Thomsen, C., Jansen, E. C., & Arlien-Soeborg, P. (2009). 1H MR spectroscopy of gray and white matter in carbon monoxide poisoning. *Journal of Neurology*, 256(6), 970-979. https://doi.org/10.1007/s00415-009-5057-y.

Lehéricy, S., Roze, E., Goizet, C., & Mochel, F. (2020). MRI of neurodegeneration with brain iron accumulation. *Current Opinion in Neurology,* 33(4), 462-473. https://doi.org/10.1097/WCO.0000000000000844.

Lim, P. J., Shikhare, S. N., & Peh, W. C. (2014). Clinics in diagnostic imaging (154). Carbon monoxide (CO) poisoning. *Singapore Medical Journal,* 55(8), 405-409, quiz 410. https://doi.org/10.11622/smedj.2014097.

Liu, X. L., & Guan, L. (2023). Research progress on head imaging features of carbon monoxide poisoning and delayed encephalopathy. *Chinese Journal of Industrial Hygiene and Occupational Diseases,* 41(1), 57-62. https://doi.org/10.3760/cma.j.cn121094-20220223-00088.

Lo, C. P., Chen, S. Y., Lee, K. W., Chen, W. L., Chen, C. Y., Hsueh, C. J., & Huang, G. S. (2007). Brain injury after acute carbon monoxide poisoning: early and late complications. *American Journal of Roentgenology,* 189(4), 205-211. https://doi.org/10.2214/AJR.07.2425.

Lo, C. P., Chen, S. Y., Chou, M. C., Wang, C. Y., Lee, K. W., Hsueh, C. J., Chen, C. Y., Huang, K. L., & Huang, G. S. (2007b). Diffusion-tensor MR imaging for evaluation of the efficacy of hyperbaric oxygen therapy in patients with delayed neuropsychiatric syndrome caused by carbon monoxide inhalation. *European Journal of Neurology,* 14(7), 777-782. https://doi.org/10.1111/j.1468-1331.2007.01854.x.

Lu, Y. Y., Tsai, S. C., Kao, C. H., & Lin, W. Y. (2012). Regional cerebral blood flow in patients with carbon monoxide intoxication. *Annals of Nuclear Medicine,* 26(10), 771-776. https://doi.org/10.1007/s12149-012-0638-8.

Mabray, M. C., & Cha, S. (2016). Advanced MR Imaging techniques in daily practice. *Neuroimaging Clinics of North America,* 26(4), 647-666. https://doi.org/10.1016/j.nic.2016.06.010.

O'Donnell, P., Buxton, P. J., Pitkin, A., & Jarvis, L. J. (2005). The magnetic resonance imaging appearances of the brain in acute carbon monoxide poisoning. *Clinical Radiology,* 55(4), 273-280. https://doi.org/10.1053/crad.1999.0369.

Ozyurt, G., Kaya, F. N., Kahveci, F., & Alper, E. (2008). Comparison of SPECT findings and neuropsychological sequelae in carbon monoxide and organophosphate poisoning. *Clinical Toxicology (Philadelphia, Pa.),* 46(3), 218-221. https://doi.org/10.1080/15563650701378704.

Pach, D., Hubalewska, A., Huszno, B., & Pach, J. (2004). Evaluation of regional cerebral perfusion using 99mTc-HmPAO single photon emission tomography (SPET) in carbon monoxide acutely poisoned patients. *Przegl Lek,* 61(4), 217-221.

Pinkston, J. B., Wu, J. C., Gouvier, W. D., & Varney, N. R. (2000). Quantitative PET scan findings in carbon monoxide poisoning: deficits seen in a matched pair. *Archives of Clinical Neuropsychology,* 15(6), 545-553.

Pracyk, J. B., Stolp, B. W., Fife, C. E., & Gray, L., Piantadosi, C. A. (1995). *Brain computerized tomography after hyperbaric oxygen therapy for carbon monoxide poisoning.* Undersea & Hyperbaric Medical Society, 22(1), 1-7.

Rissanen, E., Paavilainen, T., Virta, J., Marttila, R. J., Rinne, J. O., & Airas, L. (2010). Carbon monoxide poisoning-induced nigrostriatal dopaminergic dysfunction detected using positron emission tomography (PET). *Neurotoxicology*, 31(4), 403-407. https://doi.org/10.1016/j.neuro.2010.03.006.

Roderique, J. D., Josef, C. S., Feldman, M. J., & Spiess, B. D. (2015). A modern literature review of carbon monoxide poisoning theories, therapies, and potential targets for therapy advancement. *Toxicology,* 6, 334, 45-58. https://doi.org/10.1016/j.tox.2015.05.004.

Rose, J. J., Wang, L., Xu, Q., McTiernan, C. F., Shiva, S., Tejero, J., & Gladwin, M. T. (2017). Carbon monoxide poisoning: pathogenesis, management, and future directions of therapy. *American Journal of Respiratory and Critical Care Medicine,* 195(5), 596-606. https://doi.org/10.1164/rccm.201606-1275CI.

Saji, A. S., Raza, M. H., Anjum, A. S., Maqsood, H., Yousaf, J., & Saleem, S. (2022). Carbon monoxide poisoning with an atypical presentation on MRI: Case report and literature review. *Annals of Medicine and Surgery,* 14, 82, 104655. https://doi.org/10.1016/j.amsu.2022.104655.

Sener, R. N. (2003). Acute carbon monoxide poisoning: diffusion MR imaging findings. *American Journal of Neuroradiology,* 24(7), 1475-1477.

Silver, D. A., Cross, M., Fox, B., & Paxton, R. M. (1996). Computed tomography of the brain in acute carbon monoxide poisoning. *Clinical Radiology,* 51(7), 480-483. https://doi.org/10.1016/s0009-9260(96)80186-3.

Tengvar, C., Johansson, B., & Sorensen, J. (2004). Frontal lobe and cingulate cortical metabolic dysfunction in acquired akinetic mutism: a PET study of the interval form of carbon monoxide poisoning. *Brain Injury,* 18(6), 615-625. https://doi.org/10.1080/02699050310001622806.

Townsend, D. W., Carney, J. P., Yap, J. T., & Hall, N. C. (2004). PET/CT today and tomorrow. *Journal of Nuclear Medicine,* 45, 4-14.

Varrassi, M., Di Sibio, A., Gianneramo, C., Perri, M., Saltelli, G., Splendiani, A., & Masciocchi, C. (2017). Advanced neuroimaging of carbon monoxide poisoning. *The Neuroradiology Journal,* 30(5), 461-469. https://doi.org/10.1177/1971400916589342.

Wang, G., Zhang, C., Chen, W., Yang, X., Sun, Y., & Li, S. (2014). Correlation between diffusion tensor imaging and cognitive dysfunction in patients with delayed encephalopathy after acute carbon monoxide poisoning. *Chinese Journal of Industrial Hygiene and Occupational Diseases,* 32(10), 769-771.

Chapter 9

The Emergency Management of Carbon Monoxide Poisoning

Sevil Kuşku Kıyak*
and Yonca Senem Akdeniz
Department of Emergency Medicine, Cerrahpaşa School of Medicine,
İstanbul University-Cerrahpaşa, İstanbul, Turkey

Abstract

Carbon monoxide (CO) is a toxic, invisible gas that causes fatal consequences if not detected. The clinical manifestations are non-spesific and range from headache to unconsciousness, so they are not easy to detect. The diagnosis is based on clinical symptoms and suspicion of CO poisoning. The measurement of the level of carboxyhemoglobin (COHb) is the most important test in for a definitive diagnosis. However, negative COHb levels do not rule out the disease if the history and symptoms support it. The mainstay of treatment includes 100% normobaric oxygen administration with a non-rebreathing mask and should be started immediately after suspicion, especially in the prehospital setting. Hyperbaric oxygen therapy (HBOT) is a choice of treatment if necessary, and should also be initiated within 6 hours. If symptoms persist or the patient's clinical status gets worse despite oxygen therapy, other possible differential diagnoses should be considered. Furthermore, delayed neurological sequelae (DNS) is a serious complication that can develop after discharge, and all patients should be informed about it.

Keywords: CO poisoning, carboxyhemoglobin, emergency management

---

* Corresponding Author's Email: drsevilkusku@gmail.com.

In: Carbon Monoxide Poisoning
Editors: Seda Özkan and Afsin Ipekci
ISBN: 979-8-89113-217-7

Introduction

Carbon monoxide (CO) is a colorless, odorless, tasteless, and non-irritant gas that is produced by the incomplete burning of carbon containing materials. The concentration of CO in the atmosphere is generally low, approximately 0,03-0,20 parts per million (ppm) or less. The reason for these low levels is that CO does not occur naturally and is associated with human activities (Mattiuzzi and Lippi, 2020).

The incidence of CO poisoning in 2017 is 137 cases per million and 4.6 deaths per million worldwide. Between the years 1992-2017, a significant decrease occured in the risk of death from CO poisoning. The number of cases per million decreased from 7.2 to 4.6 even though worldwide incidence of CO poisoning did not change during the last 25 years. Thus, the mortality rate due to CO poisoning has decreased (Mattiuzzi and Lippi, 2020).

CO can be produced endogenously and exogenously.

Endogenous CO is produced in the body as a by-product of normal cellular metabolism. It is produced by the enzymatic breakdown of heme, a component of hemoglobin, myoglobin, and other heme-containing proteins. Endogenous CO plays an important role as a neurotransmitter, along with nitric oxide and hydrogen sulfide (Tomaszewski, 2011).

Exogenous CO is produced from external sources, typically from the incomplete combustion of fossil fuels such as gasoline, natural gas, and coal. Exposure to high levels of exogenous CO can be dangerous and even deadly (Tomaszewski, 2011).

In a healthy human body, carboxyhemoglobin (COHb) levels typically range from 0-5%. However, exposure to high levels of exogenous CO can increase COHb levels in the blood, leading to carbon monoxide poisoning (Tomaszewski, 2011).

CO exposure is a severe health concern, and its prevalence and causes can vary greatly depending on the society, climate, level of development, and occupation. In developed countries, industrial accidents, exhaust gases, and suicide attempts are some of the primary causes of CO exposure. In contrast, in colder countries, especially during winter, household poisonings due to the use of heating equipment such as stoves and boilers are more common. This is because of the increased use of heating equipment in such climates, which can lead to inadequate ventilation and higher concentrations of CO (Mattiuzzi and Lippi, 2020).

Certain groups are also at a higher risk of CO exposure, including firefighters, police officers, and industrial workers. The reason for this is their frequent exposure to environments where CO is produced, such as fires, industrial processes, and traffic. These work groups must take extra precautions to protect themselves from CO exposure, such as wearing proper protective equipment, monitoring CO levels, and ensuring proper ventilation in their workspaces (Ozkan and Ipekci, 2022).

Treatment of carbon monoxide poisoning is primarily supportive with the aim of reducing CO concentration and restoring normal oxygen levels. Supplemental oxygen is the mainstay of therapy and should be administered as soon as possible (Ozkan and Ipekci, 2022).

Overall, understanding the different causes and risks of CO exposure is essential to prevent its harmful effects. People should take appropriate measures to avoid exposure, including maintaining and using the correct heating equipment, installing CO detectors in homes and workplaces, and also following safety protocols in occupational settings (Ozkan and Ipekci, 2022).

Pathophysiology

CO enters the body by inhalation and can diffuse through the alveolar-capillary membrane in the lungs and enter the bloodstream, where it can rapidly bind to hemoglobin to form carboxyhemoglobin (COHb). COHb reduces the amount of hemoglobin available to carry oxygen, leading to tissue hypoxia (lack of oxygen) and ischemia (reduced blood flow to tissues). CO toxicity is the result of both tissue hypoxia-ischemia and cellular damage caused by CO, which results in multiple organ failure and cardiovascular collapse (Fan et al., 2012; Ozkan and Ipekci, 2022).

CO has a strong affinity for the heme iron moiety, a component of hemoglobin, which is responsible for carrying oxygen. Its affinity is almost 230-300 times greater than that for oxygen. CO binds to hemoglobin, forming COHb, and it can also bind to other proteins and enzymes in the body, disrupting their function. One of these proteins is cardiac myoglobin; it prevents oxidative phosphorylation in cardiac mitochondria and causes cardiac ischemia that can result in cardiogenic pulmonary edema (Teerapuncharoen et al., 2015). Futhermore, intracellular CO impairs the function of cytochrome C oxydase which is an important enzyme involved in cellular respiration. The result is hypoxia, which has an impact particularly on the central nervous system and heart because these organs are more sensitive to oxygen deprivation. Additionally, CO can cause immunological and inflammatory damage at the cellular level through various processes such as neutrophil activation, lymphocyte proliferation, mitochondrial dysfunction, and lipid peroxidation (Jüttner et al., 2021).

The severity of CO toxicity depends on the concentration and duration of exposure to CO, as well as individual factors such as age, health status, and smoking history.

Clinical Manifestations

Symptoms of CO toxicity are non-spesific and variable, so it can easily interfere with other diseases. There is no distinctive symptomatology in the literature. The symptoms commonly include headache, dizziness, fatigue, nausea, weakness, chest pain, shortness of breath, confusion, and loss of consciousness, and in severe cases, can lead to coma, brain damage, and death. Patients can be found unconscious, and a history may not be obtained. If there is no evidence of trauma, the initial physical findings include mental status deterioration, tachycardia, and tachypnea. The brain and heart need more oxygen; therefore, the effect of CO is greater on these organs (Rose et al., 2017).

Neurological symptoms at first may be mild. Headache is the most common symptom, dizziness, nausea, and weakness follow it. As the CO level increases confusion, syncope, epileptic seizures, and coma occur. Patients may also present with stroke-like symptoms (Fan et al., 2012; Ozkan and Ipekci, 2022).

As the CO level increases, there is a disequilibrium between the blood flow and the oxygen use of the myocardium. The early cardiac symptoms are due to cardiac hypoxia. Angina and exercise intolerance are the initial symptoms. In moderate to severe cases, dysrhythmias, myocardial ischemia, infarction, and cardiac arrest may occur, and thus being associated with increased mortality. Ventricular arrhythmias caused by hypoxia in the myocardium are the most important cause of death (Rose et al., 2017).

In addition, metabolic acidosis, and elevated lactate levels may occur due to tissue hypoxia (Manaker and Perry, 2021).

The other affected target system is the musculocutaneous system. The skin bullae and the cherry-red skin color can be seen. Rhabdomyolysis and acute renal failure may develop (Fan et al., 2012; Ozkan and Ipekci, 2022).

The effects of CO exposure are not only acute, delayed neuropsychiatric syndrome (DNS) is a well-documented phenomenon that mainly occurs 2-40 days after exposure (mean 20 days) and includes variable degrees of neurologic abnormalities. Cognitive deficits, amnesia, dementia, hallucinations, parkinsonism, mutism, psychosis, personality changes, movement disorders, cortical blindness, peripheral neuropathy, and focal neurological deficits may occur (Manaker and Perry, 2021). Risk factors for developing DNS include age and loss of consciousness in the acute phase of toxicity. The mechanism is poorly understood. It probably involves lipid peroxidation by reactive oxygen species generated by xanthine oxidase. Xanthine oxidase is produced *in situ* and adheres to damaged endothelial cells. During recovery, ischemia-reperfusion injury and exposure to hyperoxia may alter oxidative damage. The lesions mainly occur in the cerebral white matter, MRI studies show damage to the white matter and the hippocampus. Animal studies have shown that does not only elevated COHb concentrations cause lesions, but there must also be an episode of hypotension (Tomaszewski, 2011).

Chronic effects are also seen in patients who experienced low levels of CO exposure for a long time. These effects vary a lot, chronic fatigue, headache, dizziness, personality disorders, sleep disorders, peripheral neuropathies, recurrent infections, polycythemia can be seen. Neuropsychiatric evaluation should be performed if daily functions are altered due to these abnormalities (Rose et al., 2017).

Diagnosis

In CO poisoning, the diagnosis begins with suspicion. Detailed anamnesis is very important because it mimics different diseases. It should be questioned whether there is a source of CO at home or at work. Then the blood COHb level should be measured as a diagnostic test. The COHb level should be measured by co-oximeter devices rather than routine blood gas devices because routine blood gas devices can only measure the level of oxyhemoglobin (02Hb). The co-oximeter device also measures deoxyhemoglobin, methemoglobin, and COHb levels. Even though oxygen saturation should not be measured by pulse oximetry, it could be falsely high in CO poisoning. It is because COHb can be misinterpreted as oxyhemoglobin. Newer pulse oximeters and co-oximeters are capable of measuring COHb correctly (Tomaszewski, 2011).

The measurement of the COHb level can be made from arterial or venous blood samples. The clinical trials reveal that there is no significant difference in both samples. Even though there is a correlation between COHb levels and clinical symptoms, exposure time is also important, and serious complications can be seen in low COHb levels. On the other hand, the level of COHb decreases with time and oxygen therapy, so it may not indicate the degree of exposure (Manaker and Perry, 2021).

Table 1. Symptoms of CO poisoning

Symptoms of mild	Symptoms of severe
Headache Dizziness Nausea Vomiting Weakness Visual disturbances Flu-like symptoms	Change of consciousness Disorientation Convulsions Dyspnea Anginal Chest pain Dysrhythmias Pulmonary edema Ischemic changes in EKG Abnormality in cardiac markers Metabolic acidosis Extremely high carboxyhemoglobin levels

Additional laboratory tests may be performed in order to determine the severity of the disease. The presence of metabolic acidosis in the arterial or venous blood gas is important. Metabolic acidosis is risky in terms of exposure time, the presence of serious findings, and delayed neurological sequelae. Higher lactate levels indicate severe poisoning (Rose et al., 2017).

If there is muscle and myocardial cell damage, creatine phosphokinase and troponin levels may increase. If rhabdomyolysis occurs myoglobinuria occurs, and blood urea nitrogen and creatinine levels may increase (Rose et al., 2017).

It is difficult to distinguish mild or severe CO poisoning. Patients can be easily misdiagnosed with a viral illness if they have mild symptoms (Table 1). If a patient has a persistent headache and a group of people has the same symptoms, CO poisoning should be kept in mind. Furthermore, if a patient is found unconscious at home CO poisoning should be considered together with toxicological, metabolic, and traumatic differential diagnosis (Rose et al., 2017).

Cardiac monitoring and 12 lead electrocardiography (ECG) can reveal non-spesific changes. The ECG findings range from normal to arrhythmias and ischemia. The common electrophysiological disturbance is QT interval prolongation. In severe intoxication, non-cardiogenic pulmonary edema may occur. On chest radiographs, perihilar and peribronchial infiltrations are signs of a poor prognosis (Rose et al., 2017).

Neuropsychological evaluation should be considered, for documentation of neurologic status a mini-mental status examination can be made. Imaging modalities in CO intoxication can be used and can be helpful in determining the treatment strategy. Because mental deterioration is common, brain computed tomography (CT) and magnetic resonance imaging (MRI) can give information and show lesions. Brain CT can show acute changes within 12 hours of CO exposure. Symmetric low-density areas of globus pallidus, putamen, and caudate nuclei can be detected on brain CT. The most common MRI findings are white matter hyperintensities (WMH) and hippocampal atrophy (Rose et al., 2017; Parkinson et al., 2002). Bazal ganglia lesions are better detected by MRI. Diffusion-weighted imaging (DWI) is used to detect lesions earlier than conventional MRI. However, most studies involving DWI focus on the subacute or chronic phase of CO poisoning (Moon et al., 2018). Single photon emission tomography (SPECT) is a successful technique that shows ischemia in CO poisoning. Perfusion defects are usually associated with impairment of neuropsychological status (Gale et al., 1999).

Numerous neuropsychiatric tests are available for patients with possible neurological involvement. As a result, they were found to be effective in detecting the acute effects of CO poisoning on cortical functions.

Prehospital Management

As CO is an odorless, colorless, and tasteless gas, it is difficult to suspect at the scene. For the rescuer, it is important to recognize any threat of CO. While protecting himself, the rescuer should immediately remove the patient away from the scene.

Regardless of oxygen saturation (SpO2), oxygen administration at the highest concentration is the most necessary treatment option (Jüttner et al., 2021). The route of administration of oxygen in alert patients is 15L/min through a non-rebreather mask. If the airway is not safe, appropriate invasive airway protection techniques should be administered. The patient should be monitored, ECG should be taken, respiratory rate and blood pressure measured, and oxygen saturation monitored by pulse oximetry. Additionally, during the transportation of oxygen, the administration that has been started should continue without interruption (Jüttner et al., 2021).

For the decision of transporting the patient to the nearest suitable hospital, informing the emergency service about the patient's state of consciousness might be beneficial for the requirement of hyperbaric oxygen therapy (HBOT). Furthermore, it is important to learn the exposure time to CO (Jüttner et al., 2021).

Emergency Department Management

The initial treatment begins with stabilizing the patient's (A) airway, (B) breathing, and (C) circulation, with cardiac monitorization and intravenous access. 100% oxygen should be applied with a non-rebreathing mask. Vital signs, blood pressure, pulse, temperature, and respiratory rate should be carefully interpreted, especially if the patient has hypotension treatment with IV fluids and inotropes can be started (Manaker and Perry, 2021).

Then a neurological examination should be performed. If the patient is comatose or has altered mental status intubation should be performed without delay and 100% oxygen should be applied. Then to detect COHb, Ph, and lactate levels, blood gas analysis should be determined. A 12-lead ECG should be performed, and cardiac biomarkers (CK, CK-MB, and Troponin) should be studied if the patient has cardiac symptoms and history (Jüttner et al., 2021).

Since the symptoms of CO poisoning are non-specific, other differential diagnoses should be considered. If intoxication or substance abuse is suspected, toxicological screening can be performed. In addition, if there is no or little improvement despite treatment or is any evidence of trauma, brain imaging should be considered. In a study, nearly 1/3 of patients with intentional CO poisoning were found to have additional intoxications, especially with alcohol (Hampson and Bodwin, 2013). Some patients may develop life-threatening dysrhythmias, so standard advanced cardiac life support protocols can be followed.

The mainstay of treatment is oxygen administration. 100% normobaric oxygen therapy (NBOT) by non-rebreathing mask or if the patient is intubated by endotracheal tube. Treatment should continue until the COHb level decrease to normal (<%3) or the patient becomes asymptomatic (Jüttner et al., 2021).

Overview of Carbon Monoxide Poisoning and Emergency Management

Obtain a history if there is a potential CO exposure, patients or pets feel bad, and also the air should be tested for the presence of CO (Manaker and Perry, 2021).

Major symptoms: loss of consciousness, altered mental state, confusion, syncope, epileptic seizures, focal neurological deficit, chest pain, dyspnea, respiratory failure, ventricular dysrhythmia (Fan et al., 2012).

Common symptoms: headache, nausea, vomiting, dizziness, weakness, malaise, visual disturbances, and impaired concentration (Ozkan and Ipekci, 2022).

Physical examination mainly focuses on mental status, but surely cardiac symptoms, such as tachycardia and tachypnea, should be considered (Rose et al., 2017).

Stabilizing the airway, breathing, and circulation, in case of need intubation should be performed (Figure 1).

If the clinical status is poor, cardiac and oxygen saturation should be monitored, application of oxygen to maintain oxygen saturation>90% is important. Vascular access should be provided (Manaker and Perry, 2021).

If there is suspicion of CO poisoning, apply high-flow oxygen regardless of pulse oximetry or arterial pO2 (Jüttner et al., 2021).

Diagnostic evaluation starts with COHb level measurement with co-oximetry of arterial or venous blood. COHb>3% in non-smokers, and >10% in smokers are abnormal.

Stabilization of cardiovascular status and blood pressure is important. If hypotension occurs, it should be treated with IV fluids and inotropic agents. If life-threatening dysrhythmias occur, advanced cardiac life support can be administered (Manaker and Perry, 2021).

If the patient has major symptoms, the acid-base status should be checked from blood gas (preferably in arterial) (Jüttner et al., 2021).

In symptomatic patients, ECG should be obtained also cardiac biomarkers measured, especially if the patient has cardiac risk factors, a history of cardiac disease, or an ischemia on the ECG (Jüttner et al., 2021).

Urine and serum pregnancy should be checked tests in female patients of childbearing age.

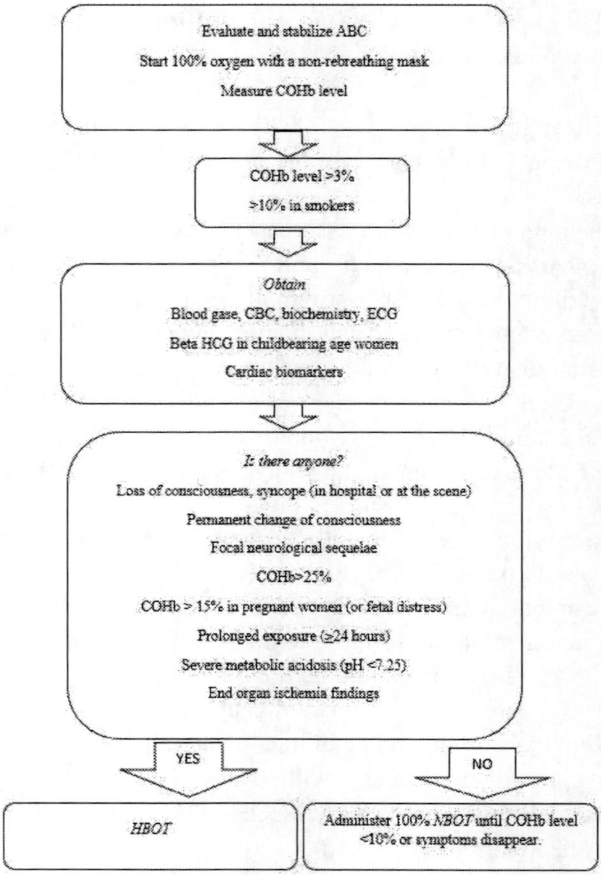

Figure 1. Emergency Department Approach Algorithm in Carbon Monoxide Poisoning.

If the diagnosis is not clear, other diagnostic tests should be performed, for example, brain CT, influenza tests, and toxicologic tests (Jüttner et al., 2021).

Treatment starts with removing the patients from the scene. The patient with smoke inhalation who has altered mental status, metabolic acidosis, hemodynamic instability, empiric treatment for cyanide poisoning with hydroxocobalamin is suggested (Manaker and Perry, 2021).

Hyperbaric oxygen (HBO) is suggested for: (Manaker and Perry, 2021)

- COHb level>25% (>15% if pregnant)
- Found unconscious at scene or hospital, if a syncope occurs
- Altered mental status (GCS<15), confusion, coma, seizure
- Severe metabolic acidosis (pH <7.25) after empiric cyanide treatment administration
- Evidence of end-organ ischemia (ECG changes, elevated cardiac biomarkers, focal neurological deficit, altered mental status, respiratory failure)
- Abnormal cerebellar function
- Fetal distress during pregnancy
- Prolonged CO exposure (≥24 hours)
- Age ≥36 years

An important point to remember is that COHb levels do not always correlate with the severity of poisoning, especially if time has passed. Any abnormally elevated levels of COHb accompanied by major symptoms should be considered significant poisoning (Jüttner et al., 2021).
The purpose of HBO is to increase the clearance of CO and also to prevent delayed neuropsychiatric syndrome. Patients can benefit from HBO up to 24 hours after exposure (Manaker and Perry, 2021).

Treatment

The main aim of the treatment of CO poisoning is to remove CO from tissues and the body as soon as possible (Jüttner et al., 2021). The current treatment for CO exposure is 100% normobaric oxygen therapy (NBOT) and hyperbaric oxygen therapy (HBOT) in 2.5-3 atmospheres (Rose et al., 2017). Oxygen removes CO from the body faster than air and prevents hypoxia. Normally, the separation time of CO from Hb in air in room is 320 minutes. When 100% NBOT is applied with a non-rebreathing reservoir mask, this time is reduced to 74 minutes. HBOT further shortens the time it takes for CO to leave Hb and can reduce this time to 20 minutes (Rose et al., 2017; Hampson et al., 2012).

Patients who are unable to maintain spontaneous breathing and protect the airway should be intubated and connected to a mechanical ventilator.

The recommended tools for use in oxygen therapy in patients with CO poisoning are:

- Non-rebreathing mask with reservoir
- High flow nasal cannula
- Non-invasive mechanical ventilation (CPAP)
- Invasive mechanical ventilation
- Hyperbaric oxygen therapy

Patients with altered mental status or with neurological or cardiovascular dysfunction may require hospitalization. It is because these patients may develop comorbidity.

Non-Rebreathing Mask with Reservoir

The initial treatment of CO poisoning starts with the administration of oxygen by a non-rebreathing mask. Traditionally, NBOT should be administered >15L/minute. Patients with mild symptoms and pregnant patients should take 100% NBOT until they are symptom-free or their COHb level falls below 3% (Jüttner et al., 2021). This is usually achieved by administering 100% NBO after 5-6 hours (approximately 375 minutes). Patients should be closely followed as long as they receive oxygen treatment, and those with heart disease should be monitored (Jüttner et al., 2021).

Patients with mild symptoms should receive oxygen treatment unless they become symptom-free. If the symptoms persist, the treatment should continue, and other causes of symptoms should be investigated (Jüttner et al., 2021).

High Flow Nasal Cannula Oxygen

In the last two decades, high-flow nasal cannula (HFNC) oxygen administration has begun to be used as an alternative respiratory support device to traditional oxygen therapy tools in critically ill patients (Kim et al., 2020; Nishimura, 2019). HFNC delivers heated (37°C) and humidified (100% RH) oxygen with a safe inspired fraction (FiO2) at 21% to 100% at a high flow rate. HFNC is a less invasive ventilation system and allows the adjustment of FiO2 regardless of the flow rate (Long et al., 2021; Rochwerg et al., 2020).

HFNC has many advantages over conventional oxygen tools that result in better physiological effects. HFNC improves oxygenation, reduces airway resistance, increases the leaching of carbon dioxide (CO2) in the anatomical dead space, provides humidified flow, and provides low levels of positive end-expiratory pressure (PEEP) through high flow rates. Based on the monitored oxygen concentration, FiO2 can be titrated up to 60 liters per minute (Tomruk et al., 2019; Kim et al., 2020; Long et al., 2021).

HFNC is used in diseases such as acute hypoxemic respiratory failure, respiratory distress syndrome, coronavirus disease 2019, interstitial lung disease, chronic obstructive pulmonary disease (COPD), pneumonia, sleep apnea, cardiogenic pulmonary edema (Tomruk et al., 2019; Long et al., 2021). The successful treatment results of HFNC in acute hypoxemic diseases in a short time have led to its trial as a treatment method in acute CO poisoning (Tomruk et al., 2019; Long et al., 2021).

Randomized controlled trials have compared HFNC with conventional normobaric oxygen in patients with acute CO exposure. It was found that HFNC reduced COHb levels significantly faster and reduce the half-life of COHb values compared to oxygen therapy with a normobaric mask (Tomruk et al., 2019; Kim et al., 2020; Yesiloglu et al., 2021; Dong et al., 2022).

In the treatment of mild to moderate acute CO poisoning, HFNC is considered to be an easy, safe, comfortable, and effective method to reduce COHb (Ozturan et al., 2019).

Noninvasive Mechanical Ventilation (NIMV)

Noninvasive mechanical ventilation (NIMV) is a method that applies positive pressure respiratory support through a mask and device without intubation in patients with spontaneous breathing. For this purpose, standard mechanical ventilators and/or portable devices produced for NIMV can be used (Roth et al., 2018; Bal et al., 2020; Turgut et al., 2020).

NIMV is used for various purposes due to its short- and long-term effects. Its short-term effects are improvement of symptoms, improvement of oxygenation, reduction of respiratory load, and prevention of intubation. Due to these effects, its use is increasing in emergency departments, especially in the treatment of hypoxic and hypercarbic respiratory failure. There are two modes used in NIMV: continuous positive airway pressure (CPAP, Continuous positive airway pressure) and bilevel positive airway pressure (BPAP, Bilevel positive airway pressure) (Roth et al., 2018; Bal et al., 2020; Turgut et al., 2020).

CPAP is the mode in which continuous positive pressure is applied at the same value in both inspiration and expiration. Equivalent to positive end-expiratory pressure (PEEP) in invasive mechanical ventilation. CPAP ventilation provides an inspiratory oxygen fraction of 1.0 compared to 0.6 using a reservoir face mask and increases gas exchange (Roth et al., 2018). It increases functional residual capacity, opens collapsed or unventilated alveoli, increases oxygenation, and reduces respiratory load and airway resistance. CPAP is useful in patients with hypoxemic respiratory failure (such as acute respiratory distress syndrome, pneumonia, and acute cardiogenic pulmonary edema) (Roth et al., 2018).

It was thought that NIMV could be effective, especially in acute CO exposure to CPAP. In studies with the use of CPAP in CO poisoning, it has been shown that CPAP treatment significantly shortens the half-life of COHb at pressures of 5-12 mbar (Roth et al., 2018; Bal et al., 2020; Turgut et al., 2020).

In CO poisoning, prehospital and emergency department use of CPAP is recommended (Roth et al., 2018; Bal et al., 2020; Turgut et al., 2020).

Invasive Mechanical Ventilation

The most sensitive organs to hypoxia are the brain and heart because of their high oxygen demand. As a result, patients with severe CO poisoning may have a loss of consciousness and ischemic cardiac changes that can result in respiratory failure. Therefore, there is a need for endotracheal intubation and mechanical ventilation. Adequate airway management should be provided in a timely manner for CO poisoning.

According to a retrospective observational study with a sample size of 796 patients diagnosed with CO poisoning, 186 were intubated, and the intubation rate of all patients with CO poisoned was 23.4%. The mean duration of mechanical ventilation was 4.3 days (range, 0.5-42) (Shen et al., 2015).

Hampson and Hauff conducted a study with 1505 patients treated with hyperbaric oxygen, 1473 patients were included. 50 patients had died within 90 days after poisoning (3.4%). In this study, the strongly associated factors with mortality were severe metabolic acidosis and the need for endotracheal intubation (Hampson and Hauff, 2008). Due to this, we can say that the need for endotracheal intubation is a poor prognostic factor.

Respiratory abnormalities suggestive of the need for mechanical ventilation: (Hyzy and McSparron, 2022)

- Apnea, stridor, severely depressed mental state, flail chest, inability to clear respiratory secretions, trauma to mandible, larynx, and trachea.
- Loss of ventilatory reserve
- Refractory Hypoxemia
- Hypoventilation periperal nervous system/respiratory muscle dysfunction (toxins, muscular dystrophy)
- Chest wall and pleural disease (kyphoscoliosis, trauma, massive pleural effusion, pneumothorax)
- Increased ventilatory demand (severe sepsis, septic shock, severe metabolic acidosis)
- Miscellaneous (airway protection)

Furthermore, the patient with cardiac arrest, respiratory arrest, swallowing impairment and multiple organ failure require mechanical ventilation.

Hyperbaric Oxygen Therapy (HBOT)

HBOT is a treatment method that 100% oxygen is administered in a pressurized chamber. The mechanism of action is to increase oxygen delivery and carbon monoxide antagonism. In an animal study, rats were exposed to CO, and those with a loss of consciousness were selected. Lipid peroxidation was not observed in the HBOT group but instead in the NBOT group (Thom, 1990). Cytochrome C oxidase is a mitochondrial enzyme whose inhibition by CO may initiate neuronal damage through mitochondrial dysfunction and cellular respiratory dysfunction, also forming oxygen radicals and reactive oxygen species. In addition, HBO prevents the adhesion of neutrophils to the brain microvascular endothelium which is mediated by β integrin. These mechanisms may explain how HBOT prevents delayed neurological sequelae (Rose et al., 2017).

HBOT decreases the half-life of COHb to 30 minutes, which is approximately 75-90 minutes with 100% normobaric oxygen (Manaker and Perry, 2021). It is recommended for those patients who have a neurological deficit, cardiac ischemia, loss of consciousness, metabolic acidosis, and respiratory insufficiency or COHb level >25. However, regardless of these indications, it is a clinical decision (Table 2). The greatest benefit is provided when treatment starts within 6 hours after CO exposure, and it is not recommended after more than 24 hours. HBOT should be performed 3 times within 24 hours (Jüttner et al., 2021). The initial session according to the Boerema Schedule corresponds to 300/90, and the second and third sessions can be performed at a pressure greater than or equal to 2.4 bar (240/90). It means that the patients should receive a treatment at 300 kPa total pressure for 90 minutes with oxygen breathing at the beginning. More sessions can be considered if the symptom persists (Jüttner et al., 2021).

Table 2. Indications of Hyperbaric Oxygen Treatment (HBOT)

Hyperbaric oxygen (HBOT) is suggested for:

- COHb level>25% (>15% if pregnant)
- Found unconscious at scene or hospital, if a syncope occurs
- Altered mental status (GCS<15), coma, focal neurological deficit
- Severe metabolic acidosis (pH <7.25) after empiric cyanide treatment administration
- Evidence of end-organ ischemia (ECG changes, elevated cardiac biomarkers, focal neurological deficit, altered mental status, respiratory failure)
- Abnormal cerebellar function
- Fetal distress during pregnancy
- Prolonged CO exposure (≥24 hours)
- Age ≥36 years

Extracorporeal Membrane Oxygenation

The ECMO is a life support machine that provides external artificial circulation. ECMO ensures that the patient's blood is cleaned of CO2 and enriched with oxygen in an external system using cannulas placed in large veins and arteries (Simonsen et al., 2019).

There are few studies on the effectiveness of ECMO in carbon monoxide poisoning. In a study in Porcine models, subjects inhaled CO until cardiac failure developed. Subsequently, venous-arterial ECMO was connected to some of the subjects, while only ventilator support was administered to some of them. Survival was higher in pigs given ECMO support (Simonsen et al., 2018). Another study published by the same team demonstrated the successful application of ECMO under long airway transfer conditions in a pig with severe CO exposure and cardiac arrest (Simonsen et al., 2019).

There are only two case reports in the literature regarding the application of ECMO in CO poisoning in humans. In the first case report, it was reported that the patient who developed ARDS and cardiovascular collapse after the severe CO poisoning was discharged after 7 days of veno-venous ECMO. It has been stated that death can be prevented with ECMO support in the early period (McCunn et al., 2000).

In the second case report, Veno-arterial ECMO was performed in a patient with severe CO exposure who developed unstable and cardiogenic shock. The patient was followed up for 6 months in terms of delayed neurological sequelae after discharge. The patient recovered without any sequelae (Teerapuncharoen et al., 2015).

As a result, ECMO reduces cardiac oxygen consumption, lowers carboxyhemoglobin levels in the blood, and returns oxygen-rich blood to the body. In this way, it allows for the rapid removal of CO from the body. The use of ECMO can be considered in patients who do not benefit from ventilatory support due to severe CO exposure or who develop cardiac failure (Teerapuncharoen et al., 2015).

Conclusion

CO poisoning is one of the most common human poisonings admitted to the emergency department. It affects people worldwide and can lead to significant morbidity and mortality. Because it affects multiple organ systems, the clinical presentation is variable, and the differential diagnosis should be considered. Early diagnosis and treatment with 100% oxygen prevent the development of sequelae. All the patients with CO poisoning should receive oxygen treatment until their COHb concentration drops to <3% or clinical symptoms disappear.

References

Bal, U., Sönmez, B. M., Inan, S., Işcanli, M. D., and Yilmaz, F. (2020). The efficiency of continuous positive airway pressure therapy in carbon monoxide poisoining in the emergency department. *European journal of emergency medicine: official journal of the European Society for Emergency Medicine*, 27(3), 217–222. https://doi.org/10.1097/MEJ.0000000000000647.

Dong, W. N., Wang, B. X., Cao, P., Zhu, Q. C., Tan, D. Y., and Ling, B. Y. (2022). Comparison of high-flow nasal cannula oxygen therapy and non-rebreather face mask in the treatment of mild carbon monoxide poisoning. *Zhonghua lao dong wei sheng zhi ye bing za zhi = Zhonghua laodong weisheng zhiyebing zazhi = Chinese journal of industrial hygiene and occupational diseases*, 40(10), 771–775. https://doi.org/10.3760/cma.j.cn121094-20211025-00513.

Fan, H. C., Juan, C. J., and Chen, S. J. (2012). Carbon monoxide: sources, uses and hazards. In D. DiLoreto, I. Corcoran (Ed.), *Carbon monoxide: sources, uses and hazards* (pp. 31-47). UK: Novthe a Science Publishers.

Gale, S. D., Hopkins, R. O., Weaver, L. K., Bigler, E. D., Booth, E. J., and Blatter, D. D. (1999). MRI, quantitative MRI, SPECT, and neuropsychological findings following carbon monoxide poisoning. *Brain injury*, 13(4), 229–243. https://doi.org/10.1080/026990599121601.

Hampson, N. B., and Bodwin, D. (2013). Toxic CO-ingestions in intentional carbon monoxide poisoning. *The Journal of emergency medicine*, 44(3), 625–630. https://doi.org/10.1016/j.jemermed.2012.08.033.

Hampson, N. B., and Hauff, N. M. (2008). Risk factors for short-term mortality from carbon monoxide poisoning treated with hyperbaric oxygen. *Critical care medicine*, 36(9), 2523–2527. https://doi.org/10.1097/CCM.0b013e31818419d8.

Hampson, N. B., Piantadosi, C. A., Thom, S. R., and Weaver, L. K. (2012). Practice recommendations in the diagnosis, management, and prevention of carbon monoxide poisoning. *American journal of respiratory and critical care medicine*, 186(11), 1095–1101. https://doi.org/10.1164/rccm.201207-1284CI.

Hyzy, R. C., and McSparron, J. I. (2022). *Overview of initiating invasive mechanical ventilation in adults in the intensive care unit.* UpToDate.

Jüttner, B., Busch, H. J., Callies, A., Dormann, H., Janisch, T., Kaiser, G., Körner-Göbel, H., Kluba, K., Kluge, S., Leidel, B. A., Müller, O., Naser, J., Pohl, C., Reiter, K., Schneider, D., Staps, E., Welslau, W., Wißuwa, H., Wöbker, G., and Muche-Borowski, C. (2021). S2k guideline diagnosis and treatment of carbon monoxide poisoning. *German medical science: GMS e-journal*, 19, Doc13. https://doi.org/10.3205/000300.

Kim, Y. M., Shin, H. J., Choi, D. W., Kim, J. M., Lee, S. W., Jeong, S. H., and Kim, H. (2020). Comparison of high-flow nasal cannula oxygen therapy and conventional reserve-bag oxygen therapy in carbon monoxide intoxication: A pilot study. *The American journal of emergency medicine*, 38(8), 1621–1626. https://doi.org/10.1016/j.ajem.2019.158451.

Long, B., Liang, S. Y., and Lentz, S. (2021). High flow nasal cannula for adult acute hypoxemic respiratory failure in the ED setting. *The American journal of emergency medicine*, 49, 352–359. https://doi.org/10.1016/j.ajem.2021.06.074.

Manaker, S., and Perry, H. (2021). Carbon monoxide poisoning. Up To Date. https://www.uptodate.com/contents/carbon-monoxide-poisoning. Last Updated Mar 02, 2023.

Mattiuzzi, C., and Lippi, G. (2020). Worldwide epidemiology of carbon monoxide poisoning. *Human and Experimental Toxicology*, 39(4), 387-392.

McCunn, M., Reynolds, H. N., Cottingham, C. A., Scalea, T. M., and Habashi, N. M. (2000). Extracorporeal support in an adult with severe carbon monoxide poisoning and shock following smoke inhalation: a case report. *Perfusion*, 15(2), 169–173. https://doi.org/10.1177/026765910001500213.

Moon, J. M., Chun, B. J., Baek, B. H., and Hong, Y. J. (2018). Initial diffusion-weighted MRI and long-term neurologic outcomes in charcoal-burning carbon monoxide poisoning. *Clinical Toxicology*, 56(3), 161-169.

Nishimura, M. (2019). High-Flow Nasal Cannula Oxygen Therapy Devices. *Respiratory care*, 64(6), 735–742. https://doi.org/10.4187/respcare.06718.

Ozkan. S., and Ipekci. A. (2022). Carbon Monoxide Poisoning. Yücel M., Güzel M., İkizceli İ., *Environmental Emergencies And İnjuries in Nature* (pp. 279-288). https://doi.org/10.52305/EMJM1370.

Ozturan, I. U., Yaka, E., Suner, S., Ozbek, A. E., Alyesil, C., Dogan, N. O., Yilmaz, S., and Pekdemir, M. (2019). Determination of carboxyhemoglobin half-life in patients with carbon monoxide toxicity treated with high flow nasal cannula oxygen therapy. *Clinical toxicology (Philadelphia, Pa.)*, 57(7), 617–623. https://doi.org/10.1080/15563650.2018.1540046.

Parkinson, R. B., Hopkins, R. O., Cleavinger, H. B., Weaver, L. K., Victoroff, J., Foley, J. F., and Bigler, E. D. (2002). White matter hyperintensities and neuropsychological outcome following carbon monoxide poisoning. *Neurology*, 58(10), 1525-1532.

Rochwerg, B., Einav, S., Chaudhuri, D., Mancebo, J., Mauri, T., Helviz, Y., Goligher, E. C., Jaber, S., Ricard, J. D., Rittayamai, N., Roca, O., Antonelli, M., Maggiore, S. M., Demoule, A., Hodgson, C. L., Mercat, A., Wilcox, M. E., Granton, D., Wang, D., Azoulay, E., Ouanes-Besbes, L., Cinnella, G., Rauseo, M., Carvalho, C., Dessap-Mekontso, A., Fraser, J., Frat, J. P., Gomersall, C., Grasselli, G., Hernandez, G., Jog, S., Pesenti, A., Riviello, E. D., Slutsky, A. S., Stapleton, R. D., Talmor, D., Thille, A. W., Brochard, L., and Burns, K. E. A. (2020). The role for high flow nasal cannula as a respiratory support strategy in adults: a clinical practice guideline. *Intensive care medicine*, 46(12), 2226–2237. https://doi.org/10.1007/s00134-020-06312-y.

Rose, J. J., Wang, L., Xu, Q., McTiernan, C. F., Shiva, S., Tejero, J., and Gladwin, M. T. (2017). Carbon Monoxide Poisoning: Pathogenesis, Management, and Future Directions of Therapy. *American journal of respiratory and critical care medicine*, 195(5), 596–606. https://doi.org/10.1164/rccm.201606-1275CI.

Roth, D., Mayer, J., Schreiber, W., Herkner, H., and Laggner, A. N. (2018). Acute carbon monoxide poisoning treatment by non-invasive CPAP-ventilation, and by reservoir face mask: Two simultaneous cases. *The American journal of emergency medicine*, 36(9), 1718.e5–1718.e6. https://doi.org/10.1016/j.ajem.2018.05.066.

Shen, C. H., Peng, C. K., Chou, Y. C., Pan, K. T., Chang, S. C., Chang, S. Y., and Huang, K. L. (2015). Predicting duration of mechanical ventilation in patients with carbon monoxide poisoning: a retrospective study. *Journal of critical care*, 30(1), 19–24. https://doi.org/10.1016/j.jcrc.2014.08.003.

Simonsen, C., Magnusdottir, S. O., Andreasen, J. J., Bleeg, R. C., Lie, C., and Kjærgaard, B. (2019). Long-Distance Transportation of Carbon Monoxide-Poisoned Patients on Extracorporeal Membrane Oxygenation Seems Possible: A Porcine Feasibility Study. *Air medical journal*, 38(3), 178–182. https://doi.org/10.1016/j.amj.2019.03.009.

Simonsen, C., Magnusdottir, S. O., Andreasen, J. J., Rohde, M. C., and Kjærgaard, B. (2018). ECMO improves survival following cardiogenic shock due to carbon monoxide poisoning- an experimental porcine model. *Scandinavian journal of trauma, resuscitation and emergency medicine*, 26(1), 103. https://doi.org/10.1186/s13049-018-0570-6

Teerapuncharoen, K., Sharma, N. S., Barker, A. B., Wille, K. M., and Diaz-Guzman, E. (2015). Successful Treatment of Severe Carbon Monoxide Poisoning and Refractory Shock Using Extracorporeal Membrane Oxygenation. *Respiratory care*, 60(9), e155–e160. https://doi.org/10.4187/respcare.03990.

Thom S. R. (1990). Antagonism of carbon monoxide-mediated brain lipid peroxidation by hyperbaric oxygen. *Toxicology and applied pharmacology*, 105(2), 340–344. https://doi.org/10.1016/0041-008x(90)90195-z.

Tomaszewski, C. (2011). Carbon monoxide. L. S. Nelson, N. A. Lewin, M. A. Howland, R. S. Hoffman, L. R. Goldfrank, N. E. Flomenbaum (Ed.), (pp. 1658-1670). New York; USA; McGraw Hill.

Tomruk, O., Karaman, K., Erdur, B., Armagan, H. H., Beceren, N. G., Oskay, A., and Bircan, H. A. (2019). A New Promising Treatment Strategy for Carbon Monoxide Poisoning: High Flow Nasal Cannula Oxygen Therapy. *Medical science monitor: international medical journal of experimental and clinical research*, 25, 605–609. https://doi.org/10.12659/MSM.914800

Turgut, K., and Yavuz, E. (2020). Comparison of non-invasive CPAP with mask use in carbon monoxide poisoning. *The American journal of emergency medicine*, 38(7), 1454–1457. https://doi.org/10.1016/j.ajem.2020.04.050.

Yesiloglu, O., Gulen, M., Satar, S., Avci, A., Acehan, S., and Akoglu, H. (2021). Treatment of carbon monoxide poisoning: high-flow nasal cannula versus non-rebreather face mask. *Clinical toxicology (Philadelphia, Pa.)*, 59(5), 386–391. https://doi.org/10.1080/15563650.2020.181.

Chapter 10

Hyperbaric Oxygen Therapy in Carbon Monoxide Poisoning

Altuğ Kanbakan*, **MD**
Clinic of Emergency Medicine,
Bakırköy Dr. Sadi Konuk Training and Research Hospital University of Health Sciences,
Istanbul, Turkey

Abstract

Carbon monoxide (CO) poisoning is a significant cause of morbidity and mortality worldwide. It is caused by inhalation of CO gas and can have lethal effects such as tissue hypoxia. For the treatment of CO poisoning, hyperbaric oxygen therapy (HBOT) is a method that is being used more frequently. With HBOT, 100% oxygen is administered in a pressurized chamber, increasing tissue oxygen supply and reducing carbon monoxide antagonism. The chapter also discusses recent studies and evidence supporting the use of HBOT in the management of CO poisoning.

Keywords: carbon monoxide, hyperbaric oxygen therapy, emergency

Introduction

In 1662, a British clergyman and doctor named Nathaniel Henshaw used organ bellows with one-way valves to change the air pressure in a sealed room called a *domicilium*. This was the first time hyperbaric therapy was known to have been used. Hyperbaric oxygen therapy (HBOT), a treatment method that

* Corresponding Author's Email: drkanbakan@outlook.com.

In: Carbon Monoxide Poisoning
Editors: Seda Özkan and Afsin Ipekci
ISBN: 979-8-89113-217-7

began to be developed in the 1830s in a modern way by French physician Junod and steam engine inventor James Watt, was first used in the treatment of carbon monoxide poisoning in the early 1960s. After doing research on animals in the 1950s and setting up a hyperbaric oxygen therapy chamber at the University of Amsterdam, the Dutch cardiac surgeon Ite Boerema came up with the idea. Smith and Sharp used HBOT in 1962 to treat people with carbon monoxide toxication. They found that it helped a lot and after the first treatment of 90 minutes at 3 atmospheres of pressure for people with carboxyhemoglobin (CO) levels above 25%, they suggested that patients get more treatments to fully recover. Boerema is known as the "Father of Modern HBOT" because he was one of the first people to use it in this way (Krishnamurti, 2020).

Carbon monoxide (CO) is an odorless, colorless, and highly poisonous gas that binds to hemoglobin more strongly than oxygen. This makes carboxyhemoglobin (COHb) and reduces the amount of oxygen that blood can carry. CO poisoning is a common cause of unintentional poisoning and death worldwide (Mattiuzzi & Lippi, 2019). While HBOT is not the first-line treatment for CO poisoning, it has been shown to reduce the risk of neurological sequelae and improve outcomes in moderate to severe cases (Gözübüyük, 2017). The therapeutic mechanism of HBOT in CO poisoning involves two key factors: increased oxygen delivery and carbon monoxide antagonism.

Hyperbaric oxygen therapy has been used to treat more than just CO poisoning. Over the past 60 years, HBOT has been recommended in these various medical scenarios. For example, it has been used to treat decompression sickness, gas gangrene, osteomyelitis, and diabetic foot ulcers. The United States Food and Drug Administration (FDA) approves these conditions to treat with HBOT: air or gas embolism, carbon monoxide poisoning, decompression sickness, clostridial myonecrosis, crush injury, traumatic ischemia, healing of wounds (including diabetic wounds), severe anemia, necrotizing soft tissue infections, refractory osteomyelitis, radiation necrosis of soft tissue and bone, compromised skin grafts and flaps (Mechem & Manaker, 2023).

Hyperbaric Oxygen Therapy

Mechanism of Action

At sea level, the normal atmospheric pressure is 760 millimeters of mercury (mmHg). This air is composed of approximately 79% nitrogen and 21% oxygen, resulting in an oxygen pressure (pO2) of approximately 160 mmHg. This atmospheric pressure corresponds to 1 absolute atmosphere (ATA). At 2 ATA with 100% oxygen, there is 1,520 mmHg of oxygen. This increases the amount of inspired oxygen and consequently, the amount of oxygen dissolved in plasma. The majority of therapeutic HBOT applications involve 3 ATA or less (Tibbles & Edelsberg, 1996).

Hemoglobin is approximately 97% oxygen-saturated, and the plasma contains a smaller amount of dissolved oxygen. Increasing inspired oxygen alone cannot improve hemoglobin delivery and breathing 100% oxygen at normal atmospheric pressure will only slightly increase the amount of oxygen dissolved in plasma. At 2.8 atmospheres, the volume of bubbles decreases by nearly two-thirds. In addition, hyperbaric oxygen accelerates the dissolution of the inert gas bubble by replacing the inert gas in the bubble with oxygen, which is metabolized rapidly by the tissues. Additionally, the use of hyperbaric oxygen prevents the formation of new bubbles (Tibbles & Edelsberg, 1996). The approximate half-life of carboxyhemoglobin (COHb) in air in the room is five hours. Under 100% oxygen supplementation (normobaric oxygen therapy [NBO]), this duration can be up to one hour. HBOT can cut down this half-life to around 30 minutes (Meade & Nelson, 2022).

Hyperbaric oxygen therapy shortens the half-life of COHb, reduces the production and concentration of oxygen free radicals, stops lipid peroxidation, and improves mitochondrial dysfunction and platelet aggregation in capillaries. Compared to normobaric oxygen therapy, HBO therapy takes less time and reduces the risk of death and the start of long-term neuropsychiatric problems (Gözübüyük, 2017).

The direct mechanical effect and hyperoxygenation are the two fundamental components of the action mechanism. Through a direct mechanical effect, HBOT reduces the size of gas bubbles. Reduces edema and tissue swelling, enhances neovascularization, and stimulates the immune system by restoring WBC functions and boosting phagocytosis and neutrophil activity with hyperoxygenation (Ustad et al., 2012; Tibbles & Edelsberg, 1996).

In carbon monoxide toxicity, the use of HBOT is based on the induction of cerebral vasoconstriction. This effect may also reduce cerebral edema and intracranial pressure. CO causes cellular asphyxiation by binding to cytochrome a-3 and myoglobin, which effectively shuts down oxidative phosphorylation, similar to nitric oxide and cyanide. This CO-mediated mitochondrial inhibition reduced the production of adenosine triphosphate (ATP) in tissues. This effect is more pronounced in tissues with a high metabolic rate, such as the brain and heart, due to the decrease in ATP (Rose et al., 2018).

It is thought that the effectiveness of this treatment is partly due to the fact that hyperbaric oxygen can separate carbon monoxide from heme proteins. In addition to these effects, HBOT could also help with neuronal death, which is caused by lipid peroxidation and the production of free oxygen radicals (Tibbles & Edelsberg, 1996).

Also, current studies indicate that neuropathology results from an inflammatory process triggered by astrocytes with myelin basic protein (MBP) and aggravated by circulating neutrophils, which eventually affects the cerebral endothelium with increased vascular permeability (Ruhela et al., 2021).

Sethuraman and Thom gave a short review of the research on seven randomized controlled trials and focused on how it is not clear if the HBO treatment is better than the NBO. They obtained their data from seven different meta-analyses. Randomized controlled studies have investigated the maximum O2 dose (ATA), HBO treatment initiation time, treatment protocols, sample sizes, and outcomes. They reported a remarkable correlation between the maximum dose of O2 and the outcomes (mortality and neurological morbidity). Specifically, they have focused on the O2 dose and emphasized that HBOT temporarily inhibits neutrophil activity at a minimum of 2.0 ATA. In addition, it has been emphasized that the effect of the treatment doses in the contradictory given may be diminished by prolonging the start time and that accompanying neuropsychiatric disorders (suicidal depressive patients) may affect the outcome. In conclusion, they determined that HBO was a necessary treatment for this toxidrome at a dose of 2.5–3.0 ATA and was beneficial for neurological disorders and DNS (Sethuraman & Thom, 2022).

Indications, Contraindications, and Complications

Current recommendations for HBOT in the emergency medicine literature are: COHb level >25% with normal clinical findings, COHb level >15% in pregnant patients (or with fetal distress), or high COHb levels with one or more of the following findings: Altered mental status (Glasgow Coma Score [GCS] < 15) Syncope, seizure, coma, abnormal cerebellar exam, prolonged exposure to CO with minor clinical findings (Meade & Nelson, 2022) The Tenth European Consensus Conference on Hyperbaric Medicine recommends HBOT for all patients with CO poisoning exhibiting altered consciousness or clinical neurological, cardiac, respiratory, or psychological symptoms, regardless of carboxyhaemoglobin level at hospital admission (Alessandro & Jacek, 2017). The American College of Emergency Physicians has reported its clinical policy on acute carbon monoxide poisoning, which states that ED physicians should use HBO2 therapy or high-flow normobaric therapy for patients with acute CO poisoning (Wolf et al., 2017).

The decision about HBO therapy should not be based on the COHb level. Although the majority of cases of acute intoxication are associated with loss of consciousness and neurological side effects, COHb levels are weakly correlated with poisoning (Manaker & Perry, 2023). There is evidence that HBO reduces the risk of delayed neuropsychiatric and neurologic effects from about 12% to less than 1%, and a meta-analysis of randomized controlled trials showed that patients who received HBO had a lower risk of memory loss than those who did not. Furthermore, compared to patients treated with normobaric oxygen, HBO patients had higher neuropsychiatric scores (Meade & Nelson, 2022).

Patients with a neurologic abnormality or cardiovascular instability may be a candidate for HBO. As a neurological abnormality, Delayed Neurological Sequelae (DNS) are the most dramatic effect of carbon monoxide intoxication. DNS after CO poisoning is not well understood, but most researchers think it has to do with demyelination, destruction, and apoptosis of neurons in the globus pallidus and white matter of the brain. Memory loss, ataxia, seizures, fecal and/or urinary incontinence, confusion, disorientation, hallucinations, psychosis, and cortical blindness are all possible symptoms of DNS (Nañagas et al., 2022). CO poisoning also causes inflammation, which can lead to neuronal damage through the release of cytokines, lipid peroxidation, mitochondrial oxidative stress, inhibition of mitochondrial function, and adaptive immune responses, among other things (Liao et al., 2021). After a period of what seems like normalcy, neurological problems can also start to appear. Up to a year after CO poisoning, about 30% of patients had long-term neurological problems caused by late encephalopathy (Lin et al., 2018). Although the majority of patients with mild CO poisoning recover completely from the acute phase, more than half of patients with severe CO poisoning develop delayed neurological sequelae within 3 to 6 weeks of the onset of CO poisoning (Gözübüyük, 2017; Manaker & Perry, 2023; Liao et al., 2021).

According to studies, a longer duration of admission, CO exposure duration >6 hours, systolic blood pressure < 90 mmHg, Glasgow Coma Scale score <9, Mini-Mental State Examination score, absence of pupil reflex, and positive Babinski reflex were associated with the occurrence of DNS or neurological sequelae (Ning et al., 2020; Pepe et al., 2011).

A small retrospective cohort study has indicated that HBOT was effective in treating DNS following a prolonged duration of time (ranging from 30 to 60 days) after acute CO poisoning. After recovering from acute carbon monoxide poisoning, all of these patients experienced neurologic and psychiatric complications. Prior to and subsequent to the commencement of HBOT, all patients underwent an electroencephalogram (EEG), Mini-Mental State Examination (MMSE), brain magnetic resonance imaging (MRI), event-related potential (ERP), and a brain perfusion scan (brain SPECT). After eight to forty sessions of hyperbaric oxygen therapy (HBOT), functional neurological tests such as event-related potentials (ERP), electroencephalography (EEG), Mini-Mental State Examination (MMSE), and brain single-photon emission computed tomography (SPECT) revealed improvements that corresponded to the patient's clinical symptoms (Chang et al., 2010).

Even though the results of randomized controlled trials (RCTs) comparing the effectiveness of normobaric oxygen therapy and hyperbaric oxygen therapy are not all the same, Sethuraman and Thom used their study to look in depth at when treatment should start (Sethuraman & Thom, 2022).

In a study conducted by Raphael et al., involving a sample size of 343, the researchers compared the efficacy of 6-hour normobaric oxygen (NBO) treatment with a combination of 2-hour hyperbaric oxygen (HBO) treatment followed by 4-hour NBO treatment, as well as 4-hour NBO treatment with 1 or 2 HBO treatment protocols, all administered under 2.0 ATA. The time to initiate treatment varied from 5.3 ± 2.3 to 6.4 ± 2.8 hours. In this study, no benefit was reported in favor of hyperbaric oxygen therapy (HBOT) in this study (Raphael et al., 1989).

Annane et al., conducted a study with 385 patients who received the same treatment at 2.0 ATA. The time of initiation of treatment ranged from 2 to 6 hours. The study findings indicate a lack of efficacy for hyperbaric oxygen therapy (HBOT) (Annane et al., 2010).

In Thom et al., (2021) investigation that involved a sample size of 65, the researchers conducted a comparison between a 6-hour administration of normobaric oxygen (NBO) and a treatment regimen consisting of 30 minutes of exposure to 2.8 ATA followed by 90 minutes of exposure to 2.0 ATA. The initiation of therapy occurred at a mean time of 2.0 ± 1.1 hours, and a favorable outcome was documented in support of hyperbaric oxygen therapy (HBOT) (Thom et al., 1995).

The study conducted by Scheinkestel et al., involved a sample size of 191 individuals. The study compared the effects of three days of normobaric oxygen (NBO) treatment versus three daily treatments of 2.8 ATA for 60 minutes with a 40-minute reduction, then three days of NBO. The treatment initiation time varied from 5.7 to 8.6 hours. There have been reports indicating a lack of efficacy for hyperbaric oxygen therapy (HBOT) (Scheinkestel et al., 1999).

Weaver et al., conducted a study with 152 people to compare the effects of 50 minutes of 3.0 ATA followed by 60 minutes of 2.0 ATA with 125 minutes of normobaric oxygen (NBO). The optimal window for commencing treatment is within 5.8 ± 2.9 hours, and Hyperbaric Oxygen Therapy (HBOT) has demonstrated potential benefits (Weaver et al., 2002).

The results may be affected by the variability of the sample sizes and the different treatment protocols utilized by these studies. Furthermore, it should not be overlooked that, while HBOT may be deemed "beneficial" or otherwise, it is merely an outcome for us clinicians. Mortality may be attributable to other neuropsychiatric factors (for example, suicide). Therefore, although it seems difficult to reach a clear conclusion without subgroup analyses in studies, we can say that the time to start the treatment and the maximum oxygen dose used are important (Sethuraman & Thom, 2022).

Due to this, patients must undergo HBOT as soon as possible, within six hours if possible (Gözübüyük, 2017; Manaker & Perry, 2023) and preferably within 24 hours of exposure, for early treatment and prevention of DNS (Zhang et al., 2022).

In the medical literature, there are not many reports that focus on how many HBOT sessions should be given during the acute stage of CO poisoning to prevent DNS. In small sample size prospective studies or case reports, the number of sessions that should be given has been reported to range from one to 40 or more sessions (Chang et al., 2010; Lo Pardo et al., 2016; Spina et al.,

2019; Pappalardo et al., 2020). In a meta-analysis of six randomized controlled trials (RCTs), Lin et al., found that hyperbaric oxygen therapy (HBOT) had an association with headache, memory impairment, difficulty concentrating, disturbed sleep, and delayed neurological sequelae. Additionally, they found that receiving two sessions of HBO increased the risk of memory impairment and difficulty concentrating compared to receiving only one session of HBO. However, it is important to point out that the researchers in this study did not calculate the scores for the neuropsychological subtests that we have just mentioned (Lin et al., 2018). In general, we can say that HBO has a lower risk of memory impairment compared to NBO, and 2 sessions of HBO treatment have a higher risk of memory impairment compared to 1 session of HBO (Wang et al., 2019).

Since the level of COHb will decrease with pulmonary elimination, the time of exposure should be taken into consideration. COHb levels are anticipated to decrease over time due to pulmonary elimination. Patients with transient loss of consciousness and confirmed CO exposure may still benefit from HBO, even if their COHb level does not accurately reflect the extent of exposure at the time of the loss of consciousness (Manaker & Perry, 2023). The most important concept is that HBO therapy should be used in asymptomatic patients with a COHb level of at least 25% and that the decision to perform it should be made in the context of transport and other medical needs, including the need for transfer to a burn center (Meade & Nelson, 2022).

Hyperbaric therapy, in general, is safe and well tolerated. The only absolute contraindication to HBOT is untreated pneumothorax. Chronic obstructive pulmonary disease, the presence of pulmonary blebs, and a recent history of the middle ear or thoracic surgery are relative contraindications to HBOT. Other relative contraindications to HBOT include a history of seizures and claustrophobia (Mechem & Manaker, 2023). Seizures caused by HBOT may be seen but are a rare side effect of oxygen toxicity (Hadanny et al., 2016). Patients with a history of epilepsy are at increased risk for central nervous system (CNS) toxicity-related complications when exposed to high oxygen concentrations. Hypoglycemia has been linked to HBO in some diabetic patients, so it should be considered in the differential diagnosis of HBO-related seizures (Roth & Weiss, 1994; Mechem & Manaker, 2023). In addition, patients using insulin, glucocorticoids, and sympathomimetic drugs may have an increased risk of seizures due to high oxygen intake. This risk increases especially in patients who receive hyperbaric oxygen therapy for longer than 90-120 minutes and at a pressure higher than 2.8-3.0 atm (Roth &

Weiss, 1994). It is important to thoroughly evaluate the patient's medical history and current condition before administering HBOT. It is thought that the pulmonary and cardiotoxic side effects of bleomycin and doxorubicin, respectively, may increase with hyperbaric oxygen therapy. Although there is not enough information to support these views, there are opinions to avoid HBO treatment during the use of these drugs. Due to the limited human studies, it would be more appropriate to evaluate HBO treatment separately for each patient during the use of these drugs (Mechem & Manaker, 2023). Nevertheless, these relative contraindications shouldn't change the choice of whether or not to use HBOT when neurological changes are life-threatening (Manaker & Perry, 2023).

The most common complications of HBOT are middle ear barotrauma and sinus barotrauma (sinus squeeze). The incidence of middle ear barotrauma is about 2% and is mostly seen in patients with multiple treatments. Valsalva maneuvers can be used to treat ear barotrauma (Enrico & Gerardo, 2014; Mechem & Manaker, 2023; Kemmer et al., 2006).

Treatment Protocols and Patient Monitoring

HBO treatment should be adjusted according to the clinical condition of the patient. Based on the previously mentioned review by Sethuraman and Thom, it can be said that treatment should be given under 2.0 ATA to suppress neutrophil activity (Sethuraman & Thom, 2022).

It should be noted that the optimal treatment duration, dose, and number of sessions in acute poisoning are not clearly determined. In general, 1 to 3- 90-minute sessions under 2.5 ATA are considered sufficient (Mathieu et al., 2006).

Pressure chambers typically range between 2.5 and 3.0 atm. While the pressure chamber in carbon monoxide intoxication is filled with 100% oxygen, nitrogen/oxygen (nitrox) or helium/oxygen (heliox) mixtures can be used in certain decompression sickness situations (e.g., neurological and vestibular accidents) (Mechem & Manaker, 2023).

HBO therapy can be used in both single-person (monoplace) and multi-person (multiplace) pressure rooms. Although single-person pressure chambers are appropriate for patients with more stable or chronic diseases, the risk of fire is higher due to the higher oxygen content of multi-person pressure chambers. The patient is alone in a monoplace chamber, and there is no direct access to the patient during the hyperbaric treatment. Multiplace chambers are designed to treat multiple sitting patients at the same time, as well as critically ill patients accompanied by attending staff. The avoidance of exposure of the health care team to hyperbaric pressures is a clear advantage of monoplace chambers, although complications due to hyperbaric exposure in attendance are rare (Kemmer et al., 2006).

The monitoring of physiological parameters during an HBO session is heavily dependent on the severity of the disease and the clinical status of the patient. The parameters measured range from simple 3-lead electrocardiography (ECG) with manual blood pressure measurement to sophisticated measurements such as pulmonary capillary wedge pressure (PCWP) or electroencephalography with direct arterial blood pressure monitoring. Also, non-invasive methods like Laser-Doppler flowmetry or more invasive monitoring like transcutaneous oxygen monitoring can be used to estimate the quality of oxygen delivery to the tissue. (Kemmer et al., 2006).

Conclusion

In conclusion, HBOT is an effective treatment for CO toxicity, especially in situations of moderate to severe toxicity or when neurological signs are present. According to the severity of the poisoning, the indications for HBOT in CO toxicity are loss of consciousness, neurologic impairments, cardiac ischemia, and a carboxyhemoglobin level greater than 25%. Patients who are not clinically ill and do not meet the criteria for HBO can usually be managed in the emergency department because high-flow oxygen will resolve most symptoms. Once CO poisoning has been diagnosed, repeated COHb levels are usually not needed because the symptoms and the first COHb level are usually enough to guide treatment. Patients who do not improve, have ECG or laboratory evidence of severe poisoning, or have other medical or social concerns should be hospitalized. With CO poisoning, the choice to employ HBOT should be tailored depending on the clinical presentation and response to initial therapy. However, further studies are needed to determine the optimal duration and pressure of HBOT in this setting.

References

Alessandro, & Jacek. (2017). *Diving and hyperbaric medicine* 47 no. *Diving and Hyperbaric Medicine*. https://doi.org/10.28920/dhm47.1.24-32.

Annane, D., Chadda, K., Gajdos, P., Jars-Guincestre, M. C., Chevret, S., & Raphael, J. C. (2010, December 2). Hyperbaric oxygen therapy for acute domestic carbon monoxide poisoning: two randomized controlled trials. *Intensive Care Medicine*, 37(3), 486–492. https://doi.org/10.1007/s00134-010-2093-0.

Chang, L., Lo, Fan, Huang, Kang, Hsieh, & Chen. (2010, January). Hyperbaric oxygen ameliorates delayed neuropsychiatric syndrome of carbon monoxide poisoning. *Undersea Hyperb Med*, 37(1), 23–33. PMID: 20369650.

Enrico & Gerardo. (2014, June). Mechanisms of action of hyperbaric oxygen therapy. *Undersea Hyperb Med*, 41(3), 247–252. PMID: 24984320.

Gözübüyük, A. A. (2017). Corbon monoxide intoxication epidemiology, pathophsiology, clinical evaluation and treatment during childhood, in newborn and fetus. *Northern Clinics of Istanbul*. https://doi.org/10.14744/nci.2017.49368.

Hadanny, M., Bechor, Fishlev, Bergan, & Efrati. (2016, January). Seizures during hyperbaric oxygen therapy: retrospective analysis of 62,614 treatment sessions. *Undersea Hyperb Med*, 43(1), 21–28. PMID: 27000010.

Kemmer, M., & Mathieu. (2006). *Chapter 3.3 - Patient Management. Handbook on Hyperbaric Medicine*, p651–669. https://doi.org/10.1007/1-4020-4448-8.

Krishnamurti, C. (2020, October 28). *Historical Aspects of Hyperbaric Physiology and Medicine. Respiratory Physiology*. https://doi.org/10.5772/intechopen.85216.

Liao, S. C., Shao, S. C., Yang, K. J., & Yang, C. C. (2021, September 28). Real-world effectiveness of hyperbaric oxygen therapy for delayed neuropsychiatric sequelae after carbon monoxide poisoning. *Scientific Reports*, 11(1). https://doi.org/10.1038/s41598-021-98539-y.

Lin, C. H., Su, W. H., Chen, Y. C., Feng, P. H., Shen, W. C., Ong, J. R., Wu, M. Y., & Wong, C. S. (2018, September). Treatment with normobaric or hyperbaric oxygen and its effect on neuropsychometric dysfunction after carbon monoxide poisoning. *Medicine*, 97(39), e12456. https://doi.org/10.1097/md.0000000000012456.

Lo Pardo, D., Amedola, D., Senatore, G., Damiano, A., Pezzuti, G., Pugliese, N., Locatelli, G., Siani, A., & Vitola, N. M. (2016, June 20). Delayed neuropsychiatric syndrome after carbon monoxide poisoning: inclusion of hyperbaric oxygen therapy in the recovery protocol. *Emergency Care Journal*, 1(1). https://doi.org/10.4081/ecj.2016.5675.

Manaker & Perry. (2023, March 2). *Carbon Monoxide Poisoning* (M. Burns & Ganetsky, Eds.). UpToDate. Retrieved March 8, 2023, from https://www.uptodate.com/contents/carbon-monoxide-poisoning.

Mathieu, D., Mathieu-Nolf, M., Linke, J. C., Favory, R., & Wattel, F. (2006). *Chapter 2.2.3 - Carbon Monoxide Poisoning. Handbook on Hyperbaric Medicine*, 239–251. https://doi.org/10.1007/1-4020-4448-8_14.

Mattiuzzi, C., & Lippi, G. (2019, December 1). Worldwide epidemiology of carbon monoxide poisoning. *Human & Experimental Toxicology*, 39(4), 387–392. https://doi.org/10.1177/0960327119891214.

Meade, W., & Nelson, S. (2022, July 20). *Rosen's Emergency Medicine: Concepts and Clinical Practice*. In R. Walls, R. Hockberger, M. Gausche-Hill, T. B. Erickson, & S. R. Wilcox (Eds.), *Chapter 148 - Inhaled Toxins* (10th ed., Vol. 2, pp. 1946–1947). Elsevier - Health Sciences Division.

Mechem, C., & Manaker. (2023, February). *Hyperbaric Oxygen Therapy* (Schwarz & Ganetsky, Eds.). UpToDate. Retrieved March 8, 2023, from https://www.uptodate.com/contents/hyperbaric-oxygen-therapy.

Nañagas, K. A., Penfound, S. J., & Kao, L. W. (2022, May). Carbon Monoxide Toxicity. Emergency Medicine *Clinics of North America*, 40(2), 283–312. https://doi.org/10.1016/j.emc.2022.01.005.

Ning, K., Zhou, Y. Y., Zhang, N., Sun, X. J., Liu, W. W., & Han, C. H. (2020). Neurocognitive sequelae after carbon monoxide poisoning and hyperbaric oxygen therapy. *Medical Gas Research*, 10(1), 30. https://doi.org/10.4103/2045-9912.279981.

Pappalardo, I., Celli, L., Arena, L., Testa, L., Giovanniello, A., Cava, M., Colla, L., Ghiazza, G., Morelli, N., & Rota, E. (2020, March). Is "delayed" hyperbaric therapy effective for "delayed" encephalopathy after carbon monoxide intoxication? *ENeurologicalSci*, 18, 100219. https://doi.org/10.1016/j.ensci.2019.100219.

Pepe, G., Castelli, M., Nazerian, P., Vanni, S., Del Panta, M., Gambassi, F., Botti, P., Missanelli, A., & Grifoni, S. (2011, March 17). Delayed neuropsychological sequelae after carbon monoxide poisoning: predictive risk factors in the Emergency Department. A retrospective study. *Scandinavian Journal of Trauma, Resuscitation and Emergency Medicine*, 19(1). https://doi.org/10.1186/1757-7241-19-16.

Raphael, J. C., Elkharrat, D., Jars-Guincestre, M. C., Chastang, C., Vercken, J. B., Chasles, V., & Gajdos, P. (1989, August). Trial Of Normobaric and Hyperbaric Oxygen for Acute Carbon Monoxide Intoxication. *The Lancet*, 334(8660), 414–419. https://doi.org/10.1016/s0140-6736(89)90592-8.

Rose, J. J., Nouraie, M., Gauthier, M. C., Pizon, A. F., Saul, M. I., Donahoe, M. P., & Gladwin, M. T. (2018, July). Clinical Outcomes and Mortality Impact of Hyperbaric Oxygen Therapy in Patients with Carbon Monoxide Poisoning. *Critical Care Medicine*, 46(7), e649–e655. https://doi.org/10.1097/ccm.0000000000003135.

Roth, R. N., & Weiss, L. D. (1994, January). Hyperbaric oxygen and wound healing. *Clinics in Dermatology*, 12(1), 141–156. https://doi.org/10.1016/0738-081x(94)90265-8.

Ruhela, D., Bhopale, V. M., Kalakonda, S., & Thom, S. R. (2021, December). Astrocyte-derived microparticles initiate a neuroinflammatory cycle due to carbon monoxide poisoning. *Brain, Behavior, & Immunity - Health*, 18, 100398. https://doi.org/10.1016/j.bbih.2021.100398.

Scheinkestel, C. D., Myles, P. S., Cooper, D. J., Millar, I. L., Tuxen, D. V., Bailey, M., & Jones, K. (1999, March). Hyperbaric or normobaric oxygen for acute carbon monoxide poisoning: a randomised controlled clinical trial. *Medical Journal of Australia*, 170(5), 203–210. https://doi.org/10.5694/j.1326-5377.1999.tb140318.x.

Sethuraman, K., & Thom, S. R. (2022, December). Hyperbaric oxygen should be used for carbon monoxide poisoning. *British Journal of Clinical Pharmacology*, 89(3), 939–941. https://doi.org/10.1111/bcp.15605.

Spina, V., Tomaiuolo, F., Celli, L., Bonfiglio, L., Cecchetti, L., & Carboncini, M. C. (2019, May 15). A Case of Carbon Monoxide-Induced Delayed Neurological Sequelae Successfully Treated with Hyperbaric Oxygen Therapy, N-Acetylcysteine, and

Glucocorticoids: Clinical and Neuroimaging Follow-Up. *Case Reports in Neurological Medicine*, 2019, 1–7. https://doi.org/10.1155/2019/9360542.

Thom, S. R., Taber, R. L., Mendiguren, I. I., Clark, J. M., Hardy, K. R., & Fisher, A. B. (1995, April). Delayed Neuropsychologic Sequelae After Carbon Monoxide Poisoning: Prevention by Treatment with Hyperbaric Oxygen. *Annals of Emergency Medicine*, 25(4), 474–480. https://doi.org/10.1016/s0196-0644(95)70261-x.

Tibbles, P. M., & Edelsberg, J. S. (1996, June 20). Hyperbaric-Oxygen Therapy. *New England Journal of Medicine*, 334(25), 1642–1648. https://doi.org/10.1056/nejm199606203342506.

Ustad, F., Ali, F. M., Ustad, T., Aher, V., M.C, P., & Suryavanshi, H. (2012, November 30). Uses of Hyperbaric Oxygen Therapy: A Review. *Journal of Evolution of Medical and Dental Sciences*, 1(5), 892–906. https://doi.org/10.14260/jemds/144.

Wang, W., Cheng, J., Zhang, J., & Wang, K. (2019, October 13). Effect of Hyperbaric Oxygen on Neurologic Sequelae and All-Cause Mortality in Patients with Carbon Monoxide Poisoning: A Meta-Analysis of Randomized Controlled Trials. *Medical Science Monitor*, 25, 7684–7693. https://doi.org/10.12659/msm.917065.

Weaver, L. K., Hopkins, R. O., Chan, K. J., Churchill, S., Elliott, C. G., Clemmer, T. P., Orme, J. F., Thomas, F. O., & Morris, A. H. (2002, October 3). Hyperbaric Oxygen for Acute Carbon Monoxide Poisoning. *New England Journal of Medicine*, 347(14), 1057–1067. https://doi.org/10.1056/nejmoa013121.

Wolf, S. J., Maloney, G. E., Shih, R. D., Shy, B. D., Brown, M. D., Brown, M. D., Byyny, R., Diercks, D. B., Gemme, S. R., Gerardo, C. J., Godwin, S. A., Hahn, S. A., Hatten, B. W., Haukoos, J. S., Ingalsbe, G. S., Kaji, A., Kwok, H., Lo, B. M., Mace, S. E., Nazarian, D. J., Proehl, J. A., Promes, S. B., Shah, K. H., Shih, R. D., Silvers, S. M., Smith, M. D., Thiessen, M. E., Tomaszewski, C. A., Valente, J. H., Wall, S. P., Wolf, S. J., Cantrill, S. V., O'Connor, R. E., Mitchell, M. A., & Whitson, R. R. Whitson, R. R. (2017, January). Clinical Policy: Critical Issues in the Evaluation and Management of Adult Patients Presenting to the Emergency Department with Acute Carbon Monoxide Poisoning. *Annals of Emergency Medicine*, 69(1), 98-107.e6. https://doi.org/10.1016/j.annemergmed.2016.11.003.

Zhang, L., Wu, D., Xu, M., Bian, Y., Wang, Y., Gao, G., & Sun, Q. (2022, February 15). Acute carbon monoxide poisoning in Shandong, China: an observational study. *Chinese Medical Journal*, 135(13), 1539–1544. https://doi.org/10.1097/cm9.0000000000001942.

Chapter 11

Carbon Monoxide Poisoning in Children

Yaşar Yusuf Can*, MD
Department of Pediatrics, Sancaktepe Sehit Prof. Dr. Ilhan Varank Egitim Arastirma Hospital, Istanbul, Turkey

Abstract

Carbon monoxide (CO) is an odorless and colorless gas created by incomplete combustion of fossil fuels, including gasoline, natural gas, propane, and coal. CO poisoning can occur in children who inhale the gas, resulting in mild to severe symptoms, including headache, dizziness, nausea, confusion, unconsciousness, and even death. Children are more susceptible to CO poisoning because they require more oxygen than adults and can be exposed to the gas for longer period of time, especially if they are sleeping in a room with gas-powered equipment or in a poorly ventilated space. CO poisoning should be promptly diagnosed and treated to prevent severe and long-lasting symptoms. Typical treatment consists of removing the child from the CO source, administering oxygen therapy, and monitoring for problems. In extreme circumstances, hyperbaric oxygen therapy may be required to raise blood oxygen levels. Prevention of CO poisoning in children involves maintaining gas-powered equipment, installing CO detectors, and educating young people about the dangers of CO and the importance of ventilation. Furthermore, it is crucial to seek immediate medical help if CO poisoning is suspected, as early treatment can dramatically reduce the risk of long-term consequences.

Keywords: Carbon Monoxide, Children, Poisoning

---

* Corresponding Author's Email: yasaryusufcan@gmail.com.

In: Carbon Monoxide Poisoning
Editors: Seda Özkan and Afsin Ipekci
ISBN: 979-8-89113-217-7

Introduction

Aside from being somewhat less thick than air, CO has no taste, no smell, and does not irritate. These qualities make it possible for exposure to go unnoticed until severe toxicity manifests itself. Carbon monoxide is naturally produced by volcanic gases, wetland gases, and coal mine emissions. CO is the second most prevalent air pollutant, after carbon dioxide, and is present anywhere carbonaceous materials are incompletely burned. It is estimated that 90% of the CO in the atmosphere comes from the combustion of fossil fuels for transportation (Jaffe, 1997). Therefore, although this is not generally known, air toxicity is potentially a significant source of exposure for metropolitan children. During the course of five years, COHb levels, pulmonary function, and immunological function were assessed in a cohort of children from an air-polluted area of Austria (Marth et al., 1996). The average concentration of COHb in the study population of 10-year-olds was 3% (no control group), and it dramatically decreased within one week of moving to an area with cleaner air (no control group). This study did not take into account the effects of exposure to passive smoking. The most common indoor air contaminant to which children are exposed is tobacco smoking. Further research is required to determine the extent to which CO in tobacco smoke contributes to these and other acute and chronic diseases, despite the fact that it has been suggested that exposed children have reduced lung capacity and a higher incidence of respiratory tract reactivity and infection (Little, 1995).

Main Body

Epidemiology

More than 20,000 people in the United States receive treatment for CO poisoning each year, and more than 400 of them pass away as a result, according to the Centers for Disease Control and Prevention (CDC). Children under the age of 14 accounts for approximately 15% of all cases of CO poisoning in the United States, and they are at increased risk for severe outcomes, including neurological damage and death (Mattiuzzi and Lippi, 2020).

The Journal of the American Medical Association (JAMA) Pediatrics released a study estimated that between 2010 and 2015, children in the United

States visited emergency departments an average of 3,175 times per year due to CO exposure (Chang et al., 2017). In respect to a report by the World Health Organization (WHO), CO poisoning causes more than 20,000 deaths annually worldwide, with the highest burden occurring in low- and middle-income nations (Mattiuzzi and Lippi, 2020).

Between 2000 and 2009, there were 1,948 hospitalizations of children under the age of 19 in Canada due to CO poisoning. Children aged 0–4 years had the highest annual hospitalization rate for CO poisoning, with a rate of 1.63 per 100,000 population. CO poisoning is estimated to cause over 400,000 nonfatal poisonings and 39,000 deaths annually on a global scale. Even though there is limited information on CO poisoning in children in many countries, it is believed that children are more susceptible than adults to this type of poisoning (Hampson and Weaver, 2007).

Children's Sources of Carbon Monoxide Exposure

Volcanic gases, wetland gases, and coal mine emissions are natural sources of carbon monoxide. CO is the second-most abundant air pollutant, after carbon dioxide, and is present wherever incomplete combustion of carbonaceous materials occurs. According to estimates, the combustion of fossil fuels for transportation causes 90% of CO in the environment. As a result, although it is not well known, air toxicity may be a significant source of exposure for urban children. Tobacco smoke is the most common indoor air contaminant to which children are exposed. The extent to which CO in cigarette smoke contributes to these and other acute and chronic diseases is unknown, despite evidence suggesting that exposed young people have decreased lung capacity and a higher incidence of respiratory tract reactivity and infection.

Children who inhale smoke are possibly exposed to carbon monoxide, hypoxia, and other toxic insults. Parish (1986) has thoroughly examined this. Zikria et al., (1972) discovered that 24% of children who died within the first 12 hours following burns had COHb levels above 50%. Furthermore, high levels of COHb were present in 39% of those who passed away within 12 hours without suffering from burns, indicating that CO is the primary killer of these fire victims.

CO poisoning is not limited to the home and vehicle. Children may be affected during recreational activities at ice rinks, on boats or water skis, in tents while camping, and while participating in athletic events (Boudreau et al., 1994). A strong index of suspicion must be maintained when children with flu-like symptoms, headaches, and syncope come into these environments.

Mechanism of Carbon Monoxide Toxicity

Hypoxic ischemia contributes significantly to the neurotoxicity caused by carbon monoxide. Its affinity for hemoglobin is much higher than that for oxygen (240 times higher) but also means that it binds slowly. At very low partial pressures of CO, oxygen-binding sites are occupied, lowering the oxygen-carrying capacity of the blood and blood oxygen levels (Gorman et al., 2003).

The typical facilitation phenomenon for additional oxygen unloading within the tissue. The end result is a left-shifted oxygen dissociation curve that is abnormally hyperbolic. The tissues most vulnerable to CO's effects are those with the highest metabolic activity. Further reductions in oxygen delivery are possible. By altering the concentration of erythrocyte diphosphoglycerate. In addition to hypoxia, carbon monoxide causes ischemia due to hypotension. The severity of damage to the central nervous system (CNS) correlates well with the severity of hypotension (Hall et al., 1993). Once it was discovered that COHb levels did not correlate with toxicity, COHb formed by non-inhalational routes did not cause the same lethal effects as inhalational exposure to CO, and delayed neuropsychiatric effects were common in people who seemed to have fully recovered from the initial CO insult, researchers have been looking for other ways that CO can be harmful. The mechanism of the delayed CO poisoning effects has been a medical enigma. There is increasing evidence for brain ischemia and reperfusion injury. Lipid peroxidation, vascular oxidative stress, neuronal excitotoxicity, and apoptosis all play important roles (Gorman et al., 2003).

Clinical Presentation

The clinical manifestation of CO poisoning in children differs depending on the amount and duration of exposure. The symptoms may range from mild to severe and may resemble other common childhood illnesses, making diagnosis difficult (Roy and Crawford, 1996). Typical symptoms of carbon monoxide intoxication are presented in Table 1.

Headache is one of the most prevalent signs of CO poisoning in children. Its severity can range from mild to severe, and it is sometimes accompanied by nausea and vomiting. Another common symptom of CO poisoning in children is dizziness. It is characterized by feelings of lightheadedness or vertigo and may be accompanied by faintness. Children may experience feelings of weakness, fatigue, and poor concentration. CO poisoning can cause dyspnea, especially during physical exertion. Even when at rest, children may feel as if they are struggling to catch their breath. Pain in the chest: CO poisoning can cause chest pain that can be described as a dull ache or sharp stabbing pain (Unsal Sac et al., 2015).

Table 1. Typical symptoms of carbon monoxide intoxication

• Headache	• Vertigo
• Dizziness	• Dyspnea
• Fatigue	• Pain in the chest
• Weakness	• Confusion, disorientation
• Impaired concentration	• Seizures
• Lightheadedness	• Coma

CO poisoning can cause confusion, disorientation, and difficulty thinking clearly. Children may appear confused, have difficulty concentrating, and be unable to recall simple information. Seizures: In extreme cases, CO poisoning can cause life-threatening seizures (Unsal Sac et al., 2015).

It is significant to remember that the symptoms of CO poisoning can be nonspecific and can vary depending on the child's age and health. Additionally, it may take hours or even days for symptoms to manifest.

Findings at Physical Examination

In up to 69% of cases (Rudge, 1993), children with CO poisoning exhibit acute neurological symptoms. In a large series, the most prevalent signs of exposure were changed state of mind, increased DTRs, a positive Babinski sign, ankle clonus, nystagmus, ataxia, amnesia, hemiplegia, and tremor. Binder and Roberts (1980) observed ataxia, extrapyramidal signs, posturing, neck stiffness, an irregular respiratory pattern, conjunctival irritation, and profuse sweating upon presentation. Similar presenting symptoms were shared by numerous smoke inhalation victims who also had CO poisoning, including lethargy, coma, syncope, ataxia or tremors, irritability or disorientation, bradypnea or apnea, abnormal vital signs and metabolic acidosis (Meert et al., 1998).

Outcome

Subsequent mortality in children has been reported to be more exposed to CO than adults. In memory impairment, personality alterations, and parietal lobe dysfunction are the higher cortical functions most frequently affected in adults and children (lack of visual perception, dyspraxia, disorder of speech and writing). Blindness, deafness, seizures, increased reflexes, hemiplegia, muscular hypertonia, extrapyramidal rigidity, akinesia, muscle atrophies, skin hyperesthesia, disorientation, confusion, decreased libido, and incontinence occur less frequently (Garland and Pearce, 1967).

Psychiatric alterations are observable. In one study, more than half of the survivors of CO poisoning reported numbness, ageusia, memory, attention span, task frustration, blurred vision, anosmia, attention deficit, anxiety, sleep disruption, headache, difficulty concentrating, depression, and family issues (Angle and Meile, 1968).

In contrast to other forms of hypoxic or ischemic brain injury, CO-hypoxia may be associated with delayed onset of neurological symptoms (DNS) in 2.8%–43.0% of the adult population exposed. Memory deficits, mental confusion, personality changes, speech impairment, forgetfulness, parietal lobe dysfunction (apraxia, agnosia, dysgraphia), and motor dysfunction are all symptoms of DNS in adults, along with the full spectrum of symptoms seen in other forms of hypoxic-ischemic damage (parkinsonism, hemiplegia) (Choi, 1983).

Diagnosis

Although the level of COHb is the most accessible diagnostic instrument for CO exposure, it does not indicate the severity of the poisoning or the likelihood of developing delayed sequelae. Important determinants of toxicity, such as duration of exposure, maximum level, and any potential delay between exposure and treatment, are not reflected in a single blood measurement.

Blood gas analysis by methods other than co-oximetry will not detect COHb, which is an important potential pitfall for the clinician to remember (Vegfors and Lennmarken, 1991). Therefore, it is essential to request that COHb levels be measured via co-oximetry; otherwise, oxygen saturation may be incorrectly reported as normal if calculated from the pO2 measurement. Other laboratory tests will not be able to determine whether a person has been exposed to carbon monoxide, but some may provide hints or help predict the outcome.

Glucose abnormalities are well-described in adults and frequently reported in pediatric CO poisonings; in fact, they are an independent risk factor for a poor outcome in adults exposed to CO. Hypoglycemia is considerably less prevalent. Other laboratory abnormalities in children in addition to serum lactate leukocytosis include hemoconcentration, elevated LDH, CPK, transaminases, proteinuria, myoglobinuria, and thrombocytopenia. (Brown et al., 1996).

Adults can have well-known ECG changes such as ischemic ST segment depression, T-wave inversion, ventricular ectopic beats, and atrial fibrillation.

Treatment

The first goal of CO poisoning treatment is to remove the patient from a toxic environment and provide oxygen therapy to reverse cellular metabolic dysfunction. Vital functions must be maintained, vascular access established, and continuous cardiopulmonary monitoring performed. Treatment for tissue hypoxia and hypovolemia should be initiated, and HBO therapy should be administered if necessary. Complications should be treated if they exist. Because CO binding to hemoglobin is reversible and binding to oxygen is competitive, rapid intervention and the delivery of an appropriate dose of oxygen form the basis of treatment (Turner et al., 1999). CO has a half-life of approximately 5 hours in room air, 1 hour in 100% oxygen, and 25 minutes during HBO treatment at 3 bar pressure. In other words, oxygen reduces the half-life of CO. In patients suffering from CO poisoning due to fire or smoke inhalation who are critically ill (i.e., those with coma, seizures, or hemodynamic compromise associated with metabolic acidosis and increased blood lactate concentration), it is recommended that hydroxocobalamin be administered to treat potential cyanide toxicity. The dose of hydroxocobalamin is 70 mg/kg intravenously (IV; 5 g is the standard adult dose) and may be repeated after 10 to 15 minutes if the patient does not experience rapid clinical improvement (Roderique et al., 2015).

The use of HBO therapy to treat CO poisoning is controversial and even pediatric toxicology specialists have differing opinions regarding the best course of action.

HBO is most effective when administered as soon as possible, preferably within six hours, in order to increase the elimination of carboxyhemoglobinemia and improve tissue oxygenation. Importantly, even if COHb levels have dropped below the recommended thresholds mentioned above, delayed HBO treatment may still be beneficial; however, it is not proven if more than 24 hours have passed since CO exposure (Leach and Rees, 1998).

Proposed Indications for HBO Therapy in Children

- Abnormal level of consciousness or mental state examination
- COHb level > 25 to 40% with no other symptoms
- Any neurological symptom other than isolated headache, including brief loss of consciousness at the scene
- Coma
- Recurrent symptomatology
- Refractory symptoms despite 100% oxygen

Conclusion

Public service messages broadcast in the mainstream media, particularly during the winter months, should emphasize the dangers of CO and advise on proper heating procedures for home and work, exhaust gases, petrochemicals, thinners, and fire. Employee health and safety must also be better regulated and monitored. Attempts should be made to include Syrian war refugees living in Turkiye in these awareness campaigns. CO poisoning can be avoided by correctly installing and using home and workplace heating systems, especially those that use gas, as well as providing adequate ventilation and performing routine maintenance. Regular maintenance and the use of catalytic converters can reduce CO levels in exhaust gases. Finally, while CO sensors do not detect low levels of CO, they are still recommended because of their ability to provide a warning.

References

Angle, C. R., McIntire, M. S., & Meile, R. L. (1968). Neurologic sequelae of poisoning in children. *The Journal of Pediatrics*, *73*(4), 531-539. https://doi.org/10.1016/S0022-3476(68)80268-9.

Binder, J. W., & Roberts, R. J. (1980). Carbon monoxide poisoning in children. Clin. Toxicol, 16, 287-295. https://doi.org/10.3109/15563658008989951.

Boudreau, D. R., Spadafora, M. P., Wolf, L. R., & Siegel, E. (1994). Carbon Monoxide Levels during Indoor Sporting Events—Cincinnati, 1992–1993, [reprint] from MMWR 43 (2): 21–23. *JAMA, Journal of the American Medical Association*, *271*(6), 419. https://doi.org/10.1001/jama.1994.03510300013006.

Brown, D. B., Golich, F. C., Tappel, J. J., Dykstra, T. A., & Ott, D. A. (1996). Severe carbon monoxide poisoning in the pediatric patient: a case report. *Aviation, space and environmental medicine*, *67*(3), 262-265.

Chang, Y. C., Lee, H. Y., Huang, J. L., Chiu, C. H., Chen, C. L., & Wu, C. T. (2017). Risk Factors and Outcome Analysis in Children with Carbon Monoxide Poisoning. *Pediatrics and neonatology*, *58*(2), 171–177. https://doi.org/10.1016/j.pedneo.2016.03.007.

Choi, S. (1983). Delayed neurologic sequelae in carbon monoxide intoxication. *Archives of Neurology*, *40*(7), 433-435. https://doi.org/10.1001/archneur.1983.04050070063016.

Garland, H., & Pearce, J. (1967). Neurological complications of carbon monoxide poisoning. *Quarterly Journal of Medicine*, *36*(144), 445-55.

Gorman, D., Drewry, A., Huang, Y. L., & Sames, C. (2003). The clinical toxicology of carbon monoxide. *Toxicology*, *187*(1), 25-38. https://doi.org/10.1016/S0300-483X(03)00005-2.

Hall, E. D., Andrus, P. K., Althaus, J. S., & Von Voigtlander, P. F. (1993). Hydroxyl radical production and lipid peroxidation paralles selective post-ischemic vulnerability in gerbil brain. *Journal of neuroscience research*, *34*(1), 107-112. https://doi.org/10.1002/jnr.490340111.

Hampson, N. B., & Weaver, L. K. (2007). Carbon monoxide poisoning: a new incidence for an old disease. *Undersea and Hyperbaric Medicine*, *34*(3), 163.

Jaffe, F. A. (1997). Pathogenicity of carbon monoxide. *The American journal of forensic medicine and pathology*, *18*(4), 406-410. https://doi.org/10.1097/00000433-199712000-00017.

Leach, R. M., & Rees, P. J. (1998). Wilmshurst PHyperbaric oxygen therapy. *BMJ*, *317*, 1140-1143. https://doi.org/10.1136/bmj.317.7166.1140.

Little, D. N. (1995). Children and environmental toxins. *Primary Care*, *22*(1), 69-79. https://doi.org/10.1016/S0095-4543(21)00501-7.

Marth, E., Haselbacher-Marko, S., & Schaffler, K. (1996). A cohort study with children living in an air-polluted region—a model for public health. *Toxicology letters*, *88*(1-3), 155-159. https://doi.org/10.1016/0378-4274(96)03731-9.

Mattiuzzi, C., & Lippi, G. (2020). Worldwide epidemiology of carbon monoxide poisoning. *Human & experimental toxicology*, *39*(4), 387–392. https://doi.org/10.1177/0960327119891214.

Meert, K. L., Heidemann, S. M., & Sarnaik, A. P. (1998). Outcome of children with carbon monoxide poisoning treated with normobaric oxygen. *Journal of Trauma and Acute Care Surgery*, *44*(1), 149-154. https://doi.org/10.1097/00005373-199801000-00020.

Parish, R. A. (1986). Smoke inhalation and carbon monoxide poisoning in children. *Pediatric Emergency Care*, *2*(1), 36-39. https://doi.org/10.1097/00006565-198603000-00010.

Roderique, J. D., Josef, C. S., Feldman, M. J., & Spiess, B. D. (2015). A modern literature review of carbon monoxide poisoning theories, therapies, and potential targets for therapy advancement. *Toxicology*, *334*, 45-58. https://doi.org/10.1016/j.tox.2015.05.004.

Roy, B., & Crawford, R. (1996). Pitfalls in diagnosis and management of carbon monoxide poisoning. *Emergency Medicine Journal*, *13*(1), 62-63. https://doi.org/10.1136/emj.13.1.62.

Rudge, F. W. (1993). Carbon monoxide poisoning in infants: treatment with hyperbaric oxygen. *Southern medical journal*, *86*(3), 334-337. https://doi.org/10.1097/00007611-199303000-00017.

Turner, M., Esaw, M., & Clark, R. J. (1999). Carbon monoxide poisoning treated with hyperbaric oxygen: metabolic acidosis as a predictor of treatment requirements. *Emergency Medicine Journal*, *16*(2), 96-98. https://doi.org/10.1136/emj.16.2.96.

Unsal Sac, R., Taşar, M. A., Bostancı, İ., Şimşek, Y., & Bilge Dallar, Y. (2015). Characteristics of Children with Acute Carbon Monoxide Poisoning in Ankara: A Single Centre Experience. *Journal of Korean medical science*, *30*(12), 1836–1840. https://doi.org/10.3346/jkms.2015.30.12.1836.

Vegfors, M., & Lennmarken, C. (1991). Carboxyhaemoglobinaemia and pulse oximetry. *BJA: British Journal of Anaesthesia*, *66*(5), 625-626. https://doi.org/10.1093/bja/66.5.625.

Zikria, B. A., Weston, G. C., Chodoff, M., & Ferrer, J. M. (1972). Smoke and carbon monoxide poisoning in fire victims. *Journal of Trauma and Acute Care Surgery*, *12*(8), 641-645. https://doi.org/10.1097/00005373-197208000-00001.

Chapter 12

Carbon Monoxide Poisoning in Pregnancy

Kübra Hamzaoğlu Canbolat[1,*], MD
and Abdullah Serdar Açıkgöz[2]

[1]Department of Obstetrics and Gynecology,
Sisli Hamidiye Etfal Training & Research Hospital, Istanbul, Turkey
[2]Department of Obstetrics and Gynecology, Division of Gynecologic Oncology,
Istanbul University-Cerrahpasa, Cerrahpasa School of Medicine, Istanbul, Turkey

Abstract

Carbon monoxide poisoning is one of the most common types of gas poisoning. The symptoms of this condition are nonspecific. Carbon monoxide binds to hemoglobin with higher affinity than oxygen, reducing oxygen distribution to tissues, and tissue hypoxia occurs. Due to the higher affinity of fetal hemoglobin for carbon monoxide, the fetus is much more affected than the mother. The fetal mortality rate in fetuses of pregnant women with carbon monoxide poisoning varies between 36-67%. Abortion, intrauterine fetal growth retardation or anatomical malformations, and neurological problems in the fetus are other effects that can be seen. Hyperbaric oxygen therapy should be considered as a treatment in pregnancy.

Keywords: carbon monoxide poisoning, hyperbaric oxygen therapy, fetal hypoxia, pregnancy outcome

---

* Corresponding Author's Email: drkubrahamzaoglu@gmail.com.

In: Carbon Monoxide Poisoning
Editors: Seda Özkan and Afsin Ipekci
ISBN: 979-8-89113-217-7

Introduction

Carbon monoxide (CO) is an odorless, colorless, and tasteless gas with a molecular weight similar to that of air. The concentration of CO in the atmosphere is usually less than 0.001%. Even a concentration of less than 0.1% can lead to mortality (Wilson and Jederlinic, 2002). The first carbon monoxide poisoning was seen in 1859, with the industrial revolution and the onset of coal gas exposure (Copel et al., 1982).

CO is released when the carbon-based fuel material is incompletely burned (Ernst and Zibrak, 1998). Smoke generated during fire, fuel-burning appliances such as stoves with poor ventilation, motor vehicles operating in poorly ventilated environments, and hookah use are the main sources of carbon monoxide (Centers for Disease Control and Prevention, 2005; Nguyen et al., 2020). CO poisonings other than intentional suicidal carbon monoxide poisonings show regional differences, mostly in the cold winter months (Centers for Disease Control and Prevention, 2001-2003). CO accounts for 80% of deaths due to smoke inhalation (Wilson and Jederlinic, 2002).

The binding affinity of CO to hemoglobin is 200 times higher than that of oxygen, and therefore the oxygen carrying capacity of hemoglobin to the tissues decreases in CO poisoning, and tissue hypoxia occurs (Ernst and Zibrak, 1998). Apart from the decrease in the oxygen capacity of the blood, due to the disruption of the cellular respiratory chain, the immunoregulatory processes continue to damage the tissue even after the carbon monoxide level decreases. Since CO also inhibits cytochrome oxidase and cytochrome p450, it can accelerate the inflammatory cascade leading to central nervous system lipid peroxidation and neurological sequelae (Rose et al., 2017). Since 10-15% of carbon monoxide is released from the circulation, it also causes effects that are not mediated by hemoglobin (Vogel et al., 1981).

CO is a common cause of domestic poisoning. It is thought that the most common cause of CO poisoning in pregnant women is accidental exposure to the home environment (Norman and Halton, 1990). Although the exact incidence of CO poisoning in pregnant women is unknown, it is estimated to be 4.6-8.5% of all patients diagnosed with CO poisoning (Palmer and Von Rueden, 2015). While the maternal mortality rate is between 19-24% in those who had CO poisoning during pregnancy, the fetal mortality rate ranges between 36-67% (Elkharrat et al., 1991).

Main Body

Although CO poisoning may show mild symptoms such as headache, flu symptoms, and visual changes, it can lead to neurological and cardiac problems, and even coma and death (Hardy and Thom, 1994). The most important long-term effects of CO poisoning are late neurocognitive disorders associated with morbidity, which can persist in 40% of patients, and myocardial injuries that are most associated with mortality. Hypocampal atrophy, changes in the pallidum, and subcortical structures were also observed as a long-term effect of carbon monoxide poisoning (Hsiao et al., 2004).

A certain amount of CO is produced physiologically in our body, and the production rate increases during pregnancy and decreases after birth. The main reason for this increase is progesterone. Progesterone increases hepatic microsomal enzymatic activity. In addition, a 30-40% increase in maternal erythrocyte mass and 15% fetal endogenous CO production are other causes of the increase in CO in pregnancy (Friedman and Stiller, 2016). CO is a gas associated with maintaining vascular tone, increasing angiogenesis, and reducing inflammation and apoptosis at physiological concentrations (Bainbridge et al., 2002; Venditti et al., 2013; Otterbein et al., 2000). Today, the most common cause of chronic CO exposure in pregnant women is smoking (Ernst and Zibrak, 1998).

Since fetal hemoglobin has a higher affinity for CO compared to maternal hemoglobin and cannot increase the fetal tidal volume or ventilation rate, the longer CO elimination time compared to adults has made the fetus more susceptible to CO poisoning (Nielsen et al., 2000). Fetal carboxyhemoglobin levels may exceed maternal levels, especially with prolonged exposure to carbon monoxide (Roderique et al., 2012). Fetal death may occur, although no serious maternal complication has been observed (Ernst and Zibrak, 1998).

Fetal COHb begins to rise later than that of the mother and peaks over a longer period of time. While the maternal half-life of CO is 2 hours, it is 7 hours in the fetus (Aubard and Magne, 2000). With the first exposure to carbon monoxide, the maternal carboxyhemoglobin level rises rapidly during the first 2-3 hours. While it continues to rise for the next 7-8 hours, fetal carboxyhemoglobin initially does not increase for the first hour. It increases at a slow rate within 4-5 hours and continues to increase for 24 hours (Longo, 1977a).

The duration of exposure to CO, and the gestational age in the week of exposure change the type of exposure of the fetus to CO. CO diffusion increases with increasing gestational age and fetal weight (Cramer, 1982). Exposure in the early stages of pregnancy may cause teratogenic effects, while exposure in the late periods may cause more fetal hypoxia and cause neurological sequelae. It has been reported that microcephaly, cardiomegaly, limb malformations, preterm birth, hypoxic ischemic encephalopathy, cerebral palsy, intrauterine growth retardation, and fetal death may occur as a result of CO poisoning (Friedman et al., 2015). In a prospective multicenter study conducted by Koren et al., no physical or neurobehavioral disorders were found after birth in 31 infants whose mothers were exposed to mild to moderate carbon monoxide poisoning in the intrauterine period (Koren et al., 1991). Towers and Corcoran investigated the fetal heart monitoring of 3 third-trimester pregnant women with carbon monoxide intoxication. While they observed fetal tachycardia and a trace with minimal variability and no deceleration-acceleration in 2 of them, they observed a trace showing minimal variability in which acceleration was not observed despite the absence of fetal tachycardia in the other. They reported that all traces returned to normal after 1 hour with 100% oxygen therapy (Towers and Corcoran, 2009).

The patient, who is thought to have CO poisoning, should be removed from the intoxication environment and normobaric oxygen therapy with 100% oxygen at 15 L/min should be started immediately. While the half-life of carboxyhemoglobin can reach 320 minutes in a patient's breathing room air, this time can be reduced to 75 minutes with high-flow oxygen (Weaver et al., 2000). Cardiac monitoring is vital for possible dysrhythmias. Transient loss of consciousness is a condition that must be questioned by the clinician and is the basic question to determine the need for hyperbaric oxygen therapy. If hyperbaric oxygen therapy is then considered, it is necessary to stabilize the patient and refer to the center where this can be done. If a patient with carbon monoxide poisoning has conditions such as unconsciousness, severe metabolic acidosis, cardiac ischemia, neurological deficit, respiratory failure, pregnancy, or very high COHb concentrations (more than 25% in normal patients, over 15% in pregnant women), a decision should be made in favor of hyperbaric oxygen therapy (Truhlář et al., 2005). By providing high oxygen pressure in the blood with hyperbaric oxygen therapy, the release of carbon monoxide from hemoglobin accelerates and the adhesion of neutrophils to the endothelium decreases (Weaver, 2009). It has been shown that starting treatment within the first 6 hours is beneficial and hyperbaric oxygen therapy reduces mortality in patients with carbon monoxide poisoning (Ziser et al., 1984; Huang et al., 2017). A patient with suspected carbon monoxide poisoning should be treated with oxygen until clinical symptoms resolve or the carboxyhemoglobin concentration drops to 3% (Hampson et al., 2012). However, the patient's symptoms and findings determine the treatment management rather than the carboxyhemoglobin level.

Hyperbaric oxygen therapy is the continuous or intermittent breathing of oxygen to the patient at pressures higher than 1 absolute atmosphere. Although there is no specific hyperbaric oxygen therapy for pregnant women in the literature, the Weaver protocol recommends 3 sessions of hyperbaric oxygen therapy within 24 hours. In another study, it was recommended that pregnant women should be given treatment 5 times longer than the oxygen therapy required to reduce their own carboxyhemoglobin levels (Longo and Hill, 1977b).

Some authors consider hyperbaric oxygen therapy in pregnancy as a definitive indication. However, in some countries, it is not used because the fetal side effects of hyperbaric oxygen therapy are not yet clear (McCrary et al., 2013). In a case report, the maternal carboxyhemoglobin level was 7% after one hour of maternal oxygen therapy, while the fetal carboxyhemoglobin level was 61% at the fetal autopsy (Truhlář et al., 2005). After fetal malformations were observed in the first animal studies in which hyperbaric oxygen therapy was applied, hyperbaric oxygen therapy, which was applied for a shorter time with lower atmosphere absolute was performed by various researchers and it was observed that there was no side effect on the fetus (Fern, 1964; Fujikura, 1964; Cho and Yun, 1982; Gilman et al., 1982). In another study in rats, hyperbaric oxygen therapy was shown to reduce the rate of spontaneous abortion (Nikkanen et al., 2011). In a study by Elkharrat et al., 3 of 5 patients with severe maternal CO poisoning received normobaric oxygen therapy, while 2 of them received hyperbaric oxygen therapy. The intrauterine injury was not detected in any of the fetuses. In addition, no adverse effects were observed in the hyperbaric oxygen therapy, which lasted for 2 hours and applied 2 atmospheres of absolute pressure (Elkharrat et al., 1991). Rodrique et al., noted that pregnant women with carbon monoxide poisoning should be transferred to a center where hyperbaric oxygen therapy is performed, and if there is no such possibility, pregnant women over the 26th gestational week should be taken to a cesarean section (Roderique et al., 2012). There are studies showing that hyperbaric oxygen therapy is also safe in infants (Koren et al., 1991; Wattel et al., 2013).

Conclusion

In mild cases of carbon monoxide poisoning, flu-like symptoms such as headache, fatigue, and dizziness may complicate the diagnosis. Every patient with suspected CO poisoning should be removed from the toxic environment and 100% oxygen support and supportive treatment should be started. Diagnosis and treatment as soon as possible are very important for maternal and fetal well-being. Pregnant women should be referred to the center where hyperbaric oxygen therapy can be performed as soon as possible, or if they cannot be referred, maternal and fetal well-being should be evaluated and the most appropriate treatment should be applied.

References

Aubard, Y., & Magne, I. (2000). Carbon monoxide poisoning in pregnancy. *British Journal of Obstetrics and Gynaecology*, *107*(7), 833-838. https://doi.org/10.1111/j. 1471-0528.2000.tb11078.x.

Bainbridge, S. A., Farley, A. E., McLaughlin, B. E., Graham, C. H., Marks, G. S., Nakatsu, K., Brien J. F., & Smith, G. N. (2002). Carbon monoxide decreases perfusion pressure in isolated human placenta. *Placenta*, *23*(8-9), 563-569. https:// doi.org/10.1053/plac.2002.0845.

Centers for Disease Control and Prevention. (2001-2003). Unintentional non-fire-related carbon monoxide exposures – United States.2005. *MMWR: Morbidity and mortality weekly report,* 54:36.

Centers for Disease Control and Prevention. (2005). Carbon monoxide poisoning from hurricane-associated use of portable generators - Florida, 2004. *MMWR: Morbidity and mortality weekly report*, *54*(28), 697-700.

Cho, S. H., & Yun, D. R. (1982). The experimental study on the effect of hyperbaric oxygen on the pregnancy wastage of rats with acute carbon monoxide poisoning. *Seoul J Med*, *23*, 67-75.

Copel, J. A., Bowen, F., & Bolognese, R. J. (1982). Carbon monoxide intoxication in early pregnancy. *Obstetrics & Gynecology*, *59*(6), 26S-28S.

Cramer, C. R. (1982). Fetal death due to accidental maternal carbon monoxide poisoning. *Journal of Toxicology: Clinical Toxicology*, *19*(3), 297-301. https://doi.org/10.3109/ 15563658209025735.

Elkharrat, D., Raphael, J. C., Korach, J. M., Jars-Guincestre, M. C., Chastang, C., Harboun, C., & Gajdos, P. (1991). Acute carbon monoxide intoxication and hyperbaric oxygen in pregnancy. *Intensive care medicine*, *17*, 289-292. https://doi. org/10.1007/BF01713940.

Ernst, A., & Zibrak, J. D. (1998). Carbon monoxide poisoning. *New England journal of medicine*, *339*(22), 1603-1608. https://doi.org/10.1056/NEJM199811263392206.

Fern, V. H. (1964). Teratogenic effects of hyperbaric oxygen. *Proc Soc Exp Biol Med.*, *116*, 975-976. https://doi.org/10.3181/00379727-116-29425.

Friedman, P., & Stiller, R. J. (2016). Winter danger Carbon monoxide poisoning during pregnancy. *Contemporary OB/GYN*, *61*(1), 27.

Friedman, P., Guo, X. M., Stiller, R. J., & Laifer, S. A. (2015). Carbon monoxide exposure during pregnancy. *Obstetrical & Gynecological Survey*, *70*(11), 705-712. https://doi.org/10.1097/OGX.0000000000000238.

Fujikura, T. (1964). Retrolental fibroplasia and prematurity in newborn rabbits induced by maternal hyperoxia. *American Journal of Obstetrics & Gynecology*, *90*(7), 854-858. https://doi.org/10.1016/0002-9378(64)90777-x.

Gilman, S. C., Greene, K. M., Bradley, M. E., & Biersner, R. J. (1982). Fetal development: effects of stimulated diving and hyperbaric oxygen treatment. *Undersea Biomedical Research*, *9*(4), 297-304.

Hampson, N. B., Piantadosi, C. A., Thom, S. R., & Weaver, L. K. (2012). Practice recommendations in the diagnosis, management, and prevention of carbon monoxide poisoning. *American journal of respiratory and critical care medicine*, *186*(11), 1095-1101. https://doi.org/10.1164/rccm.201207-1284CI.

Hardy, K. R., & Thom, S. R. (1994). Pathophysiology and treatment of carbon monoxide poisoning. *Journal of Toxicology: Clinical Toxicology*, *32*(6), 613-629. https://doi.org/10.3109/15563659409017973.

Hsiao, C. L., Kuo, H. C., & Huang, C. C. (2004). Delayed encephalopathy after carbon monoxide intoxication-long-term prognosis and correlation of clinical manifestations and neuroimages. *Acta Neurologica Taiwanica*, *13*, 64-70.

Huang, C. C., Ho, C. H., Chen, Y. C., Lin, H. J., Hsu, C. C., Wang, J. J, Su S. B., & Guo, H. R. (2017). Hyperbaric oxygen therapy is associated with lower short-and long-term mortality in patients with carbon monoxide poisoning. *Chest*, *152*(5), 943-953. https://doi.org/10.1016/j.chest.2017.03.049.

Koren, G., Sharav, T., Pastuszak, A., Garrettson, L. K., Hill, K., Samson, I., Rorem, M., King, A., & Dolgin, J. E. (1991). A multicenter, prospective study of fetal outcome following accidental carbon monoxide poisoning in pregnancy. *Reproductive toxicology*, *5*(5), 397-403. https://doi.org/10.1016/0890-6238(91)90002-w.

Longo, L. D. (1977a). The biological effects of carbon monoxide on the pregnant woman, fetus, and newborn infant. *American journal of obstetrics and gynecology*, *129*(1), 69-103. https://doi.org/10.1016/0002-9378(77)90824-9.

Longo, L. D., & Hill, E. P. (1977b). Carbon monoxide uptake and elimination in fetal and maternal sheep. *American Journal of Physiology-Heart and Circulatory Physiology*, *232*(3), H324-H330. https://doi.org/10.1152/ajpheart.1977.232.3.H324.

McCrary, B. F., Weaver, L., Marrs, K., Miller, R. S., Dicks, C., Deru, K., Close, N., & DeJong, M. (2013). Hyperbaric oxygen (HBO2) for post-concussive syndrome/chronic TBI--product summary. *Undersea & Hyperbaric Medicine: Journal of the Undersea and Hyperbaric Medical Society, Inc*, *40*(5), 443-467.

Nguyen, V., Salama, M., Fernandez, D., Sperling, J. D., Regina, A., Rivera, R., Wang, J., Friedman, B. W., & Smith, S. W. (2020). Comparison between carbon monoxide poisoning from hookah smoking versus other sources. *Clinical toxicology*, *58*(12), 1320-1325. https://doi.org/10.1080/15563650.2020.1745225.

Nielsen, D., Videbech, P., Hedegaard, M., Dalby, J., & Secher, N. J. (2000). Postpartum depression: identification of women at risk. *BJOG: An International Journal of Obstetrics & Gynaecology*, *107*(10), 1210-1217. https://doi.org/10.1111/j.1471-0528.2000.tb11609.x.

Nikkanen, H., & Skolnik, A. (2011). Diagnosis and management of carbon monoxide poisoning in the emergency department. *Emergency medicine practice*, *13*(2), 1-14.

Norman, C. A., & Halton, D. M. (1990). Is carbon monoxide a workplace teratogen? A review and evaluation of the literature. *The Annals of occupational hygiene*, *34*(4), 335-347. https://doi.org/10.1093/annhyg/34.4.335.

Otterbein, L. E., Bach, F. H., Alam, J., Soares, M., Tao Lu, H., Wysk, M., Roger, J. D., Flavell R. A., & Choi, A. M. (2000). Carbon monoxide has anti-inflammatory effects involving the mitogen-activated protein kinase pathway. *Nature medicine*, *6*(4), 422-428. https://doi.org/10.1038/74680.

Palmer, J., & Von Rueden, K. (2015). Carbon monoxide poisoning and pregnancy: critical nursing interventions. *Journal of Emergency Nursing*, *41*(6), 479-483. https://doi.org/10.1016/j.jen.2015.07.013.

Roderique, E. J. D., Gebre-Giorgis, A. A., Stewart, D. H., Feldman, M. J., & Pozez, A. L. (2012). Smoke inhalation injury in a pregnant patient: a literature review of the evidence and current best practices in the setting of a classic case. *Journal of burn care & research*, *33*(5), 624-633. https://doi.org/10.1097/BCR.0b013e31824799d2.

Rose, J. J., Wang, L., Xu, Q., McTiernan, C. F., Shiva, S., Tejero, J., & Gladwin, M. T. (2017). Carbon monoxide poisoning: pathogenesis, management, and future directions of therapy. *American journal of respiratory and critical care medicine*, *195*(5), 596-606. https://doi.org/10.1164/rccm.201606-1275CI.

Towers, C. V., & Corcoran, V. A. (2009). Influence of carbon monoxide poisoning on the fetal heart monitor tracing: a report of 3 cases. *The Journal of reproductive medicine*, *54*(3), 184-188.

Truhlář, A., Deakin, C. D., Soar, J., Khalifa, G. E. A., Alfonzo, A., Bierens, J. J. L. M., Bratteb, G., Brugger, H., Dunning, J., Hunyadi, S., Koster, R. W., Lockey, D. J., Lott, C., Pall, P., Perkins G. D., Sandroni, C. Thies, K. C., Zideman, D. A., & Nolan, J. P. (2015). Kreislaufstillstand in besonderen Situationen [Circulatory arrest in special situations]. *Notfall+ Rettungsmedizin*, *18*(8), 833-903.

Venditti, C. C., Casselman, R., Murphy, M. S., Adamson, S. L., Sled, J. G., & Smith, G. N. (2013). Chronic carbon monoxide inhalation during pregnancy augments uterine artery blood flow and uteroplacental vascular growth in mice. *American Journal of Physiology-Regulatory, Integrative and Comparative Physiology*, *305*(8), R939-R948. https://doi.org/10.1152/ajpregu.00204.2013.

Vogel, S. N., Sultan, T. R., & Ten Eyck, R. P. (1981). Cyanide poisoning. *Clinical toxicology*, *18*(3), 367-383. https://doi.org/10.3109/15563658108990043.

Wattel, F., Mathieu, D., & Mathieu-Nolf, M. (2013). Devenir des enfants intoxiqués au monoxyde de carbone en période fœtale et traités par oxygénothérapie hyperbare—Étude d'une cohorte constituée sur 25 ans de 1983 à 2008 [A 25-year study (1983-2008) of children's health outcomes after hyperbaric oxygen therapy for carbon monoxide poisoning in utero]. *Bulletin de l'Académie nationale de médecine*, *197*(3), 677-697. https://doi.org/10.1016/S0001-4079(19)31563-8.

Weaver, L. K. (2009). Carbon monoxide poisoning. *New England Journal of Medicine, 360*(12), 1217-1225. https://doi.org10.1056/NEJMcp0808891.

Weaver, L. K., Howe, S., Hopkins, R., & Chan, K. J. (2000). Carboxyhemoglobin half-life in carbon monoxide-poisoned patients treated with 100% oxygen at atmospheric pressure. *Chest, 117*(3), 801-808. https://doi.org/10.1378/chest.117.3.801.

Wilson, M., Jederlinic P. (2002). Acute inhalation injury. In Özalevli, M. (Translation Editor), *Intensive Care Handbook* (3th Ed, pp. 325-6). Adara: Nobel Medicine Bookstore.

Ziser, A., Shupak, A., Halpern, P., Gozal, D., & Melamed, Y. (1984). Delayed hyperbaric oxygen treatment for acute carbon monoxide poisoning. *British Medical Journal (Clinical Research Ed.), 289*(6450), 960. https://doi.org/10.1136/bmj.289.6450.960.

Chapter 13

The Prevention of Carbon Monoxide Poisoning

Serap Biberoğlu*
and Fatih Çakmak
Department of Emergency Medicine, Cerrahpasa Faculty of Medicine, Istanbul University Cerrahpasa, Istanbul, Türkey

Abstract

Carbon monoxide (CO) is an odorless, tasteless, and colorless gas. Every year, hundreds of people die, and thousands get sick. Many household appliances, generators, gas and oil-burning ovens, and charcoal grills produce this toxic gas. The true incidence is difficult to determine, as cases with mild symptoms usually recover quickly, and these mild symptoms can be confused with many diseases.

There are no specific symptoms of carbon monoxide poisoning, so signs and symptoms are variable. The most common symptoms are weakness, headache, dizziness, nausea-vomiting, chest pain, and altered mental status.

Governments should have prevention and disaster plans. The Cross-Governmental Group aimed to provide a common approach to gas safety and prevention of carbon monoxide poisoning. It was established with the aim of reducing death and health disorders as a result of carbon monoxide poisoning. The activities of this group are sharing information about gas safety and CO risk, discovering innovative ways to increase awareness of CO gas, reducing the risks that may occur after the use of gas and fossil fuels, reviewing industrial progress, and improving the importance and understanding of gas safety.

Keywords: carbon monoxide poisoning, prevent, CO detector, CDC

---

* Corresponding Author's Email: serap.biberoglu@istanbul.edu.tr.

In: Carbon Monoxide Poisoning
Editors: Seda Özkan and Afsin Ipekci
ISBN: 979-8-89113-217-7

Introduction

Carbon monoxide (CO), which can cause poisoning and death due to its increased concentration in ambient air, has no odor, taste, and color. This gas, which is not irritant but toxic if inhaled, can cause fatal poisoning when power outages occur in weather conditions such as hurricanes or winter storms (Table 1). So, it is an important Public Health issue. Therefore, governments should have preventive and disaster plans. Using alternative fuel or electricity sources for cooling, heating or cooking can cause CO to accumulate in the home, caravan, or garage and poison the living things inside. This is why generators, grills, camping stoves or other gas, propane, natural gas, or charcoal burning appliances should never be used in the home, inside a garage or camper, in a basement, or even outside, near an open window or window air conditioner (Centers for Disease Control and Prevention, 2018; CDC, 2022; Manaker & Perry, 2023).

Because carbon monoxide (CO) is an odorless, tasteless, and colorless gas, it can rapidly reach life-threatening levels indoors after the incomplete combustion of carbon-based fuel products (Ashcroft et al., 2019; Roca-Barceló et al., 2020). It is caused by the misuse of stoves and other gas heaters, especially in winter, due to the incomplete combustion of carbon-based fuels. It is often seen in the world by inhaling smoke from fires (CDC 2018; Ashcroft et al., 2019).

Table 1. Avoiding Carbon Monoxide Poisoning During a Power Outage (Public Service Announcements) (Centers for Disease Control and Prevention, 2018)

Power outages can occur during emergencies (such as hurricanes).	
Using gas-powered generators can cause CO to build up in the home, poisoning the people inside.	
DANGER	***CO DETECTOR***
• Carbon Monoxide	Can be stopped
• Cannot be seen	Prevent CO Poisoning:
• Cannot be smelled	Install a battery-operated CO detector in your home.
• Cannot be heard	• Use and ventilate generators and all gas-powered equipment at least 20 feet away from doors and windows.

While the normal value of the carboxyhemoglobin (COHb) level in the blood is below 3% in non-smokers, this rate increases to 10% in smokers (Manaker & Perry, 2023).

Carbon monoxide inhalation is toxic. This colorless and odorless gas is impossible to detect with the senses. Causes accidental or suicidal poisoning. Approximately 63% of CO poisonings in Turkey are caused by the stove, 30% by the water heater, and 7% by natural gas (Turkiye Public Health Institution, 2018). In the United States, national analyzes showed that intentional poisonings were more common than accidental poisonings, and fatal poisonings were higher in deliberate poisonings (Manaker &Perry, 2023).

The true incidence is difficult to determine, as cases with mild symptoms usually recover quickly, and these mild symptoms can be confused with many diseases (Olson & Smollin, 2008).

Poorly functioning heating systems (kerosene heaters, charcoal grills, camping stoves, etc.), gasoline electric generators, motor vehicles operating in poorly ventilated areas (ice rinks, parking lots, warehouses). Poisoning due to exposure to motorboat exhaust can also lead to serious consequences. Underground electrical cable fires produce large amounts of CO that can leak into adjacent buildings and homes. In the world, especially after hurricanes and in European countries such as Turkiye, poisonings are frequently seen after the southwest wind every year. Additionally, hookah use is a potential source of CO. Methylene chloride is found in lacquers, paint removers, and Christmas decorations as a bubbling liquid, inhaled and digested methylene chloride is metabolized in the liver to CO (Ozciftci & Biberoglu, 2014; Manaker & Perry, 2023).

The 'Prevention of Carbon Monoxide Poisonings in Turkey Program and Action Plan (2015-2018)' was prepared and published by the Turkish Ministry of Health, Public Health Institution (Department of Environmental Health). According to the Ministry data, the most common CO poisoning in Turkiye is stove-related poisoning (94%), and the most common death (73%) is stove poisoning. Although the rules regarding the use of stoves and other CO-source devices are detailed in the book published by the Ministry of Health, the use of detectors sensitive to carbon monoxide gas is recommended (Turkiye Public Health Institution, 2018). In addition, the United States Consumer Product Safety Commission (CPSC) recommends that every home has a CO monitor equipped with an alarm (Bean, 2015; Beckett&Sasson, 2000).

What are the Symptoms of CO Poisoning?

There are no specific symptoms of carbon monoxide poisoning, so signs and symptoms are variable. The most common symptoms are weakness, headache, dizziness, nausea, vomiting, chest pain, and altered mental status (Christensen, 2019).

The clinic of CO poisoning is the result of its underlying systemic toxicity. Its effects arise not only from impaired oxygenation but also from impaired oxygen utilization and respiration at the cellular level (especially in organs with high oxygen demand, such as the heart and brain) (Christensen, 2019; Ashcroft, 2019; Manaker & Perry, 2023).

Symptoms of CO poisoning include weakness, shortness of breath, headache, chest pain, nausea irritability, ataxia, altered mental state, other neurological symptoms, unconsciousness, coma, and death; various neurological findings including tachycardia, tachypnea, hypotension, impaired memory, cognitive and sensory disorders. Metabolic acidosis, cardiac arrhythmias, myocardial ischemia or infarction, and pulmonary edema can also affect all systems with impaired oxygenation (Ashcroft, 2019).

Infants, pregnant women, the elderly, and people with chronic heart disease, anemia, or respiratory disease are the population at particular risk for CO poisoning (Manaker & Perry, 2023).

Small Gasoline Powered Engines: Carbon Monoxide Hazards

People who operate gasoline-powered tools such as high-pressure washers, pumps, compressors, floor buffers, welding machines, and generators in semi-enclosed areas can be affected by carbon monoxide and poisoned in their work area (Centers for Disease Control and Prevention, 2023):

- Do not allow gasoline-powered engines or appliances to be used or operated inside buildings or in partially enclosed spaces unless the gasoline engines can be located away from vents.
- The use of all gasoline-powered tools in confined spaces where CO can accumulate can be fatal.
- Find out the signs and symptoms of poisoning that can occur with CO exposure: headache, nausea, weakness, dizziness, visual

disturbances, personality changes, and unconsciousness. Note that it can occur within a few minutes with the formation of a CO gas.

- Always place the pump and power unit of the high-pressure washers outdoors and away from ventilation openings. Thus, the engine exhaust does not pass into the interior. Just run the high-pressure washer line inside.
- Consider using electrical or compressed air-powered tools if they can be used and are available safely. Undoubtedly, take precautions against electric shocks.
- Use personal CO monitors indoors with the potential for CO poisoning. These monitors should have an audible alarm to alert employees when CO concentrations rise or exceed the NIOSH ceiling limit of 200 parts per million CO.

Employers also:

- Perform a workplace analysis to identify all possible sources of CO poisoning exposure.
- Educate workers about the sources of poisoning, as well as the symptoms and signs that they may encounter possible poisoning.
- Always replace it with less hazardous equipment if possible.
- Monitor the worker's CO exposure to determine the extent of the hazard.

Equipment Users Also:

- Replace it with less hazardous equipment whenever possible.
- Use power tools or power tools that can be placed outside.
- Learn to recognize and know the warning symptoms and signs of CO poisoning.
- If you have any possible symptoms, immediately turn off the equipment and go outside or go to the fresh air.
- Again, in the presence of a possible symptom, activate the emergency aid system. Call 911 or another local emergency number for assistance.
- Do not drive or use a motor vehicle - have someone else drive you to a healthcare facility.

- Do not leave the work area until the instrument is disabled and measured CO concentrations fall below accepted guidelines and standards.
- Be aware of CO toxicity and watch your coworkers for signs of it.

Tool Rental Agencies:

- Put warning labels on gasoline-powered tools.

For example:
WARNING–CARBON MONOXIDE PRODUCED DURING USE CAN KILL–DO NOT USE INDOORS OR IN OTHER SHELTERED AREAS.

- Tell tenants that these gasoline-powered appliances should NOT be used indoors and explain why.
- If available, suggest safer means for the intended use.
- Have portable, audio CO monitors for rent and encourage their use.
- Provide tenants with educational materials such as this fact sheet.

Tool Manufacturers:

- Designing vehicles that can be used safely indoors.
- Provide warning labels for gasoline-powered equipment.

For example:
WARNING–CARBON MONOXIDE PRODUCED DURING USE CAN KILL–DO NOT USE INDOORS OR IN OTHER SHELTERED AREAS.

- Make recommendations for regular maintenance of this equipment to reduce CO emissions.
- I recommend using portable audio CO monitors with these engines.

When the Power Goes Out, Keep Your Generator Outside

Portable backup generators produce the poison gas carbon monoxide (CO).

Follow these important steps to keep your family safe (CDC, 2023):

***Portable Generators

- Never use a generator inside your home or garage, even if the doors and windows are open.
- Only use generators outside, more than 20 feet away from your home, doors, and windows.

***CO-Detectors

- Install battery-operated or battery backup CO detectors near every sleeping area in your home.
- Check CO detectors regularly to make sure they are functioning properly.

Make Sure That No Toxic Gas Is Emitted When Your Furnace Is Operating

Every winter when the temperature drops, your oven can turn into a silent killer. Gas and oil-burning furnaces produce carbon monoxide (CO). CO causes thousands of people to become ill, killing hundreds of people each year. That is why it is essential to take these steps at the beginning of winter to keep your family safe (Figure 1). Have your furnace checked every year (CDC, 2023).

What Should I Do to Prevent CO Poisoning in My Home?

According to the prevention guideline (CDC, 2023), which was updated by the National Center for Environmental Health in November 2022 and shared by the CDC, you can prevent exposure to carbon monoxide (published August 2017 in the Division of Environmental Hazards and Health Effects as the National Center for Environmental Health and updated in CDC in November 2022):

- Have your gas, oil, or coal-burning appliances (heating system, water heater, and others) serviced annually by a qualified technician.
- Install a battery-operated or battery-operated CO detector in your home. Every year, when you change the clocks (every spring and fall), the battery is checked or replaced. If the detector rings, leave the house immediately and call the emergency number.

- If you have common symptoms such as dizziness, lightheadedness, or nausea and suspect CO poisoning, seek medical attention immediately.
- Do not use a charcoal grill, generator, camp stove, or other gasoline or coal-burning appliances in your home, basement, garage or near windows.

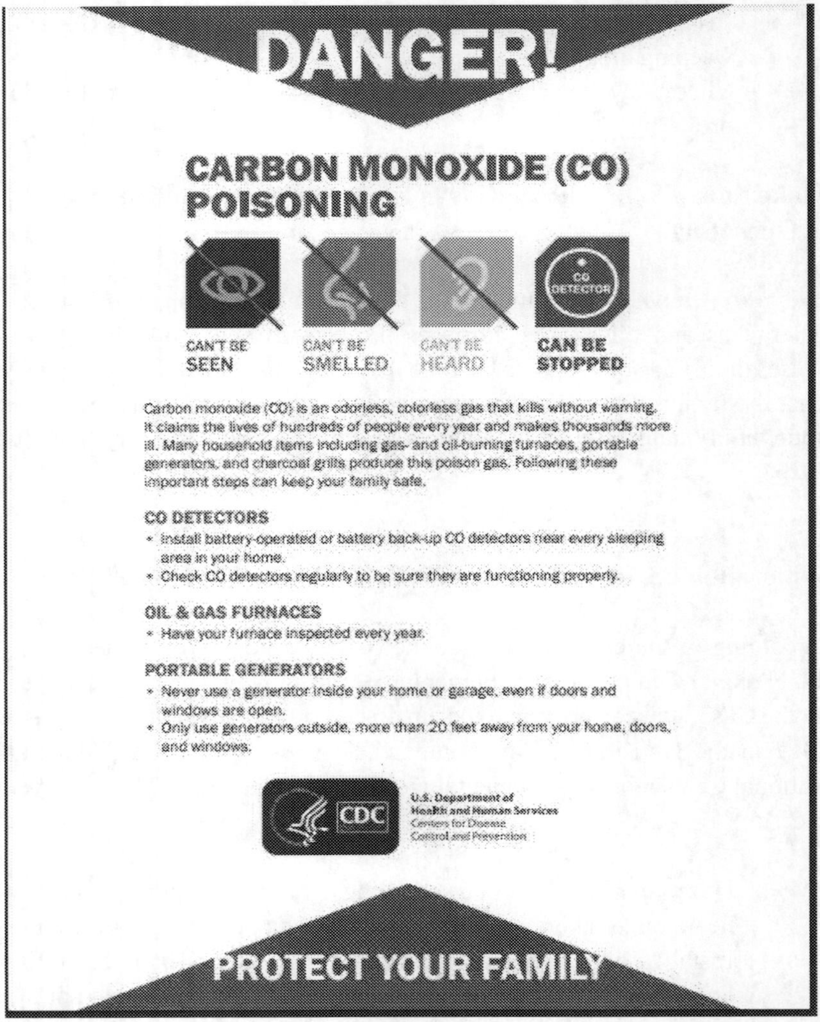

Figure 1a. Carbon monoxide factsheets, available in 9 languages on the CDC website.

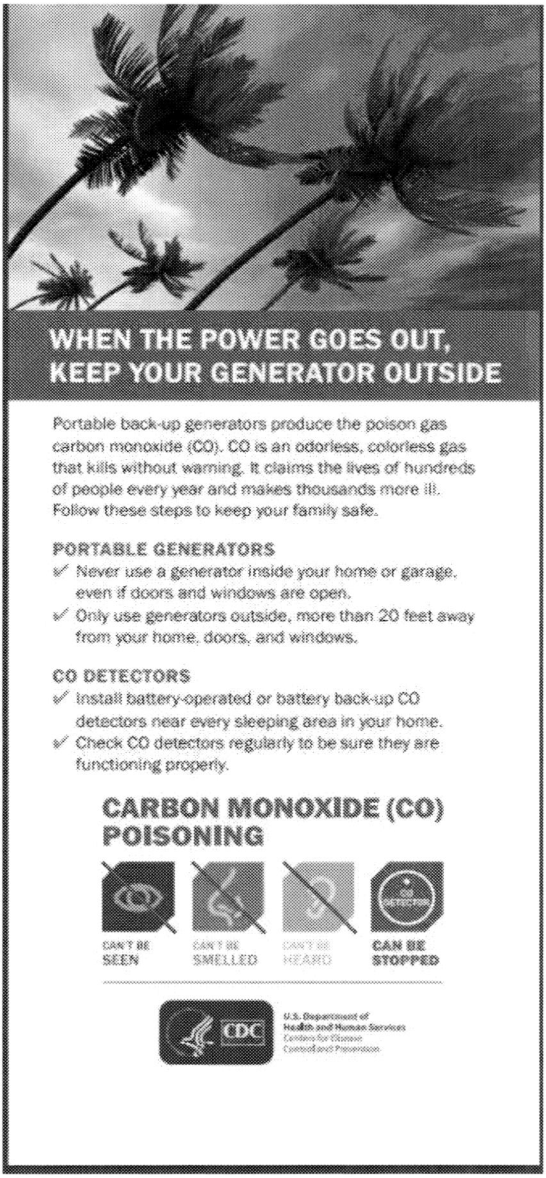

Figure 1b. Carbon monoxide factsheets, available in 9 languages on the CDC website.

- Do not start a car in a garage near your house, even if you leave the door open.
- Do not burn anything in an unventilated stove or fireplace.
- Do not use a gas stove for heating in your home.
- Use an extension cord longer than 20 feet to use the generator at a safe distance. Do not use a generator, pressure washer, or any gasoline-powered engine from any window, door, or vent closer than 20 feet (Figure 1).

Carbon Monoxide Poisoning on the Boat

Gasoline-powered engines and generators on boats can cause carbon monoxide poisoning by inhalation of excess. Because generators and engines on boats can produce carbon monoxide, a colorless, tasteless, and odorless gas, to the extent that it can cause poisoning and death. Sometimes large boats have generators that vent towards the back of the boat. This ventilation is dangerous for people on the aft deck in terms of CO poisoning. In larger boats, CO accumulates above the water platform. Thus, it can kill people in seconds with the CO gas formed in the air space below the aft deck and above the swim deck (CDC, 2022).

While traveling with these boats, low-speed operation or idling causes the accumulation of CO gas in the cabin, cockpit, and aft deck of the boat and even increases the accumulation of CO gas behind the boat with the effect of the wind (CDC, 2022).

Symptoms of CO Poisoning

Headache, nausea, dizziness, weakness, and loss of consciousness, which are common and common symptoms, can also be encountered in poisoning seen on boats. Differently, these symptoms can cause falling into the water and drowning. Even an asleep or intoxicated person can die from CO poisoning without showing any symptoms (CDC, 2018; CDC, 2022).

How to Prevent CO Poisoning on Boats (CDC, 2022):

- Inside the boat, install and maintain a CO detector listed as suitable for use by Underwriters Laboratories (UL) at sea.
- All fuel-powered engines and devices must be properly installed and maintained.
- Passengers should be educated about the signs and symptoms of CO poisoning.
- Swimming and playgrounds should be away from areas where engines discharge their exhaust.
- Children should be closely watched when playing on aft swim decks and water platforms.
- The exhaust outlets are not blocked. Blocking the outlets can result in accumulation of CO in all areas of the ship.
- If you have such a generator or engine-powered boat in your vicinity, dock at least 20 feet away, beach, or anchor because the exhaust from such nearby boats can send CO into the cabin and cockpit of your boat.

If you think someone in your boat has CO poisoning, immediately remove them from the fresh air and contact the nearest emergency room.

Gas Safety and Carbon Monoxide Awareness

The Gas Safety (Installation and Use) Regulations 1998 (GSIUR) as amended was approved, and the Implementing Rules Gas Safety (Installation and Use) (Amendment) Regulation entered into force in April 2018.

'The Cross-Government Group on Gas Safety and Carbon Monoxide Awareness Annual Report' Autumn 2020 to Autumn 2021 published in the UK (Health and Safety Executive, 2022). Members of this group are; Department for Levelling Up, Housing and Communities (DLUHC) formerly MHCLG, Department for Business, Energy & Industrial Strategy (BEIS), Health and Safety Executive (HSE), Office of Gas and Electricity Markets (Ofgem), Health and Safety Executive for Northern Ireland (HSENI), UK Health Security Agency (UKHSA) formerly PHE, Public Health Wales (PHW), Department of Health and Social Care (DHSC), Department of

Digital, Culture, Media and Sport (DCMS), Welsh Government, Scottish Government, Health Protection Scotland (HPS), Home Office (HO).

The Cross-Governmental Group aimed to provide a common approach to gas safety and prevention of carbon monoxide poisoning. It was established with the aim of reducing death and health disorders because of carbon monoxide poisoning. The activities of this group are sharing information about gas safety and CO risk, discovering innovative ways to increase awareness of CO gas, reducing the risks that may occur after the use of gas and fossil fuels, reviewing industrial progress, improving the importance, and understanding of gas safety (Gas Safety Register, 2016).

Public awareness campaigns were carried out, and for this the 'Safety Begins at Home, public awareness campaign was promoted in important TV programs through the media, radio, and television. In the reporting period, Gas Safety Week (GSW21) was also started every year. The Gas Safe Register worked with the academy to convey the message that there are no excuses when it comes to gas safety, and to make sure that your annual gas safety check is always done by experts. GSW21 featured strongly regionally on national channels (such as Times Radio, LBC news, and Sky News Radio) in nationwide broadcasts, and also featured more than 330 news items and had a total digital week reach of over 70 million.

HSENI supported Gas Safety Week 2020 with 4 posts on social media. In the Gas Safety Register, the control engineers provided encouraging messages such as CO symptoms poisoning, Homeowners' legal obligations, and CO alarms.

Britain reported its alert requirements as follows (DLUHC, Expands Carbon Monoxide Alert Requirements (UK);

- Smoke alarms will be mandatory in all social rental homes.
- Carbon monoxide alarms will be mandatory in rooms with any fixed combustion appliances (except gas stoves) in both private and social rental homes.
- Carbon monoxide alarms will also be mandatory when any fixed combustion system is installed.
- (except for gas hobs) at all times of use according to building regulations.
- Homeowners will be expected to repair or replace alarms after they are reported as defective.

Finally, this report was created to describe the government's joint work to improve gas safety and address the risks of CO from all fuels (UK gas supply explainer-GOV.UK (www.gov.uk) English Housing Survey - English Housing Survey: headline report 2020-21 (publishing.service.gov.uk). (Health and Safety Executive, 2022; Gentile et al., 2021; Department for Levelling Up, Housing and Communities and Ministry of Housing, Communities & Local Government, 2020).

Surveillance of Carbon Monoxide Poisoning

Carbon monoxide poisoning is a critical health concern for public health surveillance, due to its frequency, severity, and preventability, as well as the effectiveness of simple preventive measures such as the establishment of a carbon monoxide alarm. Establishing state-based public health surveillance for CO poisoning is a viable prevention. Surveillance is required for guidance and control efforts. It should be further investigated, as the result is that more than 20% of poisoning cases are classified as occupational (Graber JM, Smith AE 2007).

In the study, which was analyzed at the Wisconsin Poison Center (WPC) and published in 2019, 3703 people were exposed to CO poisoning between 2006 and 2016 in the United States, it was determined that despite public health efforts to reduce CO exposure, CO poisoning continues to affect the residents of Wisconsin. The most common sources of exposure were found to be ovens, water heaters, and fire. Efforts to prevent large-scale CO poisoning should focus on awareness of the risk in public or occupational settings, as well as CO exposure in the home. In addition, these efforts should focus on improving the use of CO detectors in all environments to avoid exposure (Christensen GM, 2019).

The surveillance of CO cases is generally limited to the most affected geographical area where the disaster occurred and excludes populations in less affected areas. In the past, although many states had extensive power outages for a long time after Hurricane Katrina, only five Gulf coast states (Alabama, Mississippi, Louisiana, Texas, and Florida) had reported cases of CO poisoning due to severe Katrina damage (CDC 2005; CDC 2006; Cox R. 2008; CDC 2006). Similarly, during an ice storm in Kentucky in 2009, CO poisoning surveillance focused on areas the most affected (Lutterloh EC, 2011).

Regarding the effectiveness of carbon monoxide detectors in reducing poisoning, individuals exposed to CO in the absence of a CO detector were more likely to be poisoned and have more serious medical consequences than those with an alarming CO detector (Christensen GM, 2020).

In a study examining 28 journal articles on disaster-related CO poisoning cases in the United States between 1991 and 2009. It found that charcoal grills are a major source of exposure as methods of exposure during winter storms, with 67% of fatal cases caused by generator placement indoors. Most deaths (94%) occurred at home. Approximately 89% of fatal cases and 53% of non-fatal cases occurred within 3 days of the onset of the disaster (Iqbal et al., 2012).

Most undesirable exposures can be avoided with the use of CO detectors and proper ventilation and maintenance of the burning appliances. The fact that a high proportion of household appliances are generally unsafe and not installed by competent people (Smollin and Olson, 2008; Penney et al., 2010; Gas Safety Record, 2016) suggests that more precautions can be taken. Unintentional CO poisoning continues to be an important cause of preventable morbidity and mortality worldwide (Stearns and Sircar, 2019; Khadem-Rezaiyan and Afshari, 2016; Lavigne et al., 2015; Braubach et al., 2013; Fisher et al., 2013, Fisher et al., 2014; Yari et al., 2012; Barceló AR et al., 2020).

The Global Burden of Disease (GBD) added its estimates due to CO poisoning in 2017, resulting in 35,500 (95% CI: 25,700–38,800) deaths and 1462.4 (95% CI: 1,073,000; 1,613,600) deaths worldwide for that year. reported an adjusted life year (Roth et al., 2018). In addition to fatal exposures, CO poisoning can have significant short- or long-term health effects (depending on inhaled concentration, exposure time, and physical condition) (Ashcroft et al., 2019; Smollin and Olson, 2008).

Carbon Monoxide Detectors: Types and How Do They Work?

There are many different types and brands of CO detectors available, and they can be grouped according to whether they are powered by household electricity or batteries (Office of the State Fire Commissioner, n.d.).

Home current detectors periodically self-clean and resample for CO, a type of solid-state sensor.

Battery-operated detectors, on the other hand, have a passive sensor that responds to prolonged exposure to carbon monoxide gas.

The common feature of both types is that they must comply with minimum sensitivity and alarm standards. A CO detector that is not Underwriters Laboratory (UL) approved should not be purchased. Each detector type has its own advantages and disadvantages. The types household currents need to be connected to electrical wiring.

Some detectors last 5-10 years, others 2-3 years, so the batteries need to be changed periodically. Some continuously show a CO level, while others only alarm when set levels are reached. Some reset when the CO problem is resolved, and others need the sensor package removed (Office of the State Fire Commissioner, n.d.).

How Many CO Detectors Are Required and Where Should They Be Installed?

The Consumer Product Safety Commission makes its recommendations as follows:

- A detector in each flat of the residences,
- At least 1 detector per sleep floor
- Additional detectors in large fuel-burning appliances such as ovens, kettles, or wood stoves
- It should be installed high, close to the ceiling.
- Placing within 1.5 meters of gas appliances, wood stoves, bathing or cooking areas
- The correctly placed detectors will ensure that alarms are heard in all sleeping areas (Office of the State Fire Commissioner, n.d.).

What Should You Do If Your CO Detector Sounds an Alarm?

- First, be calm.
- Most CO detector activations are not life-threatening.
- If asked if anyone is feeling sick, experiencing flu-like headaches, nausea, fatigue, dizziness, or drowsiness and answers yes to any of the symptoms, IMMEDIATELY evacuate the building to a safe place and call 9-1-1 (Office of the State Fire Commissioner, n.d.).

Conclusion

Carbon monoxide poisoning is a type of poisoning that affects public health and is important because it is a preventable poisoning. Governments in countries have published prevention programs against these poisoning hazards.

Since it can be encountered in all areas of our lives, the importance of people acting in accordance with these national and international guidelines and regulations is increasing day by day.

Precautions and precautions to be taken about this gas, which insidiously causes poisoning, are summarized in this chapter titled "Prevention of Carbon Monoxide Poisoning".

References

Ashcroft, J., Fraser, E., Krishnamoorthy, S., and Westwood-Ruttledge, S. (2019). Carbon monoxide poisoning. *BMJ (Clinical research ed.)*, 365, l2299. https://doi.org/10.1136/bmj.l2299.

Beckett, K., and Sasson, T. (2000). *The politics of injustice: Crime and punishment in America*. Thousand Oaks, CA: Pine Forge Press.

Braubach, M., Algoet, A., Beaton, M., Lauriou, S., Héroux, M. E., and Krzyzanowski, M. (2013). Mortality associated with exposure to carbon monoxide in WHO European Member States. *Indoor air*, 23(2), 115–125. https://doi.org/10.1111/ina.12007.

Christensen, G. M., Creswell, P. D., and Meiman, J. G. (2019). Carbon Monoxide Exposure and Poisoning Cases in Wisconsin, 2006-2016. *WMJ: official publication of the State Medical Society of Wisconsin*, 118(1), 21–26.

Christensen, G. M., Creswell, P. D., Theobald, J., and Meiman, J. G. (2020). Carbon monoxide detector effectiveness in reducing poisoning, Wisconsin 2014-2016. *Clinical toxicology (Philadelphia, Pa.)*, 58(12), 1335–1341. https://doi.org/10.1080/15563650.2020.1733592.

Centers for Disease Control and Prevention (CDC) (2005). Carbon monoxide poisoning after hurricane Katrina--Alabama, Louisiana, and Mississippi, August-September 2005. *MMWR. Morbidity and mortality weekly report*, 54(39), 996–998.

Centers for Disease Control and Prevention (CDC) (2006). Carbon monoxide poisonings after two major hurricanes--Alabama and Texas, August-October 2005. *MMWR. Morbidity and mortality weekly report*, 55(9), 236–239.

Centers for Disease Control and Prevention (CDC) (2006). Mortality associated with Hurricane Katrina--Florida and Alabama, August-October 2005. *MMWR. Morbidity and mortality weekly report*, 55(9), 239–242.

Centers for Disease Control and Prevention (CDC) (2018). Prevent Carbon Monoxide (CO) Poisoning. Retrieved from www.cdc.gov/CO.

Centers for Disease Control and Prevention (CDC) (2022). Carbon Monoxide Poisoning on the Boat. Retrieved from https://www.cdc.gov/niosh/topics/coboating/.

Centers for Disease Control and Prevention (CDC) (2018) *Prevent Carbon Monoxide (CO) Poisoning* YouTube. Retrieved from https://www.cdc.gov/co/videos/Prevent-CO-Poisoning-Transcript-082118-508.pdf.

Centers for Disease Control and Prevention (CDC) (2023). *Preventing Carbon Monoxide Poisoning from Small Gasoline-Powered Engines & Tools (96-118a) | NIOSH | CDC.* Retrieved from https://www.cdc.gov/niosh/topics/co/.

Centers for Disease Control and Prevention (CDC) (2023). *Carbon Monoxide Poisoning, Frequently Asked Question.* Retrieved from https://www.cdc.gov/co/faqs.htm.

Cox, R., Amundson, T., and Brackin, B. (2008). Evaluation of the patterns of potentially toxic exposures in Mississippi following Hurricane Katrina. *Clinical toxicology (Philadelphia, Pa.)*, 46(8), 722–727. https://doi.org/10.1080/15563650701455379.

Department for Levelling Up, Housing and Communities and Ministry of Housing, Communities & Local Government (2020). *Consultation outcome Domestic smoke and carbon monoxide alarms: proposals to extend regulations – government response.* Retrieved from https://www.gov.uk/government/consultations/domestic-smoke-and-carbon-monoxide/alarms/outcome/domestic-smoke-and-carbon-monoxide-alarms-proposals-to-extend/regulations-government-response.

Gas Safety Register (2016). *2.7 million Retners at Risk from Dangerous Gas Appliances*. Retrieved from https://www.gassaferegister.co.uk/about-us/news/news-2016/renters-at-risk-from-dangerous-gas-appliances/.

GBD 2017 Causes of Death Collaborators (2018). Global, regional, and national age-sex-specific mortality for 282 causes of death in 195 countries and territories, 1980-2017: a systematic analysis for the Global Burden of Disease Study 2017. *Lancet (London, England)*, 392(10159), 1736–1788. https://doi.org/10.1016/S0140-6736(18)32203-7.

Gentile, D., Adams, R., Klatka, M., Bradberry, S., Gray, L., Thanacoody, R., Jackson, G., and Sandilands, E. A. (2022). Carbon monoxide exposures reported to the UK National Poisons Information Service: a 4-year study. *Journal of public health (Oxford, England)*, 44(3), 565–574. https://doi.org/10.1093/pubmed/fdab132.

Graber, J. M., and Smith, A. E. (2007). Results from a state-based surveillance system for carbon monoxide poisoning. *Public health reports* (Washington, D.C.: 1974), 122(2), 145–154. https://doi.org/10.1177/003335490712200203.

Health and Safety Executive (2022). *The Cross-Government Group on Gas Safety and Carbon Monoxide Awareness. Annual Report*, Autumn 2020 To Autumn 2021. Retrieved from https://www.hse.gov.uk/gas/domestic/cross-government-group-2021.pdf.

Jones, S. J., Horton, A., Brunt, H., and Shankar, G. (2019). Preventing carbon monoxide poisoning. *BMJ (Clinical research ed.)*, 366, l4613. https://doi.org/10.1136/bmj.l4613.

Iqbal, S., Clower, J. H., Boehmer, T. K., Yip, F. Y., and Garbe, P. (2010). Carbon monoxide-related hospitalizations in the U.S.: evaluation of a web-based query system for public health surveillance. *Public health reports* (Washington, D.C.: 1974), 125(3), 423–432. https://doi.org/10.1177/003335491012500311.

Iqbal, S., Clower, J. H., Hernandez, S. A., Damon, S. A., and Yip, F. Y. (2012). A review of disaster-related carbon monoxide poisoning: surveillance, epidemiology, and opportunities for prevention. *American journal of public health*, 102(10), 1957–1963. https://doi.org/10.2105/AJPH.2012.300674.

Iqbal, S., Law, H. Z., Clower, J. H., Yip, F. Y., and Elixhauser, A. (2012). Hospital burden of unintentional carbon monoxide poisoning in the United States, 2007. *The American journal of emergency medicine*, 30(5), 657–664. https://doi.org/10.1016/j.ajem.2011.03.003.

Khadem-Rezaiyan, M., and Afshari, R. (2016). Carbon monoxide poisoning in Northeast of Iran. *Journal of forensic and legal medicine*, 41, 1–4. https://doi.org/10.1016/j.jflm.2016.04.002.

Lavigne, E., Weichenthal, S., Wong, J., Smith-Doiron, M., Dugandzic, R., and Kosatsky, T. (2015). Mortality and hospital admission rates for unintentional nonfire-related carbon monoxide poisoning across Canada: a trend analysis. *CMAJ open*, 3(2), E223–E230. https://doi.org/10.9778/cmajo.20140122.

Lutterloh, E. C., Iqbal, S., Clower, J. H., Spiller, H. A., Riggs, M. A., Sugg, T. J., Humbaugh, K. E., Cadwell, B. L., and Thoroughman, D. A. (2011). Carbon monoxide poisoning after an ice storm in Kentucky, 2009. *Public health reports* (Washington, D.C.:1974), 126 Suppl 1(Suppl 1), 108–115. https://doi.org/10.1177/00333549111260S114.

Manaker, S., and Perry, H. (2023). Carbon monoxide poisoning Literature review current through: Mar 2023. | UpToDate. Mar 02, 2023. https://www.uptodate.com/contents/carbon-monoxide-poisoning?source=mostViewed_widget#H17.

Office of the State Fire Commissioner (n.d.). *Carbon Monoxide Poisoning Prevention.* https://www.osfc.pa.gov/FireSafety/Pages/Carbon-Monoxide-Poisoning-Prevention.aspx.

Olson, K., and Smollin, C. (2008). Carbon monoxide poisoning (acute). *BMJ clinical evidence*, 2008, 2103.

Ozçiftçi, S., and Biberoğlu., S. (2014). Approach to Carbon Monoxide Intoxication. *Ortadoğu Tıp Dergisi* [*Middle East Journal of Medicine*], 6, 86-89.

Penney, D., Benignus, V., Kephalopoulos, S., Kotzias, D., Kleinman, M., and Verrier, A. (2010). Carbon monoxide. In: *WHO Guidelines for Indoor Air Quality: Selected Pollutants*. Geneva: World Health Organization. https://www.ncbi.nlm.nih.gov/books/NBK138710/.

Roca-Barceló, A., Crabbe, H., Ghosh, R., Freni-Sterrantino, A., Fletcher, T., Leonardi, G., Hoge, C., Hansell, A. L., and Piel, F. B. (2020). Temporal trends and demographic risk factors for hospital admissions due to carbon monoxide poisoning in England. *Preventive medicine*, 136, 106104. https://doi.org/10.1016/j.ypmed.2020.106104.

Smollin, C., and Olson, K. (2010). Carbon monoxide poisoning (acute). *BMJ clinical evidence*, 2010, 2103.

Stearns, D., and Sircar, K. (2019). National unintentional carbon monoxide poisoning estimates using hospitalization and emergency department data. *The American journal of emergency medicine*, 37(3), 421–426. https://doi.org/10.1016/ j.ajem.2018.06.002.

Torre Cantalapiedra, E. (2018). Bean, Frank D., Susan K. Brown y James D. Bachmeier (2015), Parents without papers: The progress and pitfalls of Mexican-American integration, Nueva York, Russell Sage Foundation. *Estudios Demográficos y Urbanos* [*Demographic and Urban Studies*], 33(1), 267–272. https://doi.org/10.24201/edu.v33i1.1744.

Turkiye Public Health Institution (2018). *Turkiye Carbon Monoxide Poisoning Prevention Program and Action Plan.* Retrieved from https://hsgm.saglik.gov.tr/depo/birimler/cevre-sagligi/2-ced/karbonmonoksit-zehirlenmesi/.

Chapter 14

New and Promising Treatment Options in Carbon Monoxide Poisoning

Seda Özkan*, **MD**
Department of Emergency Medicine, İstanbul University-Cerrahpaşa, İstanbul, Turkey

Abstract

Carbon monoxide poisoning is a common and deadly public health problem worldwide. Carbon monoxide binds to hemoglobin in the blood, reducing the amount of oxygen that can be carried to the body's tissues, leading to hypoxia and tissue damage, particularly in the brain and heart. The traditional treatment of patients with carbon monoxide poisoning is normobaric and hyperbaric oxygen therapy. Severe carbon monoxide poisonings have persistent neurological effects and high morbidity rates. As the pathophysiology of carbon monoxide poisoning is understood, new treatment methods are being researched and developed. These new and promising treatment methods are: antidote treatments aiming at preventing oxidative stress and inflammation, neuroprotective drugs, treatments that prevent the binding of carbon monoxide to heme-containing proteins, and methods that increase the separation of carbon monoxide from hemoglobin, are treatment methods that have the ability to regenerate and repair damaged tissues.

Keywords: carbon monoxide, poisoning, treatment

* Corresponding Author's Email: seda.ozkan@iuc.edu.tr.

In: Carbon Monoxide Poisoning
Editors: Seda Özkan and Afsin Ipekci
ISBN: 979-8-89113-217-7

Introduction

The toxic effects of carbon monoxide (CO) begin with its binding to hemoglobin in the blood. CO competes with oxygen to bind to Hb. The affinity of CO for hemoglobin is 300 times higher than for oxygen. The oxygen-carrying capacity of hemoglobin decreases with the binding of CO to Hb. In addition, carbon monoxide shifts the oxyhemoglobin dissociation curve to the left, impairing the release of oxygen to the tissues. Thus, hypoxia occurs in all tissues. In addition to hemoglobin, CO is bound to other heme-containing proteins (myoglobin and cytochrome c oxidase). Global hypoxia, ischemia, free oxygen radicals, and inflammation are responsible for damage to the brain, heart, and other organs in CO poisoning (Xiang et al., 2014; Xue & Wang, 2014; Rose et al., 2017; Zhao et al., 2018; Zhang et al., 2020; Rose et al., 2020).

In the traditional treatment of CO poisoning, normobaric and hyperbaric oxygen are used. Although hyperbaric oxygen therapy significantly reduces the lasting effects of CO poisoning, some survivors still have significant morbidity (Rose et al., 2017).

Delayed neurological sequelae (DNS) after CO exposure are the most important complications of CO poisoning. Studies are continuing to prevent DNS. The pathophysiology of DNS is not yet fully understood. It is thought to result of neuron death resulting from inflammation, mitochondrial oxidative stress, inhibition of mitochondrial function, lipid peroxidation, apoptosis, and adaptive immunological responses. Studies continue to explain the pathophysiology of CO poisoning (O'Donnell et al., 2000; Lo et al., 2007; Pearce et al., 2017; Zhao et al., 2018; Tabrizian et al., 2018; Rose et al., 2020).

As the pathophysiology of CO poisoning is understood, studies trying new treatment methods are increasing. These studies include antidote treatments to prevent oxidative stress and inflammation, neuroprotective drugs, anti-apoptotic drugs, treatments to prevent the binding of CO to heme proteins, methods to increase the separation of CO from hemoglobin, and treatment methods that have the ability to regenerate and repair damaged tissues.

In this chapter, these new and promising treatment methods researched in CO poisoning will be explained.

High-Flow Nasal Cannula Oxygen

In the last two decades, the administration of high-flow nasal cannula (HFNC) oxygen has begun to be used as an alternative respiratory support device to traditional oxygen therapy tools in critically ill patients (Kim et al., 2020; Nishimura, 2019). The HFNC delivers heated (37 °C) and humidified (100% RH) oxygen with a safe inspired fraction (FiO2) at 21% to 100% at a high-flow rate. HFNC is a less invasive ventilation system and allows adjustment of FiO2 regardless of flow rate (Long et al., 2021; Rochwerg et al., 2020).

HFNC has many advantages over conventional oxygen tools that result in better physiological effects. HFNC; It improves oxygenation, reduces airway resistance, increases the leaching of carbon dioxide (CO2) in the anatomical dead space, provides humidified flow, and provides low levels of positive end-expiratory pressure (PEEP) through high flow rates. Based on the monitored oxygen concentration, FiO2 can be titrated up to 60 liters per minute (Tomruk et al., 2019; Kim et al., 2020; Long et al., 2021).

The use of HFNC is increasing day by day. It is used in diseases such as acute hypoxemic respiratory failure, respiratory distress syndrome, coronavirus disease 2019, interstitial lung disease, chronic obstructive pulmonary disease (COPD), pneumonia, sleep apnea, cardiogenic pulmonary edema (Tomruk et al., 2019; Long et al., 2021). The successful results of the HFNC treatment in acute hypoxemic diseases in a short period of time have led to its trial as a treatment method in acute CO poisoning.

Randomized controlled trials have compared HFNC with conventional normobaric oxygen in patients with acute CO exposure. It was found that HFNC reduced COHb levels significantly faster and reduced the half-life of COHb values compared to oxygen therapy with a normobaric mask (Tomruk et al., 2019; Kim et al., 2020; Yesiloglu et al., 2021; Dong et al., 2022).

In the treatment of mild to moderate acute CO poisoning, HFNC is considered an easy, safe, comfortable, and effective method to reduce COHb (Ozturan et al., 2019).

Extracorporeal Membrane Oxygenation

The frequency of use of extracorporeal membrane oxygenation (ECMO) in cardiac and respiratory failure is increasing day by day. The ECMO is a life support machine that provides external artificial circulation. ECMO ensures that the patient's blood is cleaned of CO2 and enriched from oxygen in an external system using cannulas placed in large veins and arteries (Simonsen et al., 2019).

There are few studies on the effectiveness of ECMO in carbon monoxide poisoning. In a study in Porcine models, subjects inhaled CO until cardiac failure developed. Afterwards, venous-arterial ECMO was connected to some of the subjects, while only ventilator support was given to some of them. Survival was higher in pigs given ECMO support (Simonsen et al., 2018). Another study published by the same team demonstrated the successful application of ECMO under long airway transfer conditions in a pig with severe exposure to CO and cardiac arrest (Simonsen et al., 2019).

There are only two case reports in the literature regarding the application of ECMO in CO poisoning in humans. In the first case report, it was reported that the patient who developed ARDS and cardiovascular collapse after severe CO poisoning was discharged after 7 days of veno-venous ECMO. It has been stated that death can be prevented with ECMO support in the early period (McCunn et al., 2000).

In the second case report, veno-arterial ECMO was performed in a patient with severe CO exposure who developed unstable and cardiogenic shock. The patient was followed up for 6 months in terms of delayed neurological sequelae after discharge. The patient recovered without any sequelae (Teerapuncharoen et al., 2015).

As a result, ECMO, reduces cardiac oxygen consumption, lowers carboxy hemoglobin levels in the blood, and returns oxygen-rich blood to the body (Teerapuncharoen et al., 2015). In this way, it allows the rapid removal of CO from the body. The use of ECMO can be considered in patients who do not benefit from ventilatory support due to severe exposure to CO or who develop cardiac failure.

Phototherapy

Studies aiming to increase the elimination of CO by separating CO from hemoglobin with phototherapy are also promising developments for future use. It has long been known that light breaks the CO bond and does not touch the oxygen while removing the CO (Rose et al., 2015).

In an experimental study, blood was drawn from the subject using an ECMO, the blood was irradiated, and the blood was given back to the subject. With this method, called extracorporeal photodynamic blood illumination, more CO dissociation from hemoglobin was achieved and survival was higher (Rose et al., 2017).

Direct phototherapy was performed after open thoracotomy on laboratory rats. The half-life of carboxyhemoglobin was reduced by more than 50% with phototherapy. The same team additionally applied transesophageal pulmonary phototherapy with fiber optic placed in the esophagus and found that the carbon monoxide elimination rate increased (Zazzeron et al., 2015).

Especially if phototherapy is developed with a non-invasive method, it may be an effective treatment method that can be applied in the future for patients with severe CO exposure.

N-Acetylcysteine

N-acetylcysteine (NAC), the precursor of L-cysteine, is an antioxidant widely used in mucolytic therapy. NAC destroys free oxygen radicals before they cause damage to cells. NAC acts as a cysteine source for glutathione synthesis and increases cysteine/glutathione levels in cells. It provides the regeneration of glutathione consumed by free radicals, scavenges reactive oxygen species (ROS), and restores the antioxidant potential in cells (Spina et al., 2019; Tardiolo et al., 2018).

NAC acts as a glutathione precursor in paracetamol overdose. Thus, it prevents liver damage by inhibiting the binding of N-acetyl-p-benzo-quinone imine (NAPQI) to hepatic macromolecules. NAC helps prevent cellular damage in the body by increasing the production of glutathione, neutralizing free radicals, reducing oxidative stress, improving microcirculation blood flow, and increasing tissue oxygenation (Chiew & Buckley, 2021).

NAC also has weak anti-inflammatory effects by reducing Nuclear Factor-kB activation. As an anti-inflammatory agent, NAC can limit the release of cytokines in the early stages of immune proliferation (Spina et al., 2019, Tardiolo et al., 2018, Omara et al., 1997).

NAC has been shown to effectively cross the blood-brain barrier by increasing glutathione levels in the brain. It has been hypothesized that NAC may be a very important factor in the treatment of neurological disorders in which variations in glutathione levels and redox pathways are observed (Tardiolo et al., 2018).

Due to the properties of NAC, mentioned above, it was considered that it would be useful to prevent tissue damage after CO poisoning. Spina et al. used high-dose NAC (12 g/day) and low-dose prednisone (25 mg/day) in addition to HBOT in the treatment of a young woman with neurological sequelae after CO poisoning. In the patient's MRI study, they observed a progressive and sustained clinical improvement in motor, cognitive, and behavioral symptoms, along with a reduction in the size of the white matter abnormalities (Spina et al., 2019).

In another study in rats, melatonin and NAC were used. Both NAC and melatonin have been shown to reduce brain and lung tissue damage caused by CO poisoning (Kekec et al., 2010).

It is thought that the combination of HBOT with antioxidant and anti-inflammatory drugs may create a positive synergistic effect. More research is needed to clarify the role of antioxidants in therapy and the duration of persistent neurological changes that occur after CO poisoning (Spina et al., 2019).

Dexamethasone

Delayed neuropsychiatric sequelae are the main complications of carbon monoxide poisoning. Although the pathophysiology of DNS is not exactly understood, CO is thought to trigger brain oxidation and inflammation. It is thought that transient intramyelin edema or inflammation resulting from lipid peroxidation causes white matter involvement (Lo et al., 2007; O'Donnell et al., 2000). Persistent neuropathology has been associated with an immunological response to the modified myelin basic protein (Thom et al., 2004; Spina et al., 2019).

It has been suggested that corticosteroids, such as dexamethasone, may modulate neurological damage after carbon monoxide poisoning through anti-inflammatory effects and immune response inhibition (Kim et al., 2023).

In a study in rats, it was revealed that inflammation resulting from acute CO poisoning plays an important role in delayed encephalopathy. It has been reported that dexamethasone may weaken the development of delayed encephalopathy by protecting myelin from damage by the inflammatory response (Xiang et al., 2014; Xue & Wang, 2014). In addition, the authors stated that 30 mg/kg of dexamethasone per day could significantly reduce the mortality rate of CO-poisoning rats.

Atalay et al. reported that the addition of dexamethasone to treatment in CO-poisoning rats could affect brain tissue lipid peroxidation (Atalay et al., 2006).

In another animal (rat) study, it was shown that early dexamethasone treatment could prevent delayed encephalopathy after carbon monoxide poisoning (DEACMP) by blocking lipid oxidation and myelin basic protein (MBP)-related immune response, reducing ischemia and hypoxic cell swelling, reducing permeability, and inhibiting the inflammatory response (Li et al., 2015). In the study, serum myelin basic protein levels were measured after 18 days of dexamethasone treatment was administered to rats. Dexamethasone was found to decrease the level of serum myelin basic protein, which causes delayed neurological encephalopathy (Li et al., 2015).

In a clinical study conducted in 2017, it was reported that the combined administration of dexamethasone and HBOT resulted in better functional recovery from DNS compared to HBOT alone, as assessed by the mini-mental state examination (MMSE) score and the National Institutes of Health Stroke Scale (NIHSS) score (Xiang et al., 2017).

In another clinical study investigating whether corticosteroids prevent delayed neuropsychiatric sequelae due to CO poisoning, IV dexamethasone was given to 99 patients. The rate of development of delayed neuropsychic-atric sequelae (16%) in patients who received dexamethasone was significantly lower than in patients who did not receive dexamethasone (38%). Therefore, the authors reported that early dexamethasone treatment was associated with a decreased incidence of delayed neuropsychiatric sequelae (Kim et al., 2023).

The results of studies show that the addition of dexamethasone to HBOT has potential benefits and can provide a better cognitive and neurological function (Xu et al., 2019). However, more clinical studies are needed to determine the appropriate dose and use of dexamethasone in the treatment of CO poisoning.

N-Butylphthalide

N-Butylphthalide (NBP) is a compound that is a plant extract and has long been used in traditional Chinese medicine. Dl-3-N-butylphthalide obtained from celery seeds is the main ingredient of NBP. NBP is a cerebral ischemia drug that is lipid-soluble and has good blood-brain barrier permeability (Diao et al., 2015). Soft NBP capsules were developed to improve cerebral artery thrombosis in cerebrovascular disease. Since NBP has antioxidant and neuroprotective properties, it is thought that it can also be used in the treatment of delayed encephalopathy due to CO poisoning (Zhang et al., 2020).

The efficacy of NBP in the treatment of CO poisoning has been studied in several studies. Although the effect of NBP on the treatment of CO poisoning has not been proven yet, the research is promising.

In the first study conducted in humans in 2016, combined treatment of butylphthalide and mesenchymal stem cell (MSC) transplantation was more successful than MSC transplantation and hyperbaric oxygen therapy alone. Combined treatment of MSC with butylphthalide was found to be superior to MSC transplantation alone in improving cognitive function, activities of daily living, and rate of neurological recovery. Butylphthalide has been reported to be safe and effective in the treatment of DEACMP (Wang et al., 2016).

In a study conducted in China, a combination of NBP and high-pressure oxygen was used in 84 patients with CO poisoning. As a result, it was stated that the duration of the coma of the patients was shortened and their recovery accelerated (Han et al., 2017).

In the clinical study conducted by Xiang et al. in 2017, it was shown that the combined administration of N-Butylphthalide and HBO can significantly improve the cognitive function of patients with DEACMP and produce better clinical efficacy. It has been shown that patients treated with N-Butylphthalide and HBO can significantly increase the MMSE score, decrease the NIHSS score, and achieve a significantly higher RR in DEACMP patients with cognitive dysfunction, compared to patients treated with HBO alone (Xiang et al., 2017).

It was observed that the cognitive and motor functions of patients who were given NBP and dexametaxazone in addition to HBO treatment improved without significant side effects (Zhang et al., 2020).

The possible mechanisms of action of NBP on DEACMP are as follows (Zhang et al., 2020):

- NBP selectively inhibits physiological and pathological processes mediated by arachidonic acid and its metabolites. It inhibits platelet aggregation and reverses microvasospasm to reduce thrombosis.
- It increases the fluidity of the mitochondrial membrane in nerve cells in areas of cerebral ischemia. It activates the complex IV enzyme in the respiratory chain. It increases the activity of antioxidant enzymes. It decreases the production of free oxygen radicals.
- It maintains the complete structure of the microvessels and increases the number of microvessels. It improves microcirculation by creating

collateral circulation in areas of cerebral ischemia. Thus, it significantly increases regional cerebral blood flow.

- It reduces intracellular calcium concentration by inhibiting glutamate release. It develops resistance to oxidative stress, thereby attenuating the inflammatory response and cell apoptosis after brain ischemia. NBP, therefore, exerts a significant neuroprotective effect, attenuating nerve damage and reducing disability or death rates in patients with DEACMP.
- NBP increases axon, synapse, and nerve regeneration in the subventricular space after cerebral ischemia and hypoxia. It improves the survival rate of new cells and regulates their differentiation into mature neurons. It enhances the memory function of certain nerve cells and effectively reverses or ameliorates cognitive impairment.

In a meta-analysis published in 2023; it is reported that NBP can stably bind Albumin, estrogen receptor 1, epidermal growth factor receptor, Heat Shock Protein 90α (HSP90AA1), and other targets. NBP modulates lipid and atherosclerosis, Interleukin-17 (IL-17), mitogen-activated protein kinase, forkhead box O, and phosphatidylinositol 3'-kinase signaling pathways. Thus, NBP may play a role in neuroprotection in patients with DEACMP (Song et al., 2023).

Studies on the clinical applicability of the combined application of N-Butylphthalide and HBOT are promising for the future and show that it can be an effective option in the treatment of CO poisoning. However, future studies involving more patients from different centers are needed to confirm and support the efficacy of this method (Zhang et al., 2020).

Stem Cell Treatment

Stem cells are undifferentiated cells capable of self-renewal and multi-lineage differentiation. Stem cells can be induced in vitro or in vivo to differentiate into specific tissue cells. Thus, they have the potential to regenerate damaged tissues and support tissue repair for treatment purposes (Jeong et al., 2004). In the context of CO poisoning, it has been hypothesized that stem cells can repair damage caused by hypoxia and oxidative stress in the brain, heart, and other organs.

Studies have shown that mesenchymal stem cells (MSCs) can be induced into neurons or glial cells under certain conditions (Jeong et al., 2004; Crigler et al., 2006; Jin et al., 2008; Kim et al., 2009). According to these studies, stem cells have the following functions:

- In the microenvironment of the central nervous system (CNS), they secrete brain-derived neurotrophic factors and essential fibroblast growth factors.
- They can secrete multiple neurotrophic factors and activate endogenous neural stem cells.
- They can differentiate into neural cells to replace damaged cells, which is the endogenous pathway of neural repair.
- They can differentiate into vascular endothelial cells and promote angiogenesis. In hypoxia, they mediate microvascular endothelial cell migration and vasculogenesis.

Experimental research has shown that stem cell-based therapy after severe CO poisoning can play an effective role in improving brain damage and function after severe acute CO poisoning. Thus, it was presented as a new approach model for the treatment of severe CO poisoning patients with delayed neurological sequelae (Jiang et al., 2009).

A combined treatment consisting of umbilical cord blood (UCB) stem cell transplantation, nicholine injection, and intranasal insulin inhalation was applied to a patient who presented with severe CO poisoning. It was stated that the neurological findings of the patient regressed with this treatment. The authors suggested that incorporating human UCB stem cell transplantation into DNS therapy of CO poisoning improves neurological regeneration (Yom et al., 2020).

In a clinical study, combined MSC transplantation and butylphthalide therapy in CO poisoning was shown to significantly improve MMSE and Barthel scores compared to MSC transplantation or hyperbaric oxygen therapy alone. Mesenchymal stem cell transplantation was found to be superior to HBO treatment. In addition, the authors reported that combined treatment of MSC with butylphthalide was superior to MSC transplantation alone in improving cognitive function, activities of daily living, and rate of neurological recovery. They suggested that MSCs differentiate into undamaged nerve cells by activating endogenous neural stem cells. They stated that butylphthalidine, as a lipid-soluble drug, may have helped MSCs to cross the blood-brain barrier (Wang et al., 2016).

More research is needed to fully understand the therapeutic potential of stem cells.

Hidroxokobalamin (B12r)

It has been shown in experimental studies that hydroxocobalamin (B12) increases brain oxygenation, reduces total cell number loss, and improves demyelination and myoglial damage (Roderique et al., 2015; Del Moral-Barbudo et al., 2020).

In a preclinical study, a solution consisting of hydroxocobalamin (OHCbl), an FDA-approved antidote, and ascorbic acid (vitamin C), a potent reducing agent, was recommended for the treatment of CO poisoning (Roderique et al., 2015). Reduced hydroxocobalamin (B12r) converted CO to CO_2 in simple solutions in vitro. In this study, ascorbic acid-reduced hydroxocobalamin produced a CO_2 outgassing at levels 5 to 8 times higher than in the control group. The half-life of carboxyhemoglobin was reduced from 33 minutes to 15 minutes when the combination of oxygen (O_2) and B12r was used. It is obvious that more benefits will emerge with the synergistic effect in cases where high flow or HBO treatment and B12r are used together (Roderique et al., 2015).

The reduced hydroxocobalamin is considered to have great potential as an injectable antidote for CO poisoning.

Hemin

The neuroglobin activator hemin is a heme chloride with a high absorption rate. It is a good source of iron and can combine with oxygen to improve the oxygen-carrying capacity of the blood. Neuroglobin plays a role in protecting neurons from hypoxic damage. It helps to transport and store oxygen in neurons and increases the partial oxygen pressure within the cell. Because of these properties, it was thought that hemin could be used in the treatment of hypoxia in CO poisoning (Li et al., 2017).

There are two experimental studies on the use of hemin in CO poisoning. The results of these studies are promising.

The first study investigated the effects of hemin on the induction of hemoxygenase 1 (HO-1) activity in rats with severe hippocampal damage after CO exposure. As a result, a higher elevation of HO-1 was detected in the hippocampus (Guan et al., 2009). HO-1, a heme oxygenase isoform, regulates the levels of blood proteins by breaking down the heme in free iron and biliverdin. It is a protein that protects the cell against oxidative stress (Del Moral-Barbudo et al., 2020). In the study by Guan et al., rats pretreated with hemin had significantly higher survival rates at 24-h. Up-regulation of HO-1 was achieved with hemin pretreatment. On the other hand, a significant decrease was observed in hippocampal malondialdehyde (MDA) and proapoptotic caspase-3 levels, which are a marker of oxidative stress. They reported that hemin pretreatment decreased both the CO-induced increase in water content in the hippocampus and the number of damaged neurons in the hippocampus. In conclusion, they suggested that up-regulation of endogenous HO-1 expression plays a very important protective role in CO neurotoxicity. They did not elucidate the exact mechanisms of these hemin-related effects. However, they attributed neuroprotection to antioxidant and anti-apoptotic effects resulting from the activity of the HO-1 enzyme (Guan et al., 2009).

The second study was also conducted on mice. Mortality rates were significantly reduced by the administration of Hemin in mice exposed to CO gas. COHb levels and MDA levels, an indicator of blood oxidative stress, were found to be significantly lower in those treated with hemin compared to those who did not. In addition, histopathological examination revealed inflammation in the cells in the hippocampal region and a decrease in the number of pyramidal cells in untreated cases. On the other hand, it was determined that these pathologies resolved in patients treated with hemin. As a result, the authors reported that hemin has protective effects in reducing mortality and alleviating hippocampal edema in acute exposure to CO. They also attributed potential protective mechanisms to the reduction in HbCO level, inhibition of lipid peroxidation, and reduction of free oxygen radicals (Li et al., 2017).

Neuroglobin Mutation (Ngb-H64QCCC)

Recent research shows that a carbon monoxide antidote called "Ngb-H64QCCC" has been developed as a new treatment option for carbon monoxide poisoning. "Ngb-H64QCCC" is a form of a protein called neuroglobin produced by a specific mutation. This mutation causes the protein to bind more strongly to carbon monoxide molecules. In exposure to carbon monoxide, CO binds to all heme-containing proteins, including myoglobin and cytochrome c oxidase. Myoglobin is mostly found in the heart and muscle tissue. Cytochrome c oxidase (CcO; complex IV) is involved in the electron transport chain of the mitochondria as the terminal respiratory complex (Rose et al., 2020).

Neuroglobin (Ngb) secreted from the brain and retina is a cellular hemoprotein that has protective effects against ischemia and reperfusion injury. It is assumed that the cell-protective property of Ngb is formed by the reduction of cytochrome c or the reduction of nitrite to form nitric oxide (NO) (Raychaudhuri et al., 2010; Tiso et al., 2011). Hemoglobin and myoglobin (Mb) are five coordinate globins. These globins have a high affinity for CO. Ngb is a six-coordinate hemoprotein, and heme iron is coordinated by two histidine residues. The researchers mutated the distal histidine residue (H64) to produce Ngb-H64Q-CCC, a five-coordinate heme protein. With this mutation, they hypothesized that Ngb molecules could bind oxygen and CO with a very high affinity (similar to and more than Hb and Mg) (Dewilde et al., 2001; Nienhaus et al., 2004; Azarov et al., 2016).

In a study performed both in vitro and in vivo, rapid CO transfer from carboxy-hemoglobin to Ngb-H64Q-CCC was detected. Ngb-H64Q-CCC has been observed to bind to CO approximately 500 times stronger than hemoglobin. Ngb-H64Q-CCC has been reported to reduce the half-life of carboxy-hemoglobin (100% CO saturated hb) in room air from "≥ 200 minutes" to 0.11 and 0.41 minutes. As a result of the infusion of Ngb-H64Q-CCC into CO-poisoning mice; It has been reported that CO excretion from red blood cells increases, heart rate and blood pressure are restored, and survival increases. CO-bound Ngb-H64Q-CCC was rapidly eliminated by renal (Azarov et al., 2016).

CO binds to hemoglobin, reducing oxygen delivery. It suppresses oxidative phosphorylation by inhibiting mitochondrial cytochrome c oxidase. In their second study, the same team tested whether Ngb-H64QCCC could scavenge CO from cytochrome c oxidase (CcO) and reduce CO-induced inhibition of mitochondrial respiration. In conclusion, the authors reported that Ngb-H64Q-CCC reversed the effects of CO on mitochondria and improved systemic oxygen delivery (Rose et al., 2020).

These studies indicate that Ngb-H64QCCC as a CO scavenger may be a promising option for the treatment of carbon monoxide poisoning. However, clinical studies are needed.

Methane

Methane is the simplest aliphatic hydrocarbon and the main gas energy. Exogenous methane has anti-apoptotic, anti-oxidative, and anti-inflammatory effects. It has been shown that exogenous methane significantly ameliorates the histological damage caused by ischemia/reperfusion by affecting important events in oxidative and nitrosative stress caused by ischemia/reperfusion. Thus, methane has a potential therapeutic effect on oxidative stress pathologies (Fan et al., 2016).

Fan et al. in their experimental study on rats; showed that intraperitoneal injection of methane-rich saline improved the outcomes of DNS induced by CO exposure. Methane improved learning ability and reduced neuronal damage (Fan et al., 2016). In their second study, they confirmed the neuroprotective effect of methane-rich saline (MRS) histologically. The findings showed that methane-rich saline treatment ameliorated neuronal damage and reduced MDA, 3-NT, and 8-OHdG compared to normal saline-treated rats. Thus, they stated that methane-rich saline may protect the brain against damage caused by acute CO poisoning through its anti-oxidative and anti-inflammatory activities (Shen et al., 2016).

Acetylcholinesterase Inhibitors

The mechanism of action of acetylcholinesterase inhibitors on the neuropathological effects induced by CO is not exactly known (Del Moral-Barbudo et al., 2020). However, dysfunction of nicotinic acetylcholinergic neurons in the hippocampus has been demonstrated in animal models of delayed encephalopathy due to CO poisoning (Ochi et al., 2014). Based on this, Yanagiha et al. reported that they treated two patients with DNS who did not respond to HBOT using acetylcholinesterase inhibitors (Yanagiha et al. 2017).

It is thought that acetylcholinesterase inhibitors prevent CO-induced delayed neuronal death by enhancing hippocampal acetylcholinergic neuron function (Ochi et al., 2014). In addition, acetylcholinesterase inhibitors have antiapoptotic effects, increase Bcl-2 protein expression, stimulate nicotinic acetylcholine receptors, and suppress glycogen synthase kinase-3. Thus, they reveal neuroprotective effects (Yanagiha et al., 2017; Del Moral-Barbudo et al., 2020).

Methylene Blue

Methylene blue (MB) is used in the treatment of diseases such as malaria, methemoglobinemia, vasoplegic syndrome, surgical staining, and ifosfamide neurotoxicity (Tucker et al., 2018; Zhao et al., 2018).

It is known that methylene blue can reduce the formation of amyloid plaques and neurofibrillary tangles and partially protect mitochondrial function (Oz et al., 2009; Atamna et al., 2010; Zhao et al., 2018).

Recent studies have discovered that methylene blue strengthens mitochondria and acts as a recycling antioxidant. Methylene blue reduces the generation of free oxygen radicals through its effects on mitochondria (Ryou et al., 2015; Tucker et al., 2018; Zhao et al., 2018). In addition, in vitro studies have shown that methylene blue protects astrocytes under ischemic conditions (Roy Choudhury et al., 2015).

Due to the anti-inflammatory and newly discovered neuroprotective properties of methylene blue, it is thought that it can prevent the symptoms of intoxication and permanent neurological disorders that occur in CO exposure.

In a study conducted in rats exposed to acute CO gas, methylene blue was started to be administered to subjects after 1 hour with a subcutaneously implanted pump and continued for 7 days. The authors reported that proinflammatory cytokine levels were decreased, oxidative damage was suppressed, mitochondrial function was preserved, neuronal apoptosis was reduced in the hippocampus, and cognitive impairment was alleviated in rats with severe CO poisoning (Zhao et al., 2018).

It seems that more studies are needed to prove the effects of methylene blue on CO poisoning.

Allopurinol

Xanthine oxidase metabolizes hypoxanthine to xanthine and then xanthine to uric acid. Thus, it produces reactive oxygen species such as superoxide and hydrogen peroxide, which are required for lipid peroxidation. It has been stated that xanthine oxidase is a key component in the formation of reactive oxygen species after CO poisoning (Dong et al., 2015).

Allopurinol is an inhibitor of xanthine oxidase. Allopurinol has anti-inflammatory properties and also reduces oxidative stress. In a study conducted in rats, it was shown that allopurinol may have protective effects against delayed neurological sequelae caused by CO toxicity (Dong et al., 2015). After exposure to CO, rats were given 50 mg/kg of Allopurinol intraperitoneally six times. It has been found to suppress the expression of proinflammatory factors, including tumor necrosis factor-α, intercellular adhesion molecule-1, ionized calcium-binding adapter molecule 1, and impaired myelin essential protein. As a result, the authors emphasized that Allopurinol alleviates neuronal damage due to severe CO poisoning and reduces neuronal death by weakening inflammation and demyelination (Dong et al., 2015). This experimental study is the first preclinical study performed with Allopurinol in CO poisoning.

Erythropoietin

Recently, erythropoietin, a hematopoietic cytokine produced by the kidney in response to hypoxia, has been extensively investigated as an anti-ischemic and tissue-preserving agent with its cardioprotective effect independent of its erythropoietic property (Favory et al., 2006; Hara et al., 2007; Rezaee et al., 2016; Moallem et al., 2015). This novel effect of erythropoietin is thought to be mediated by erythropoietin receptors located in non-hematopoietic regions such as endothelial cells, neurons, astrocytes, oligodendrocytes, cardiac myocytes, and vascular smooth cells. Studies have also supported them (Asgharian Rezaee et al., 2012; Del Moral-Barbudo et al., 2020).

The effects of erythpoetin against neurological and cardiac pathologies due to CO poisoning are being investigated. In the first study, erythropoietin was shown to increase survival after CO exposure. It was concluded that erythropoietin can relatively prevent the occurrence of neurotoxicity. It has also been shown that CO poisoning causes a significant increase in serum glial fibrillary acidic protein (GFAP), possibly due to astrocyte damage and hypoxia, but erythropoietin reduces this increase (Moallem et al., 2015).

Erythropoietin has been shown to improve cardiac hemodynamic functions, reduce infarct size, inhibit myocardial apoptosis, and normalize the hypertrophic index. In vivo and in vitro studies have shown that the anti-apoptotic mechanism plays a major role in the tissue protective effect of erythropoietin (Rezaee et al., 2016; Hara et al., 2007; Iheagwara et al., 2007).

It has been shown that erythropoietin can reduce ischemic ECG changes caused by severe CO poisoning in rats. In moderate to severe CO poisoning in rats, ST segment elevation/depression, T wave inversion, and first-degree AV block were detected on the ECG. The authors reported that these ischemic

ECG changes were significantly reduced in those treated with EPO (Asgharian Rezaee et al., 2012).

CO exposure has been shown to cause myocardial apoptosis. Regression of myocardial apoptosis was detected with the administration of erythropoietin (Rezaee et al., 2016).

In a randomized prospective clinical study in 103 patients with CO poisoning, it was shown that the early administration of erythropoietin improves the neurological outcomes of the patients and reduces the incidence of DNS (Pang et al., 2013).

In conclusion, with its anti-oxidative, anti-apoptotic, anti-inflammatory, and anti-ischemic properties, erythropoietin can reduce neurological and cardiological pathologies secondary to CO exposure.

Magnesium Sulfate

Recent research shows that magnesium sulfate (MgSO4) reduces brain cell necrosis, apoptosis, and oxidative stress levels. Magnesium sulfate has been widely used for many years in the treatment of preeclampsia, eclampsia and torsade de pointes (Pearce et al., 2017).

Considering its effects on ischemia/reperfusion, magnesium sulfate may also reduce the hypoxic effects of CO exposure.

Magnesium sulfate reduced the rates of necrosis and apoptosis in cardiomyocytes as a result of CO exposure in a preclinical study. It reduced the ST-segment depression, ST-segment elevation, and T-wave inversion seen on the ECG due to CO exposure. Also, magnesium sulfate dilates blood vessels and lowers heart rate. Magnesium sulfate can be developed as a new treatment method due to its cardioprotective effects (Tabrizian et al., 2018).

The effects of magnesium sulfate on CO-induced brain injury in rats were also studied. Magnesium sulfate decreased oxidative stress, apoptosis, and cell necrosis, while increasing Akt protein levels, which contribute to survival, in a dose-dependent manner (Bagheri et al., 2019).

Granulocyte Colony Stimulating Factor (G-CSF)

Granulocyte colony stimulating factor (G-CSF) is a cytokine that increases the production of granulocytes in the bone marrow by mobilizing them from stem cells. Granulocyte colony stimulating factor is considered to have anti-apoptotic and neuroprotective properties (Hashemzaei et al., 2016; Ghorbani et al., 2017).

It was determined that the number of apoptotic neurons and Caspase 3 protein levels in the brain of rats given G-CSF after CO exposure was significantly reduced (Ghorbani et al., 2017). In addition, G-CSF reduces brain cell damage through remyelination. It lowers the levels of related biomarkers such as S100β and GFAP (Ghorbani et al., 2013). A single dose of G-CSF immediately after CO poisoning significantly reduces CO neurotoxicity through different mechanisms (Ghorbani et al., 2017).

The effects of G-CSF on cardiac damage in rats with CO poisoning were also investigated due to its anti-apoptotic properties (Mohamadpour et al., 2012; Hashemzaei et al., 2016). In a study conducted in 2012, the frequencies of ischemic changes in the ECG due to CO exposure decreased significantly after G-CSF treatment. In addition, some cardiac arrhythmias (eg, atrioventricular block types 1 and 2) that occur after CO poisoning were suppressed. However, G-CSF did not show a protective effect on cardiomyocyte pathological outcomes in CO-poisoning rats. These results showed that G-CSF could protect against ECG changes after cardiac ischemia secondary to CO, but did not affect pathological changes (Mohamadpour et al., 2012). In the second study on cardiac effects, it was reported that the levels of phosphorylated proteins such as p-JAK2, p-STAT3, and p-Akt1, which stimulate the anti-apoptotic pathway, were significantly increased in G-CSF groups (Hashemzaei et al., 2016).

G-CSF is still at the level of preclinical studies. More studies are needed to fully understand its role in CO poisoning.

Hydrogen-Rich Saline Solutions

In experimental studies with rats, it has been found that hydrogen-rich saline solutions have antioxidant effects, improve cognitive deficits, and reduce the degree of necrosis, apoptosis, and cell autophagy (Sun et al., 2011; Wang et al., 2013).

Peritoneal injection of hydrogen-rich saline provides a histological and functional improvement in encephalopathy due to acute CO poisoning. It is thought that the therapeutic effects of hydrogen-rich saline may be related to antioxidant and anti-inflammatory effects (Sun et al., 2011; Wang et al., 2013).

Conclusion

Currently, the treatment of patients with CO poisoning consists of oxygen and supportive therapy. HBOT is applied to those with neurological and cardiological effects. Mechanical ventilator support is applied to patients who develop respiratory failure. However, these treatments are insufficient to prevent complications after poisoning.

As a result, as the pathophysiology of CO poisoning is understood, new treatment methods will continue to be studied. The results of studies including antidote treatments that prevent oxidative stress and inflammation, neuroprotective drugs, anti-apoptotic drugs, treatments that prevent the binding of CO to heme-containing proteins, methods that increase the separation of CO from Hb, and treatment methods that have the ability to repair damaged tissues are promising. However, most of the studies are in the preclinical stage. More clinical studies are needed to use these methods in clinical practice.

References

Asgharian Rezaee, M., Moallem, S. A., Imenshahidi, M., Farzadnia, M., & Mohammadpour, A. H. (2012). Effects of erythropoietin on electrocardiogram changes in carbon monoxide poisoning: an experimental study in rats. *Iranian journal of pharmaceutical research: IJPR, 11*(4), 1191–1199.

Atalay, H., Aybek, H., Koseoglu, M., Demir, S., Erbay, H., Bolaman, A. Z., & Avci, A. (2006). The effects of amifostine and dexamethasone on brain tissue lipid peroxidation during oxygen treatment of carbon monoxide-poisoned rats. *Advances in therapy, 23*(2), 332–341. https://doi.org/10.1007/BF02850138

Atamna, H., & Kumar, R. (2010). Protective role of methylene blue in Alzheimer's disease via mitochondria and cytochrome c oxidase. *Journal of Alzheimer's disease: JAD, 20 Suppl 2*, S439–S452. https://doi.org/10.3233/JAD-2010-100414

Azarov, I., Wang, L., Rose, J. J., Xu, Q., Huang, X. N., Belanger, A., Wang, Y., Guo, L., Liu, C., Ucer, K. B., McTiernan, C. F., O'Donnell, C. P., Shiva, S., Tejero, J., Kim-Shapiro, D. B., & Gladwin, M. T. (2016). Five-coordinate H64Q neuroglobin as a ligand-trap antidote for carbon monoxide poisoning. *Science translational medicine, 8*(368):368ra173. https://doi.org/10.1126/scitranslmed.aah6571

Bagheri, G., Rezaee, R., Tsarouhas, K., Docea, A. O., Shahraki, J., Shahriari, M., Wilks, M. F., Jahantigh, H., Tabrizian, K., Moghadam, A. A., Bagheri, S., Spandidos, D. A., Tsatsakis, A., & Hashemzaei, M. (2019). Magnesium sulfate ameliorates carbon monoxide-induced cerebral injury in male rats. *Molecular medicine reports, 19*(2), 1032–1039. https://doi.org/10.3892/mmr.2018.9771

Chiew, A. L., & Buckley, N. A. (2021). Acetaminophen Poisoning. *Critical care clinics,* 37(3), 543–561. https://doi.org/10.1016/j.ccc.2021.03.005

Crigler, L., Robey, R. C., Asawachaicharn, A., Gaupp, D., & Phinney, D. G. (2006). Human mesenchymal stem cell subpopulations express a variety of neuro-regulatory molecules and promote neuronal cell survival and neuritogenesis. *Experimental neurology, 198*(1), 54–64.

Del Moral-Barbudo, B., Blancas, R., Ballesteros-Ortega, D., Quintana-Díaz, M., & Martínez-González, Ó. (2020). Current and research therapies for the prevention and treatment of delayed neurological syndrome associated with carbon monoxide poisoning: A narrative review. *Human & experimental toxicology, 39*(6), 765–772. https://doi.org/10.1177/0960327120901572

Dewilde, S., Kiger, L., Burmester, T., Hankeln, T., Baudin-Creuza, V., Aerts, T., Marden, M. C., Caubergs, R., & Moens, L. (2001). Biochemical characterization and ligand binding properties of neuroglobin, a novel member of the globin family. *The Journal of biological chemistry, 276*(42), 38949–38955. https://doi.org/10.1074/jbc.M106438200

Diao, X. X., Zhong, K., Li, X. L., Zhong, D. F., & Chen, X. Y. (2015). Isomer-selective distribution of 3-n-butylphthalide (NBP) hydroxylated metabolites, 3-hydroxy-NBP and 10-hydroxy-NBP, across the rat blood-brain barrier. *Acta pharmacologica Sinica, 36*(12), 1520–1527. https://doi.org/10.1038/aps.2015.64

Dong, G., Ren, M., Wang, X., Jiang, H., Yin, X., Wang, S., Wang, X., & Feng, H. (2015). Allopurinol reduces severity of delayed neurologic sequelae in experimental carbon monoxide toxicity in rats. *Neurotoxicology, 48*, 171–179. https://doi.org/10.1016/j.neuro.2015.03.015

Dong, W. N., Wang, B. X., Cao, P., Zhu, Q. C., Tan, D. Y., & Ling, B. Y. (2022). Comparison of high-flow nasal cannula oxygen therapy and non-rebreather face mask in the treatment of mild carbon monoxide poisoning. *Zhonghua lao dong wei sheng zhi ye bing za zhi = Zhonghua laodong weisheng zhiyebing zazhi = Chinese journal of industrial hygiene and occupational diseases*, *40*(10), 771–775. https://doi.org/10.3760/cma.j.cn121094-20211025-00513

Fan, D. F., Hu, H. J., Sun, Q., Lv, Y., Ye, Z. H., Sun, X. J., & Pan, S. Y. (2016). Neuroprotective effects of exogenous methane in a rat model of acute carbon monoxide poisoning. Brain research, 1633, 62–72. https://doi.org/10.1016/j.brainres.2015.12.019

Favory, R., Lancel, S., Tissier, S., Mathieu, D., Decoster, B., & Nevière, R. (2006). Myocardial dysfunction and potential cardiac hypoxia in rats induced by carbon monoxide inhalation. *American journal of respiratory and critical care medicine, 174*(3), 320–325. https://doi.org/10.1164/rccm.200601-117OC

Ghorbani, M., Moallem, S., Abnous, K., Tabatabaee Yazdi, S. A., Movassaghi, A. R., Azizzadeh, M., & Mohamadpour, A. H. (2013). The effect of granulocyte colony-stimulating factor administration on carbon monoxide neurotoxicity in rats. Drug and chemical toxicology, 36(1), 102–108. https://doi.org/10.3109/01480545.2012.737802

Ghorbani, M., Mohammadpour, A. H., Abnous, K., Movassaghi, A. R., Sarshoori, J. R., Shahsavand, S., Hashemzaei, M., & Moallem, S. A. (2017). G-CSF administration attenuates brain injury in rats following carbon monoxide poisoning via different mechanisms. *Environmental toxicology, 32*(1), 37–47. https://doi.org/10.1002/tox.22210

Guan, L., Wen, T., Zhang, Y., Wang, X., & Zhao, J. (2009). Induction of heme oxygenase-1 with hemin attenuates hippocampal injury in rats after acute carbon monoxide poisoning. *Toxicology, 262*(2), 146–152. https://doi.org/10.1016/j.tox.2009.06.001

Han, Q., Guo, X. T., Zhang, H. H., Tian, R., Gao, X., & Zhang, Z. Q. (2017). Clinical effect of high pressure oxygen and Butylphthalide in the recovery of cerebral metabolism after carbon monoxide poisoning. *Chinese journal of industrial hygiene and occupational diseases, 35*(8), 591–593. https://doi.org/10.3760/cma.j.issn.1001-9391.2017.08.009

Hara, S., Mukai, T., Kurosaki, K., Mizukami, H., Kuriiwa, F., & Endo, T. (2007). Role of nitric oxide system in hydroxyl radical generation in rat striatum due to carbon monoxide poisoning, as determined by microdialysis. *Toxicology, 239*(1-2), 136–143. https://doi.org/10.1016/j.tox.2007.07.008

Hashemzaei, M., Imen Shahidi, M., Moallem, S. A., Abnous, K., Ghorbani, M., & Mohamadpour, A. H. (2016). Modulation of JAK2, STAT3 and Akt1 proteins by granulocyte colony stimulating factor following carbon monoxide poisoning in male rat. *Drug and chemical toxicology, 39*(4), 375–379. https://doi.org/10.3109/01480545.2015.1123267

Iheagwara, K. N., Thom, S. R., Deutschman, C. S., & Levy, R. J. (2007). Myocardial cytochrome oxidase activity is decreased following carbon monoxide exposure. *Biochimica et biophysica acta, 1772*(9), 1112–1116. https://doi.org/10.1016/j.bbadis.2007.06.002

Jeong, J. A., Gang, E. J., Hong, S. H., Hwang, S. H., Kim, S. W., Yang, I. H., Ahn, C., Han, H., & Kim, H. (2004). Rapid neural differentiation of human cord blood-derived mesenchymal stem cells. *Neuroreport, 15*(11), 1731–1734. https://doi.org/10.1097/01.wnr.0000134846.79002.5c.

Jiang, G., Gao, J., Xu, Y., Ma, Y., Jiang, G., & Yan, W. (2009). Structural and functional improvement of injured brain after severe acute carbon monoxide poisoning by stem cell-based therapy in rats. *Critical care medicine, 37*(4), 1416–1422. https://doi.org/10.1097/CCM.0b013e31819d6821

Jin, G. Z., Cho, S. J., Choi, E. G., Lee, Y. S., Yu, X. F., Choi, K. S., Yee, S. T., Jeon, J. T., Kim, M. O., & Kong, I. K. (2008). Rat mesenchymal stem cells increase tyrosine hydroxylase expression and dopamine content in ventral mesencephalic cells in vitro. *Cell biology international, 32*(11), 1433–1438. https://doi.org/10.1016/j.cellbi.2008.08.014

Kekec, Z., Seydaoglul, G., Sever, H., & Ozturk, F. (2010). The effect of antioxidants (N-acetylcysteine and melatonin) on hypoxia due to carbonmonoxide poisoning. *Bratislavske lekarske listy, 111*(4), 189–193.

Kim, S., Choi, S., Ko, Y., Lee, C. A., Kim, G. W., Moon, J. E., Nah, S., & Han, S. (2023). Dexamethasone therapy prevents delayed neuropsychiatric sequelae after carbon monoxide poisoning: a prospective registry-based study. *Clinical toxicology (Philadelphia, Pa.), 61*(2), 98–103. https://doi.org/10.1080/15563650.2023.2169707

Kim, Y. J., Park, H. J., Lee, G., Bang, O. Y., Ahn, Y. H., Joe, E., Kim, H. O., & Lee, P. H. (2009). Neuroprotective effects of human mesenchymal stem cells on dopaminergic neurons through anti-inflammatory action. *Glia, 57*(1), 13–23. https://doi.org/10.1002/glia.20731

Kim, Y. M., Shin, H. J., Choi, D. W., Kim, J. M., Lee, S. W., Jeong, S. H., & Kim, H. (2020). Comparison of high-flow nasal cannula oxygen therapy and conventional reserve-bag oxygen therapy in carbon monoxide intoxication: A pilot study. *The American journal of emergency medicine*, *38*(8), 1621–1626. https://doi.org/10.1016/j.ajem.2019.158451

Li, H. M., Shi, Y. L., Wen, D., Luo, H. M., Lin, X., & Xiao, F. (2017). A novel effective chemical hemin for the treatment of acute carbon monoxide poisoning in mice. *Experimental and therapeutic medicine, 14*(5), 5186–5192. https://doi.org/10.3892/etm.2017.5157

Li, Q., Song, J. J., Zhang, H. Y., Fu, K., Lan, H. B., & Deng, Y. (2015). Dexamethasone therapy for preventing delayed encephalopathy after carbon monoxide poisoning. *Biotechnic & histochemistry: official publication of the Biological Stain Commission, 90*(8), 561–567. https://doi.org/10.3109/10520295.2015.1019565

Lo, C. P., Chen, S. Y., Lee, K. W., Chen, W. L., Chen, C. Y., Hsueh, C. J., & Huang, G. S. (2007). Brain injury after acute carbon monoxide poisoning: early and late complications. *AJR. American journal of roentgenology*, *189*(4), W205–W211. https://doi.org/10.2214/AJR.07.2425

Long, B., Liang, S. Y., & Lentz, S. (2021). High flow nasal cannula for adult acute hypoxemic respiratory failure in the ED setting. *The American journal of emergency medicine*, *49*, 352–359. https://doi.org/10.1016/j.ajem.2021.06.074

McCunn, M., Reynolds, H. N., Cottingham, C. A., Scalea, T. M., & Habashi, N. M. (2000). Extracorporeal support in an adult with severe carbon monoxide poisoning and shock following smoke inhalation: a case report. *Perfusion, 15*(2), 169–173. https://doi.org/10.1177/026765910001500213

Moallem, S. A., Mohamadpour, A. H., Abnous, K., Sankian, M., Sadeghnia, H. R., Tsatsakis, A., & Shahsavand, S. (2015). Erythropoietin in the treatment of carbon monoxide neurotoxicity in rat. *Food and chemical toxicology: an international journal published for the British Industrial Biological Research Association*, *86*, 56–64. https://doi.org/10.1016/j.fct.2015.09.015

Mohamadpour, A. H., Moallem, S. A., Hashemzaei, M., Abnous, K., Tabatabaee Yazdi, S. A., & Imenshahidi, M. (2012). Effects of granulocyte colony-stimulating factor on electrocardiogram changes after carbon monoxide poisoning in rats. *Drug and chemical toxicology,* 35(4), 353–360. https://doi.org/10.3109/01480545.2011.627863

Nienhaus, K., Kriegl, J. M., & Nienhaus, G. U. (2004). Structural dynamics in the active site of murine neuroglobin and its effects on ligand binding. *The Journal of biological chemistry*, *279*(22), 22944–22952. https://doi.org/10.1074/jbc.M401561200

Nishimura M. (2019). High-Flow Nasal Cannula Oxygen Therapy Devices. *Respiratory care*, *64*(6), 735–742. https://doi.org/10.4187/respcare.06718

Ochi, S., Abe, M., Li, C., Mori, Y., Ishimaru, T., Yoshino, Y., Yamazaki, K., Mori, T., Fukuhara, R., Tanimukai, S., Matsuda, S., Yoshida, K., & Ueno, S. (2014). The nicotinic cholinergic system is affected in rats with delayed carbon monoxide encephalopathy. *Neuroscience letters, 569*, 33–37. https://doi.org/10.1016/j.neulet.2014.03.054

O'Donnell, P., Buxton, P. J., Pitkin, A., & Jarvis, L. J. (2000). The magnetic resonance imaging appearances of the brain in acute carbon monoxide poisoning. *Clinical radiology*, *55*(4), 273–280. https://doi.org/10.1053/crad.1999.0369

Omara, F. O., Blakley, B. R., Bernier, J., & Fournier, M. (1997). Immunomodulatory and protective effects of N-acetylcysteine in mitogen-activated murine splenocytes in vitro. *Toxicology*, *116*(1-3), 219–226. https://doi.org/10.1016/s0300-483x(96)03520-2

Oz, M., Lorke, D. E., & Petroianu, G. A. (2009). Methylene blue and Alzheimer's disease. *Biochemical pharmacology, 78*(8), 927–932. https://doi.org/10.1016/j.bcp.2009.04.034

Ozturan, I. U., Yaka, E., Suner, S., Ozbek, A. E., Alyesil, C., Dogan, N. O., Yilmaz, S., & Pekdemir, M. (2019). Determination of carboxyhemoglobin half-life in patients with carbon monoxide toxicity treated with high flow nasal cannula oxygen therapy. *Clinical toxicology (Philadelphia, Pa.)*, *57*(7), 617–623. https://doi.org/10.1080/15563650.2018.1540046

Pang, L., Bian, M., Zang, X. X., Wu, Y., Xu, D. H., Dong, N., Wang, Z. H., Yan, B. L., Wang, D. W., Zhao, H. J., & Zhang, N. (2013). Neuroprotective effects of erythropoietin in patients with carbon monoxide poisoning. *Journal of biochemical and molecular toxicology*, *27*(5), 266–271. https://doi.org/10.1002/jbt.21484

Pearce, A., Lockwood, C., van den Heuvel, C., & Pearce, J. (2017). The use of therapeutic magnesium for neuroprotection during global cerebral ischemia associated with cardiac arrest and cardiac surgery in adults: a systematic review. *JBI database of systematic reviews and implementation reports*, *15*(1), 86–118. https://doi.org/10.11124/JBISRIR-2016-003236

Raychaudhuri, S., Skommer, J., Henty, K., Birch, N., & Brittain, T. (2010). Neuroglobin protects nerve cells from apoptosis by inhibiting the intrinsic pathway of cell death. *Apoptosis: an international journal on programmed cell death*, *15*(4), 401–411. https://doi.org/10.1007/s10495-009-0436-5

Rezaee, M. A., Mohammadpour, A. H., Imenshahidi, M., Mahmoudi, M., Sankian, M., Tsarouhas, K., Tsakalof, A., Tsatsakis, A. M., & Moallem, S. A. (2016). Protective effect of erythropoietin on myocardial apoptosis in rats exposed to carbon monoxide. *Life sciences*, *148*, 118–124. https://doi.org/10.1016/j.lfs.2016.02.007

Rochwerg, B., Einav, S., Chaudhuri, D., Mancebo, J., Mauri, T., Helviz, Y., Goligher, E. C., Jaber, S., Ricard, J. D., Rittayamai, N., Roca, O., Antonelli, M., Maggiore, S. M., Demoule, A., Hodgson, C. L., Mercat, A., Wilcox, M. E., Granton, D., Wang, D., Azoulay, E., Ouanes-Besbes L, Cinnella G, Rauseo M, Carvalho C, Dessap-Mekontso A, Fraser J, Frat JP, Gomersall C, Grasselli G, Hernandez G, Jog S, Pesenti A, Riviello ED, Slutsky AS, Stapleton RD, Talmor D, Thille AW, Brochard L, & Burns, K. E. A. (2020). The role for high flow nasal cannula as a respiratory support strategy in adults: a clinical practice guideline. *Intensive care medicine*, *46*(12), 2226–2237. https://doi.org/10.1007/s00134-020-06312-y

Roderique, J. D., Josef, C. S., Newcomb, A. H., Reynolds, P. S., Somera, L. G., & Spiess, B. D. (2015). Preclinical evaluation of injectable reduced hydroxocobalamin as an antidote to acute carbon monoxide poisoning. *The journal of trauma and acute care surgery, 79*(4 Suppl 2), S116–S120. https://doi.org/10.1097/TA.0000000000000740

Rose, J. J., Xu, Q., Wang, L., & Gladwin, M. T. (2015). Shining a Light on Carbon Monoxide Poisoning. *American journal of respiratory and critical care medicine, 192*(10), 1145–1147. https://doi.org/10.1164/rccm.201508-1579ED

Rose, J. J., Wang, L., Xu, Q., McTiernan, C. F., Shiva, S., Tejero, J., & Gladwin, M. T. (2017). Carbon Monoxide Poisoning: Pathogenesis, Management, and Future Directions of Therapy. *American journal of respiratory and critical care medicine, 195*(5), 596–606. https://doi.org/10.1164/rccm.201606-1275CI

Rose, J. J., Bocian, K. A., Xu, Q., Wang, L., DeMartino, A. W., Chen, X., Corey, C. G., Guimarães, D. A., Azarov, I., Huang, X. N., Tong, Q., Guo, L., Nouraie, M., McTiernan, C. F., O'Donnell, C. P., Tejero, J., Shiva, S., & Gladwin, M. T. (2020). A neuroglobin-based high-affinity ligand trap reverses carbon monoxide-induced mitochondrial poisoning. *The journal of biological chemistry, 295*(19):6357-6371. https://doi.org/10.1074/jbc.RA119.010593.

Roy Choudhury, G., Winters, A., Rich, R. M., Ryou, M. G., Gryczynski, Z., Yuan, F., Yang, S. H., & Liu, R. (2015). Methylene blue protects astrocytes against glucose oxygen deprivation by improving cellular respiration. *PloS one, 10*(4), e0123096. https://doi.org/10.1371/journal.pone.0123096

Ryou, M. G., Choudhury, G. R., Li, W., Winters, A., Yuan, F., Liu, R., & Yang, S. H. (2015). Methylene blue-induced neuronal protective mechanism against hypoxia-reoxygenation stress. *Neuroscience, 301*, 193–203. https://doi.org/10.1016/j.neuroscience.2015.05.064

Shen, M., Fan, D., Zang, Y., Chen, Y., Zhu, K., Cai, Z., Liu, Y., Sun, X., Liu, J., & Gong, J. (2016). Neuroprotective effects of methane-rich saline on experimental acute carbon monoxide toxicity. *Journal of the neurological sciences, 369*, 361–367. https://doi.org/10.1016/j.jns.2016.08.055

Simonsen, C., Magnusdottir, S. O., Andreasen, J. J., Bleeg, R. C., Lie, C., & Kjærgaard, B. (2019). Long-Distance Transportation of Carbon Monoxide-Poisoned Patients on Extracorporeal Membrane Oxygenation Seems Possible: A Porcine Feasibility Study. *Air medical journal, 38*(3), 178–182. https://doi.org/10.1016/j.amj.2019.03.009

Simonsen, C., Magnusdottir, S. O., Andreasen, J. J., Rohde, M. C., & Kjærgaard, B. (2018). ECMO improves survival following cardiogenic shock due to carbon monoxide poisoning - an experimental porcine model. *Scandinavian journal of trauma, resuscitation and emergency medicine, 26*(1), 103. https://doi.org/10.1186/s13049-018-0570-6

Song, H., Yue, A., Zhou, X., Han, W., & Li, Q. (2023). Evidence of clinical efficacy and pharmacological mechanism of N-butylphthalide in the treatment of delayed encephalopathy after acute carbon monoxide poisoning. *Frontiers in neurology, 14,* 1119871. https://doi.org/10.3389/fneur.2023.1119871

Spina, V., Tomaiuolo, F., Celli, L., Bonfiglio, L., Cecchetti, L., & Carboncini, M. C. (2019). A Case of Carbon Monoxide-Induced Delayed Neurological Sequelae Successfully Treated with Hyperbaric Oxygen Therapy, N-Acetylcysteine, and Glucocorticoids:

Clinical and Neuroimaging Follow-Up. *Case reports in neurological medicine*, *2019*, 9360542. https://doi.org/10.1155/2019/9360542

Sun, Q., Cai, J., Zhou, J., Tao, H., Zhang, J. H., Zhang, W., & Sun, X. J. (2011). Hydrogen-rich saline reduces delayed neurologic sequelae in experimental carbon monoxide toxicity. *Critical care medicine*, *39*(4), 765–769. https://doi.org/10.1097/CCM.0b013e318206bf44

Tabrizian, K., Khodayari, H., Rezaee, R., Jahantigh, H., Bagheri, G., Tsarouhas, K., & Hashemzaei, M. (2018). Magnesium sulfate protects the heart against carbon monoxide-induced cardiotoxicity in rats. *Research in pharmaceutical sciences*, *13*(1), 65–72. https://doi.org/10.4103/1735-5362.220969

Tardiolo, G., Bramanti, P., & Mazzon, E. (2018). Overview on the Effects of N-Acetylcysteine in Neurodegenerative Diseases. *Molecules (Basel, Switzerland)*, *23*(12), 3305. https://doi.org/10.3390/molecules23123305

Teerapuncharoen, K., Sharma, N. S., Barker, A. B., Wille, K. M., & Diaz-Guzman, E. (2015). Successful Treatment of Severe Carbon Monoxide Poisoning and Refractory Shock Using Extracorporeal Membrane Oxygenation. *Respiratory care*, *60*(9), e155–e160. https://doi.org/10.4187/respcare.03990

Thom S. (2009). Stem cell rescue for carbon monoxide poisoning?. *Critical care medicine*, *37*(4), 1520–1521. https://doi.org/10.1097/CCM.0b013e318196fd6e

Thom, S. R., Bhopale, V. M., Fisher, D., Zhang, J., & Gimotty, P. (2004). Delayed neuropathology after carbon monoxide poisoning is immune-mediated. *Proceedings of the National Academy of Sciences of the United States of America*, *101*(37), 13660–13665. https://doi.org/10.1073/pnas.0405642101

Tiso, M., Tejero, J., Basu, S., Azarov, I., Wang, X., Simplaceanu, V., Frizzell, S., Jayaraman, T., Geary, L., Shapiro, C., Ho, C., Shiva, S., Kim-Shapiro, D. B., & Gladwin, M. T. (2011). Human neuroglobin functions as a redox-regulated nitrite reductase. *The Journal of biological chemistry*, *286*(20), 18277–18289. https://doi.org/10.1074/jbc.M110.159541

Tomruk, O., Karaman, K., Erdur, B., Armagan, H. H., Beceren, N. G., Oskay, A., & Bircan, H. A. (2019). A New Promising Treatment Strategy for Carbon Monoxide Poisoning: High Flow Nasal Cannula Oxygen Therapy. *Medical science monitor: international medical journal of experimental and clinical research*, *25*, 605–609. https://doi.org/10.12659/MSM.914800

Tucker, D., Lu, Y., & Zhang, Q. (2018). From Mitochondrial Function to Neuroprotection-an Emerging Role for Methylene Blue. *Molecular neurobiology*, *55*(6), 5137–5153. https://doi.org/10.1007/s12035-017-0712-2

Wang, H., Li, Y., Wu, Q., Xu, C., & Liu, Q. (2016). Combination of butylphthalide with umbilical mesenchymal stem cells for the treatment of delayed encephalopathy after carbon monoxide poisoning. *Medicine*, *95*(49), e5412. https://doi.org/10.1097/MD.0000000000005412

Wang, W., Tian, L., Li, Y., Wang, X., Xia, F., Li, L., Li, J., & Zhang, Z. (2013). Effects of hydrogen-rich saline on rats with acute carbon monoxide poisoning. *The Journal of emergency medicine*, *44*(1), 107–115. https://doi.org/10.1016/j.jemermed.2012.01.065

Xiang, W. P., Xue, H., & Wang, B. J. (2014). Delayed encephalopathy of acute carbon monoxide intoxication in rats: potential mechanism and intervention of dexamethasone. *Pakistan journal of pharmaceutical sciences, 27*(6 Suppl), 2025–2028.

Xiang, W., Xue, H., Wang, B., Li, Y., Zhang, J., Jiang, C., & Pang, J. (2017). Efficacy of N-Butylphthalide and Hyperbaric Oxygen Therapy on Cognitive Dysfunction in Patients with Delayed Encephalopathy After Acute Carbon Monoxide Poisoning. *Medical science monitor: international medical journal of experimental and clinical research, 23,* 1501–1506. https://doi.org/10.12659/msm.899499

Xiang, W., Xue, H., Wang, B., Li, Y., Zhang, J., Jiang, C., Liang, F., Pang, J., & Yu, L. (2017). Combined application of dexamethasone and hyperbaric oxygen therapy yields better efficacy for patients with delayed encephalopathy after acute carbon monoxide poisoning. *Drug design, development and therapy, 11*, 513–519. https://doi.org/10.2147/DDDT.S126569

Xu, X. M., Luo, H., Rong, B. B., Zheng, X. M., Wang, F. T., Zhang, S. J., & Li, Z. X. (2019). Management of delayed encephalopathy after CO poisoning: An evidence-based narrative review. *Medicine, 98*(49), e18199. https://doi.org/10.1097/MD.0000000000018199

Yanagiha, K., Ishii, K., & Tamaoka, A. (2017). Acetylcholinesterase inhibitor treatment alleviated cognitive impairment caused by delayed encephalopathy due to carbon monoxide poisoning: Two case reports and a review of the literature. *Medicine, 96*(8), e6125. https://doi.org/10.1097/MD.0000000000006125

Yesiloglu, O., Gulen, M., Satar, S., Avci, A., Acehan, S., & Akoglu, H. (2021). Treatment of carbon monoxide poisoning: high-flow nasal cannula versus non-rebreather face mask. *Clinical toxicology (Philadelphia, Pa.), 59*(5), 386–391. https://doi.org/10.1080/15563650.2020.1817477

Yom, D. Y., Hwang, S. K., Jon, S. G., & Ri, R. (2020). Delayed neuropsychiatric syndrome of acute carbon monoxide poisoning from oak burning gas cured by therapy combined with transplantation of human umbilical cord blood stem cell, injection of nicholine, and intranasal inhalation of insulin. *Neurocase, 26*(1), 64–68. https://doi.org/10.1080/13554794.2019.1706748

Zhang, J., Guo, Y., Li, W., Li, G., & Chen, Y. (2020). The Efficacy of N-Butylphthalide and Dexamethasone Combined with Hyperbaric Oxygen on Delayed Encephalopathy After Acute Carbon Monoxide Poisoning. *Drug design, develop-ment and therapy, 14*, 1333–1339. https://doi.org/10.2147/DDDT.S217010

Zhao, N., Liang, P., Zhuo, X., Su, C., Zong, X., Guo, B., Han, D., Yan, X., Hu, S., Zhang, Q., & Tie, X. (2018). After Treatment with Methylene Blue is Effective against Delayed Encephalopathy after Acute Carbon Monoxide Poisoning. *Basic & clinical pharmacology & toxicology, 122*(5), 470–480. https://doi.org/10.1111/bcpt.12940

Index

A

B

C

D

E

F

G

H

I

L

M

N

O

P

S